Exemplary Research for Nursing and Midwifery

Although nurses make up the largest clinical group in the health care workforces of most developed countries, research into what nurses do, how effective they are and how their interventions work, is seriously underdeveloped. In many countries, national funding for nursing research is negligible compared with the vast budgets available for medical research. Partly because of this, nursing research has been seen as small scale, low quality and unsystematic. This book, however, tells a different story.

Exemplary Research for Nursing and Midwifery incudes nineteen classic and influential accounts of nursing research selected by a panel of senior nurse researchers and teachers. Each paper is accompanied by editorial commentary explaining:

- the significance of the research in question
- how it relates to the research tradition
- its influence and impact.

Organised under three headings – research classics, conceptualising practice and clinical effectiveness – *Exemplary Research for Nursing and Midwifery* provides an invaluable tool for any nurse or midwife embarking on the research process.

Anne Marie Rafferty is Director and **Michael Traynor** Lecturer, both at the Centre for Policy in Nursing Research, London School of Hygiene and Tropical Medicine.

Exemplary Research for Nursing and Midwifery

Edited by

Anne Marie Rafferty

and

Michael Traynor

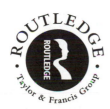

ROUTLEDGE
ROUTLEDGE
Taylor & Francis Group

London and New York

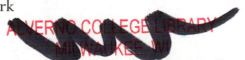

First published 2002
by Routledge
11 New Fetter Lane, London EC4P 4EE

Simultaneously published in the USA and Canada
by Routledge
29 West 35th Street, New York, NY 10001

Routledge is an imprint of the Taylor & Francis Group

Typeset in Bell Gothic and Perpetua by M Rules
Printed and bound in Great Britain by TJ International Ltd, Padstow, Cornwall

British Library Cataloguing in Publication Data
A catalogue record for this book is available from the British Library

Library of Congress Cataloging in Publication Data
Exemplary research for nursing and midwifery / edited by Anne Marie Rafferty
and Michael Traynor.
     p. cm.
Includes bibliographical references and index.
1. Nursing–Research. 2.Midwives–Research. I. Rafferty, Anne Marie.
II. Traynor, Michael, 1956–
RT81.5 .E95 2001
610.73′07′2–dc21   2001040811

ISBN 0-415-24162-6 (hbk)
ISBN 0-415-24163-4 (pbk)

Contents

Foreword

There is probably no other major area of public spending in the UK that is based on such a thin research base as nursing, midwifery and health visiting. While investment in research and development in health services generally is notoriously low compared with manufacturing industries and most other service industries, little of that investment is devoted to increasing our knowledge and understanding of the main workforce and the activities they undertake. Nursing consumes 3 per cent of the UK Gross Domestic Product which, with a largely publicly funded health system, means nurses are one of the largest occupational groups as regards government expenditure. Combine this with the realisation that the most crucial current issue facing health policy-makers is that of workforce recruitment, retention and skill-mix, it is astonishing how little investment has been and continues to be made in research on nursing, midwifery and health visiting.

One explanation often offered in defence of the situation is that the quality of nursing research has not been impressive enough to invest more, focusing, as much of it has, on the process of nursing itself. While many leading advocates and exponents of nursing research would not demur from this (at least in private), they would, correctly, point out the 'chicken and egg' dilemma which they confront. It is really little use for critics to bemoan the plethora of nurse researchers who devote their attention to the nature of nursing or the philosophy of nursing education when traditionally nurses have been denied research access to patients and health services (often by doctors who do not want their research territory invaded). It is, therefore, not surprising that nursing research has ended up (like several other health care groups with relatively little power) in a ghetto, divorced from mainstream health services research. And the few leading health services research groups that include nurses in their ranks, all too often see them as low-cost, clinically trained data collectors rather than as equal partners providing a unique, complementary perspective.

Although this is a somewhat disheartening picture, there are encouraging signs for the future. Some of these can be found in this excellent collection of fine examples of what nursing research can and has achieved. It should provide hope and encouragement to those committed to or planning on entering nursing research. The examples illustrate the breadth and sophistication of what can be achieved. They also demonstrate how slowly policies and practice change. Some of the contributions could have been written today, leaving this reader feeling ambivalent – impressed by the insight of nurse researchers several decades ago, but conscious of how little we have advanced in the intervening years.

The editors, Anne Marie Rafferty and Michael Traynor, have provided us not only with a highly informed selection of work that ranges across the full breadth of international nursing research, but also guidance as to how to approach each contribution. The introductions to each article help us to understand the context in which the research was conducted. This serves to explain why the topics were selected for study, where the research was undertaken, why particular research methods were employed, and what influence, if any, the research had on practice or policy.

As the editors point out, the aim of much research is to de-stigmatise and enhance the status of neglected areas of health care. This book makes a major contribution to enhancing nursing, midwifery and health visiting research. Practitioners should be proud of these past achievements and researchers should be inspired to build on such a foundation. It should provide researchers with a nursing background with the confidence not only to expand their study of nursing, but to 'pull back the curtain' and study health care in all its complexity. Nursing research will have arrived only when researchers with a nursing background study the work of their medical colleagues with the same level of confidence as non-nurses study nursing.

Nick Black
Professor of Health Services Research
London School of Hygiene and Tropical Medicine
July 2001

Preface

WHY RESEARCH?

Many people think of research as a rarefied activity, one that is far removed from day-to-day practice. But research influences practice in many different ways. Sometimes that influence is clear-cut and direct. Sometimes it is more vague. Indeed, it may even become such an automatic part of our thinking that we hardly even notice it. The aim of this book is to 'showcase' research in nursing and midwifery at its best, studies that have changed clinical practice and the way we think about clinical care. Not all the studies were carried out by nurses or midwives, and some are pioneering efforts in the field. What they all have in common is their impact upon clinical practice or the political and philosophical underpinnings of care. We hope you will find in this collection an impressive range of topics, methods and organisational models of research. Included are randomised controlled trials, qualitative and discursive studies, single-author and multi-disciplinary approaches. Sometimes the focus has been on a specific nursing, midwifery or health visiting procedure or service, sometimes it has been on far broader organisational structures or policies. Whatever the emphasis, all the articles, we believe, reveal research at its best.

But why research? For some, such as pioneer Lisbeth Hockey, research is driven by a deep curiosity about why things are the way they are and whether they could be better if changed. The purpose of this collection is to celebrate research in nursing and midwifery with examples of excellence. To do this, we invited key opinion-leaders in the field to identify an exemplary piece of research. We gave them one criterion; choose a piece of research which is influential, either for the profession or for you personally. What emerged shows an impressive diversity and depth. We hope it will locate research in nursing, midwifery and health visiting as part of a longer, and broader, intellectual tradition.

Our panel was international in character, drawn from the UK, USA and Australia.

Selected studies fell into three broad categories; classics, conceptualising practice and clinical effectiveness. Each contributes in a distinctive way to theory, method and clinical practice. Given the broad spectrum of skills and expectations that span education in nursing, midwifery and health visiting this collection of readings is intended as a vehicle for understanding the characteristics of exemplary research. Before each article within the themed sections is an introduction in which we set out the context and summarise the main ideas in the paper or its implications for us today. Some articles are presented verbatim while others have been edited and abstracted for reasons of brevity.

CLASSICS

The term 'classic' has many meanings. Margaret Drabble, in the *Oxford Companion to English Literature*, defines a literary classic as: 'a work considered first rate or excellent of its kind, therefore standard, fit to be used as a model or imitated' (Drabble, 2000). A number of the studies presented here can certainly be included in this category. The programme of research inaugurated by *The Proper Study of the Nurse* (McFarlane, Chapter 1 of this volume) and the studies associated with it (Stockwell, Chapter 2) have a timeless quality. Many of the issues and challenges associated with measuring the quality of care are as relevant today. There is a sense in which *The Proper Study of the Nurse* can be considered the godmother of nursing research, for it articulates in microcosm the problems and aspirations of nursing's research agenda since. Its reputation as a classic is owed to the impact it made not only upon its own generation but upon its successors. Within this tradition Stockwell and Hayward (Chapter 3) both broke new ground, demonstrating that nurses' attitudes influenced the quality of care (Stockwell), but also that they could intervene to bring about quality improvement and better outcomes (Hayward).

While some of these studies may be regarded as methodological models, others can be considered classics in that they create a sense of wonder when one considers the limitations within which researchers then had to work. The sweep and scope of the studies by Norton *et al.*, Clark *et al.* and Menzies (Chapters 4–6) retain this capacity to impress and inspire, and part of this derives from the sense of ingenuity and imagination that they embody. We should also remember just how bold and brave it must have been to venture into research when there were so few role models and sources of support. For many it must have been an exotic escapade and a leap into the unknown with few career prospects beyond the fledgling academic departments of nursing. Menzies stands out in the depth and insights of her analysis and the furore that followed the study's publication. Rarely does research create such a rumpus. We still see traces of her contribution in the debates surrounding reflective practice and clinical supervision. Such studies are classics in the sense that they retain a freshness, news that remains news.

CONCEPTUALISING PRACTICE

The second category consists of contributions to theory and method in the realm of practice. Patricia Benner's study (Chapter 7) contributes on both counts. Through the use of phenomenology, which has become something of a cottage industry in nursing, Benner unearths different levels of expertise. She develops a framework within which it can be conceptualised and impacted upon continuing education programmes. Trudy Rudge (Chapter 8) uses ethnography to explore the duality of the research 'field' as a site of clinical and surgical nursing practice from the different vantage points of the nurse as a researcher and as a nurse–researcher in relation to patients and fellow clinicians. Rudge's research explores reactions to wound dressing in patients who have undergone skin-grafting for burns in plastic surgery wards. Jocalyn Lawler (Chapter 9) plays on the duality of the body in her piece in her discussion of knowledge of the body and bodies of knowledge. In this, Lawler argues that the manner in which we conceptualise the body and its implications for health care institutions relies upon a language and disciplines of knowledge that screen out the meaning for the patient. Nurses, Lawler argues, have colluded with these practices in an attempt to gain credence for their work, but ironically in doing so have helped to erase the emotional from such value and reward schemes. Insofar as 'body work' for many is the work of women, Lawler's critique comes from a feminist position, arguing for a feminist approach to knowledge of bodies and bodies of knowledge. Continuing a more philosophical approach, the theme of feminism and the value systems that underpin the canon of research in terms of its content and contributors is taken up by David Allen (Chapter 10). He explores the territory that researchers enter when they question the idea that disinterested knowledge is possible. Both Davina Allen and Nolan et al. (Chapters 11 and 12) deal with different aspects of the division of labour and boundaries between workers and carers, but in radically different ways. Allen uses ethnography to explore the manner in which professional groups define themselves by policing the permeability of the boundaries between themselves and other workers. She argues that boundaries are not fixed or stable, but shaped by negotiation through policy and political pressures. Such processes force into sharp relief the logic of claims about occupational expertise. The issue of boundaries and the relational aspects of caring are tackled in almost a literal way by Mike Nolan and colleagues who examine the intimate subtleties of family care giving, and through its different expressions and components hold a mirror up to professional caring.

CLINICAL EFFECTIVENESS

The final section demonstrates the clinical effectiveness of nursing, midwifery and health visiting interventions. A number of these papers derive from advanced practice (Marks, Brooten et al., Naylor et al., Chapters 13–15), others from more conventional roles (Luker, Sleep et al., Aiken et al., Chapters 16–18), or the analysis of existing datasets (Robinson, Chapter 19). Each in many ways represents an example of the extent to which nursing, midwifery or health visiting can make a measurable difference to patient care, or, in the case of Robinson, uncover variations in outcome that may be attributable to clinical care. Research has played an important role in legitimising advanced practice roles for nurses, an initiative launched in the UK by Isaac Marks and colleagues in the field of psychiatry. Interestingly, expanding nursing expertise also took root in the USA in what are considered (by doctors) under-served populations, such as the elderly (Naylor) and single mothers (Brooten). Research in nursing, midwifery and health visiting often suffers form the lack of a sound survey or analytic basis upon which to build evaluative studies. But, as many of these examples demonstrate, robust and sophisticated randomised and controlled trials are not the preserve of medicine and can be powerful tools with which to demonstrate effectiveness. Some studies involved a cross-over component (Luker, Naylor) adding weight and strength to the impact of interventions. Midwifery, relatively speaking, probably has a stronger tradition of trials than nursing or health visiting through its historical association with the Perinatal Epidemiology Unit in Oxford, as in the paper by Jennifer Sleep and colleagues. Karen Luker's evaluation of health visiting is exemplary in breaking new ground and in its boldness in testing the value of health visiting practice, with all its attendant complexities and subtleties. Research may also deliver negative news reflecting poorly upon the professions (Robinson). The study by Linda Aiken and colleagues, on the other hand, has been particularly influential in debates within policy arenas on the value of nursing. Unusually too, it uses a case-control design to demonstrate the contribution that nurses can make to reducing mortality of medical and surgical patients in so-called 'magnet' hospitals, known for good nursing care.

CONCLUSION

What this collection demonstrates is the diversity of topics and methodologies deployed in studies regarded as exemplifying quality and impact in nursing, midwifery and health visiting. Many were conducted before there was any government funding for research, and exemplify the entrepreneurial skill and zeal with which pioneers pursued their agendas. Many undertook research without much support from their peers within the profession. Often it was necessary to draw upon the expertise of those beyond the profession, both to gain training and access to supervision as in *The Proper Study of the Nurse*, or to build alliances with professionals in others fields and constituencies to collaborate on research (Norton *et al.*). And there *is* something to celebrate. Nursing and midwifery are gaining strength as fields of research and publication. A recent study of outputs from biomedical research revealed that although nursing and midwifery are small sub-fields they are the fastest growing of the 26 sub-specialisms studied (Dawson *et al.*, 1998). Taking nursing alone, Britain's publication performance has increased between 1991 and 1996, as has its share of the international publication market. Indeed, its growth rate exceeds that of any other country studied, including the USA and Australia. The period is also marked by rise in the number of nursing journals. A 1995 RCN study found that 40 per cent of the 37 existing journals had started publication within the past 5 years and of these 15 new titles, 5 had been published for no more than 2 years. Funding patterns, however, reveal that the largest source of funding acknowledged in research (70 per cent) is no funding, from which we may infer self-funding. Initiatives are underway at the time of writing to change the funding for research in nursing and midwifery. So, although much has been accomplished, much remains to be done. We believe the studies presented here, classic and contemporary, compare favourably with those in other fields. Mark Twain defined a classic as a 'book which nobody wants to read but everybody wishes to have read'. We hope that this book proves him wrong – if only just this once!

REFERENCES

Dawson, G., B. Lucocq, R. Cottrell and G. Lewison (1998) *Mapping the Landscape: national biomedical research outputs 1988–95*. London, The Wellcome Trust.

Drabble, M. (ed.) (2000) *Oxford Companion to English Literature*, Oxford, Oxford University Press.

Acknowledgements

This book grew out of discussions with a number of people, particularly Patricia Lynne, RCN Professor of Nursing at the University of Wales, Cardiff.

We would like to express our gratitude to those we approached for advice about the contents of this collection: Linda Aiken, Claire Fagin, Jocalyn Lawler, Alison Kitson, Maggie Pearson, Karen Luker, Judy Lumby, Senga Bond, Alison Tierney, Jenny Wilson-Barnett, Sally Redfern, Jane Robinson, David Thompson, Judith Parker, Lisbeth Hockey, Patricia Lyne, Tony Butterworth, Kevin Gournay and Mary Renfrew.

We would also like to thank Nick Black, Christine Hancock, Alison Kitson and John Wyn Owen for on-going encouragement and support for the Centre for Policy in Nursing Research, and the Nuffield Trust for funding us.

We also thank Edwina Welham at Routledge for her continued support of our work and for not giving up on us: we promise to be on time in the future.

Finally, gratitude to David Spiegelhalter, statistician, healer.

Our thanks also to the following publishers who have granted permission to reproduce their material. (A full acknowledgement and details of the source appears at the head of each article or extract.) Chapters 1–3, Royal College of Nursing; Chapter 4, Churchill Livingstone; Chapter 5, *Nursing Times*; Chapter 6, The Tavistock Institute; Chapter 7, Prentice-Hall; Chapter 8, Blackwell Science; Chapter 9, Churchill Livingstone; Chapter 10, Jones & Bartlett Publishers; Chapter 11, Sage Publications; Chapter 12, Open University Press; Chapters 13 and 17, BMJ Publishing Group; Chapter 14, Massachusetts Medical Society; Chapter 15, American Medical Association; Chapter 16, John Wiley & Sons; Chapter 18, J.B. Lippincott; Chapter 19, Nelson Thornes.

PART ONE

Research classics

Chapter 1

The proper study of the nurse

JEAN KENNEDY MCFARLANE

Introduction

The Proper Study of the Nurse occupies a seminal place in the history of nursing research. Not only does it represent in microcosm some of the prevailing dilemmas of measurement in nursing research, but the studies themselves have come to form part of the early 'canon' of nursing research. Some of the studies cited are presented within the present volume (Stockwell, Norton *et al.*, Chapters 2 and 4). The brainchild of Marjorie Simpson, it sets out the challenge for research in nursing with a clarity of vision and an agenda that remains relevant today. Marjorie Simpson was appointed to the pioneering post of Nursing Officer (Research) within the then Department of Health and Society Security (DHSS). A visionary and graduate of LSE, Miss Simpson proposed a programme of research around which a team of researchers based at the Royal College of Nursing (RCN) in London would develop measures of the quality of nursing care. The work is also significant as the first programme of research which recognised and integrated training and supervision for nurse researchers.

The 'Study of Nursing Care' as it became known was stimulated by studies within the Ministry of Health between 1963 and 1965 which examined the deployment of nursing staff in acute hospitals. These studies revealed that, even when hospital staffing figures were standardised for factors normally taken into account in the deployment of staff, wide variations in staffing remained in institutions that were otherwise similar. While differences in quality of care might be one of the effects of differences in staffing patterns, no measures were available to test any claims in this regard. If we sometimes find it an uphill struggle to persuade funders of the value of nursing research today, can you imagine the enormity of the task in the late 1960s with little in the way of track record to argue from?

The work began in 1967, and the lack of experienced researchers within nursing led to a search for supervision and registration for higher degrees in cognate fields, such as occupational psychology and sociology. The intention of the studies was to develop measuring devices to serve as indicators of quality in nursing care. It was recognised, however, that a direct analogy could not be drawn between the nature of work in industrial settings and health care. Nevertheless, the complexity of the measurement task in health care raised many more questions, especially those related to outcomes. What were the goals of performance? What counted as 'cure'? How could one identify a therapeutic relationship? These and related questions have exercised the minds of many a researcher since. Significantly, it was recognised at the time that nurses were not alone in their definitional dilemma; doctors, social workers, teachers and managers faced a similar challenge. To cope with the different layers and levels of complexity, a multi-disciplinary team approach was adopted to take the problem forward.

The objectives of the programme were ambitious. Techniques for measuring the quality of nursing care were combined with a training programme enabling nurses to participate in and understand research processes and procedures. The programme ran over six years, with six nurse research assistants recruited to form teams of investigators. It was guided by a multi-disciplinary steering committee, but an overall leader oversaw day-to-day management. Notably, so novel was the venture that reservations were expressed at the time about recruiting someone of university standing within the UK. An experienced nurse tutor with wide nursing experience was appointed. That person was Jean McFarlane, later the first Professor of Nursing in England at the University of Manchester. The recruitment procedure for research assistants was arduous, involving the contemporary fashion for administering psychological tests and intensive interviewing. The pool for selection appears to have been buoyant and the team selected included many who would later assume leadership positions in nursing research. A final feature of the programme was the pioneering role that it played in capacity building. A training syllabus was drawn up by the steering group, including research methods in the clinical sciences, social sciences and statistical methods.

The programme was managed to the degree that broad topic areas were identified by students to maximise 'ownership', but guided and shaped by a steering group. Inevitably perhaps, there was a certain degree of self-consciousness about the pioneering status of the studies, and an awareness that rigour and high standards needed to be upheld in training as well as the research projects themselves. The studies covered a wide range of topics and methodologies, and have come to be regarded as classics of nursing research. Characteristically, each project critiqued and challenged some aspect of the received wisdom and ritual in nursing practice, such as preoperative fasting or that associated with bowel function. Others exposed the gulf between the rhetoric and reality of care, such as that evidenced in teaching procedures as taught and those that were subsequently practised. Others still drew attention to unmet needs of patients, be that for preoperative information to alleviate anxiety or the impact on hospitalised children of separation from their mothers. Findings sometimes painted an unflattering portrait of practice. Nurses were judgemental and their behaviour had significant implications for their attitudes towards 'difficult' patients.

Many of the findings have a contemporary feel that challenges any glib notion of linear progress. The study searched for solutions not only across the Atlantic, but in other organisations. The studies show an impressive sensitivity to the methodological challenges associated with measuring quality of care. It is also possible to see the tension that was created by attempts to derive staffing norms and to deliver measurable standards of service. The search for such a formula proved largely elusive on account of the complexity of the nursing role, its variability in different contexts for different actors and the lack of any direct causal link with patient welfare. Much conceptual confusion surrounded the criteria for quality in nursing care. There is a refreshing openness to challenging cherished assumptions, even the sacrosanct notion that good nursing care implied an improvement in health status. A sound and admirable scepticism was demonstrated in relation to methodologies of measurement. Similarly, it was recognised that it was not possible to isolate the specifically nursing contribution to patient welfare from that of other factors such as the hospital or medical contributions. There was a strong sensitivity to contextualising findings within a systems framework, and conducting experimental studies of different models of service delivery. In doing so the study demonstrates a prescience that is both timely and expresses the durability of 'quality' in research itself.

MCFARLANE, J.K. (1970)

The Proper Study of the Nurse*

PREFACE

This account of the setting up of the Research Project 'The Study of Nursing Care' provides an introduction to the thinking behind the initiation of the Project and to the reports of the individual studies carried out by the Research Assistants during the first four years of the Project. It serves to emphasise that whilst each study isolates a critical area in nursing care and establishes facts in that area, none of the studies can alone achieve the aims of the Project. It is hoped that the studies will lead to the development of measuring devices which when brought together will serve as indicators of quality in nursing care.

The nurse reader is interested in the findings of research projects. The findings of individual studies in this Project will be published as separate reports in the first instance. What the first six studies have contributed to the objectives of the Project is summarised in Chapter 2 of Part I. For the reader wishing to have a summary of progress this is the essential chapter. The other chapters in Part I give an outline of the administrative aspects of setting up and conducting the Project. The second six studies are in progress and reports on them will be published as they become available.

The first six studies have developed more than 20 research instruments from which some will later be selected to be tested on a wider scale and validated as measures of quality. Methods have been found for looking at a variety of aspects of nursing care, including organisational aspects of nursing, nurse performance, patient reaction, nurse and patient attitudes. Additionally, methods have been found for looking at work relations. Some of the studies deal with nursing care initiated by doctors, others with care initiated directly by nurses.

The studies cover many aspects of patient need, physical, emotional, social, thera-peutic, and they investigate a range of aspects of nurse performance which affect the quality of care given. The six studies make a creditable start in developing tools to mea-sure the quality of nursing care.

THE PROBLEM AND THE PROJECT

The problem

Many fundamental research studies have their origin in a management problem. The research project 'The Study of Nursing Care' was set up in response to a need to estab-lish criteria or standards of quality of nursing care.

The then Ministry of Health in 1963/65 carried out studies of the deployment of nursing staff in acute hospitals in the National Health Service. These demonstrated that even when hospital staffing figures were standardised for factors normally taken into account in the deployment of staff within a hospital, wide differences in the staffing of apparently similar hospitals remained unaccounted for.

Whereas many nurses would be ready to assert that alterations in staffing patterns and ratios would affect the quality of nursing care, no measures of quality existed with which such assertions could be verified or disproved. It was recognised that quality of care might be one of the factors influencing the variations in staffing and whilst the deployment study was still in progress negotiations started for a study of quality of nursing care.

It was known that studies to establish criteria for the quality of nursing care had been carried out in North America over a considerable period of time. From the review of these in Part II it will be seen that no final answer had been found to the problem. Moreover, work carried out in North America might well not be relevant in the United Kingdom where the content and context of nursing work is different.

The significance of the problem

Studies of quality of nursing care are intrinsically valuable for the light they throw on nursing practice. They are important because all changes made in nursing services and in nursing practice have as their ultimate objective improvements in patient care and the success or otherwise of changes needs to be assessed. They are basic to all aspects of manpower evaluation.

Manpower considerations

The manpower model is an aid to the analysis of the effective use of manpower in any working situation. It has two complementary aspects – 'fitting the man to the job' and 'fitting the job to the man'. Figure 1.1 shows that each aspect is conveniently analysed under three subheadings. The effectiveness of manpower strategy in any of these areas can only be measured in terms of the effectiveness with which the JOB is performed.

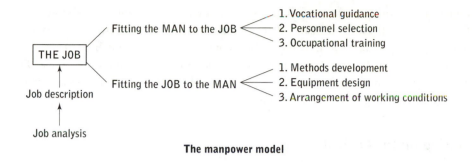

The manpower model

Figure 1.1   The manpower model

Thus, measures of the quality of performance of the JOB are crucial to the evaluation of any manpower strategy.

Thus, measures of the effectiveness of manpower strategies in nursing can only be measured adequately in terms of the quality of nursing care which they enable. These include strategies for recruitment, selection and training, the methods of performing nursing tasks, the nursing equipment used and all aspects of the working conditions, including the management structure, the payment system or off-duty rotas.

The unique function of the nurse is to give nursing care. To this function both nursing management and nursing education are in a service relationship. Their excellence can only be judged by the excellence of nursing care which they enable.

To date, no tools have been developed with which effective deployment or any other manpower strategy can be measured.

The complexity of the problem

If it were possible to measure the effectiveness of manpower strategies in nursing by quantitative means, the task would be relatively easy and well tested methods are available. Establishing criteria of quality is a highly complex task. Part of the complexity lies in the complexity of nursing itself. (This problem is elaborated in the discussion of the literature.)

Where a simple production task is involved in an industrial setting, it is comparatively easy to state acceptable criteria for performance in precise terms. The performance of an operator can be defined in measures to a thousandth of an inch or the number of unacceptable pieces per batch can be laid down. The caring professions have established no such precise goals. In medicine and in social work fundamental questions remain about the goals of performance. What is a cure? What is a therapeutic relationship? The answers may be relative and personal to the patient or client.

Standards of performance in motor skills may be laid down, e.g. the accuracy with which a prescribed dose of a drug should be drawn up for injection, but standards of performance in human relationship skills are far less easily defined and the quality of care exercised in the nurse/patient relationship is an integral part of the unique function of the nurse. This problem of establishing criteria of quality where the task entails human relationships is one which faces all the caring professions and the literature from these professions indicates that we share a common dilemma with teachers, doctors, managers and social workers. If the complexity of the problem seems at times to be insurmountable it is reassuring to know that other professions share these difficulties and this emphasises the value of multi-disciplinary teams or at least a sharing of approaches to the problem in research.

Setting up the Project

Conscious of the centrality of the need to establish criteria of quality for nursing care if manpower strategies are to be assessed, the Department of Health and Social Security decided to finance a research project over a six-year period to develop such measures. Miss H. M. Simpson, Nursing Officer (Research) at the Department of Health and Social Security, was involved in the scheme from its inception and guided much of the thinking. A Working Group of nurses, doctors, sociologists and Department representatives was called together in 1966.

From the earliest discussions it was accepted that nurses themselves should be fully involved in the Project. But nursing research was in its infancy in the United Kingdom and few were adequately prepared to undertake such work. Nevertheless, it was decided that even though the primary work of the Project might be delayed by this, it was desirable that nurses should be involved and a subsidiary aim of the Project became an educational one – to give nurses an introduction to research methods in a short programme of preparation. Thus, at an early stage Miss M. F. Carpenter, Director of Education of the Royal College of Nursing and the National Council of Nurses, was asked to join the Working Group. A formal request was made to the Council of the Rcn, who readily agreed that the Project should be administered by the Education Division where the programme of preparation could most suitably take place and where the library facilities necessary to the Project were located. Miss A. M. C. Thompson was at that time Librarian. In her custody the Library of Nursing had become a unique repository of nursing literature. Her special interest in the literature of nursing research gave those working on the Project a magnificent start and her personal interest in the needs of individual research assistants was a continuing encouragement.

Objectives

The objectives of the Project were thus established:

1   To develop techniques for measuring the quality of nursing care.
2   To involve nurses fully in the studies.
3   To develop a pattern for this type of preparation of nurses to take part in and understand research procedures.

Organisation and administration

It was agreed that the objectives of the Project could best be achieved by appointing teams of 4–6 nurse investigators as research assistants for two-year periods. This would allow for three teams during the six-year project which was budgeted for accordingly.

Besides a programme of preparation the nurse investigators would need guidance from experienced research workers. A multi-disciplinary Committee now including a statistician as well as the disciplines involved in the Working Group was set up to act as a selection panel for the nurse investigators and as a steering committee for the Project. In this role it had the delegated responsibilities for preparing advertisements and particulars for recruiting the nurse investigators, for preparing syllabuses for the course of training and laying down procedures which would launch the study.

The terms of reference of the Steering Committee were:

> To undertake the continuing task of advising on all aspects of the Project, individually and collectively helping the Royal College of Nursing officers to deal with problems as they arise in the course of the Project and receiving progress reports, commenting upon them and reporting back to the Working Group.

Since the Project would be administered by the Royal College of Nursing, it was deemed appropriate that the Chair of the Steering Committee should be taken by the Director of Education.

A Project Committee took the place of the original Working Group at the Department of Health. Its terms of reference are:

> To keep the progress of the Project under regular review, receiving annual progress reports and reviewing the programme for the following year; to advise as necessary on the development of the Project.

The Committee had an agreed membership of five Department of Health and Social Security members, two Royal College of Nursing members, the Director in the Education Division and the Project Leader, and the research advisers from the Steering Committee. Subsequently the Chairman of the Council of the Royal College of Nursing and the Chairman of the General Nursing Council were invited to join the Committee. The Department's Chief Nursing Officer is the Committee's Chairman.

THE PROJECT TEAM

The steering committee

As outlined in the previous chapter, the Steering Committee of the Project was conceived as an essential part of the team. On an individual and group basis, the members contributed to the total thinking of the Project and guided individual studies. The committee was multi-disciplinary and was able to make available to the research assistants expert advice from different fields of research. Where further advice was required, this was freely taken and was invariably freely given. The Project has thus grown by help and advice from many experienced research workers. Additionally, members of the Steering Committee contributed the main series of lectures and seminar sessions in the introductory training programme.

The Project Leader

The Working Group early reached the conclusion that there should be a full-time Project Leader. Preferably, this should be someone with sufficient knowledge and experience of research to help the nurse investigators plan and carry through their studies. This implied someone at university lecturer level and it was recognised that such a person might be difficult to recruit in the United Kingdom. It was known that the nurse investigators would need advice on research techniques from more than one discipline. It was decided, therefore, that advice should come as outlined in the previous paragraph and that the Project Leader should be a graduate nurse with wide experience in nursing.

The first Project Leader appointed was an experienced nurse tutor with wide nursing experience. She was given leave of absence for a year to complete a degree which was felt to be essential to her ability to lead the team of research assistants.

In time, the following aspects of the role of the Project Leader emerged:

1   Project Committee and Steering Committee

Servicing the Project Committee and Steering Committee, including the Selection Committee.

2   Course planning and tutorial work

Planning and organising the introductory course. Participating in a tutorial capacity and conducting seminars. Arranging additional tuition for individual research assistants in connection with their studies.

3   Individual studies

Guiding and supervising the individual studies in consultation with members of the Steering Committee and other specialists and completing a study on her own account which would contribute to the Project as a whole.

4   Co-ordination

Co-ordinating the individual studies in the Project in consultation with the Steering Committee so that the total aims of the Project are met.

5   Supervision for higher degrees

In some instances acting as supervisor for higher degrees on a collaborative basis with universities.

6   Publication

Working with the editor, Steering Committee and research assistants to produce reports on the study which would be suitable for publication.

7   Final report

Bringing together the work of the research assistants into a battery of tests of quality and taking responsibility for preparation and publication of a final report.

8   General

Contributing to the appreciation of research in the Royal College of Nursing and in the profession nationally and internationally.

The research assistants

The first team of research assistants was recruited to start work in October 1967. Advertisements were placed in the general and nursing press the previous November and much interest was shown. Candidates were normally required to be general trained nurses with a good general education. They were required to have not less than three years' experience in nursing or in some allied work or educational programme before or after training. Over 200 enquiries were made and particulars of the Project and application forms were sent out. Of 27 firm applications, 15 candidates were short-listed and called for interview before the final team of six research assistants was selected.

Selection was made on the basis of educational background, professional qualifications and experience, professional and social references. Candidates were asked to state on their application form whether they had any previous research experience or published projects. They were also asked to 'State briefly why you are interested in taking part in this project and what use you plan to make of the experience'. A whole day was spent in selection. Each candidate received two individual interviews, one from an experienced nurse, the other from an academic research worker. Personnel and deductive reasoning tests as used by Professor Woodward for Master's Degree applicants in the Department of Mechanical Engineering at Imperial College of Science and Technology were administered in a modified way. Grades were allotted for the candidates' performance in all these aspects so that a profile of the candidates' attainments and potentialities was built up and a final grading awarded. In this way, the Selection Committee (Steering Committee) made a final selection of six candidates and the full Committee then interviewed them together as a team.

Conditions of service

The conditions under which the research assistants should receive scholarships or be employed was discussed in great detail. After wide consultation it was agreed that they should be seconded from the Health Service on full salary. Where their present salary fell below that mid-way up the ward sister's grade their starting salary was made up to that level. By this system of secondment, superannuation rights were maintained and Whitley Council conditions of service could be applied. In this way, the Project could hope to attract experienced nurses of good calibre who would not be at a disadvantage whilst participating in the Project, and who could then readily return to the service after two years or proceed to further research if their qualifications and inclinations lay that way.

The programme of work

A projected programme for the two years of a research assistantship was mapped out.

1　The first three months (October–December)

The research assistants would primarily be occupied in the introductory training programme. Towards the end of this period they would select an area of study and read round it in the literature. A record was kept of all literature searched and reports under the analytical framework given in Appendix III were recorded.

2　Second three months (January–March)

The necessary research tools for the study would be developed, e.g. questionnaires, observation schedules, etc.

3　Third three months (April–June)

A pilot study would be mounted in which the tools and method would be tested.

End of first year (June–September). The pilot study would be completed and written up and the tools revised as necessary.

Second year. The full studies would be mounted, followed by analysis of the findings and writing up.

Higher degrees

From the start it was hoped that certain of the research assistants who were graduates would register for higher degrees on the basis of their work. In these cases an extension of time might be granted for writing up for a Master's Degree and in other cases an extra year could be granted for work towards a doctorate.

The training programme

The Steering Committee drew up a syllabus in three aspects of research method:

1   Research methods in the clinical sciences.
2   Research methods in the social sciences.
3   Statistical method.

The syllabus is given in Appendix 1 in which completed studies of nursing research were analysed and particular attention paid to the method used. The list of studies initially used is given in Appendix 2. These were followed by discussions with research workers who had recently completed nursing studies. Each study was analysed using a modified form of the headings used by Dr. J. MacGuire in analysing the studies in 'Threshold to Nursing'. These exercises developed a skill in the critical evaluation of research studies which was later applied to the design of the work undertaken by the research assistants themselves. The list of analytical headings is given in Appendix 3.

Late in the first term and early in the second, seminars were held on some of the American studies which had developed criteria of quality for nursing care. A selection of the studies was made to illustrate a variety of approaches. These are listed in Appendix 4. It was hoped that one of these studies might provide a model of nursing on which the present Project could be based. The group were not, however, convinced that any of the American models used were valid for the purpose of the Project. In Appendix 5 illustrations of American models are given.

At this time, the research assistants received additional information and training in research methods from a variety of specialists on both an individual and group basis. For example, the North East Metropolitan Regional Hospital Board co-operated in giving a week's training in work study methods of observation.

THE FIRST SIX STUDIES

Selection of topics for studies

Towards the end of their training programme the first six research assistants were encouraged to select for study some aspect of nursing care which interested them or which they felt was critical to the quality of such care. The studies were thus selected by a group of nurses with a wide variety of experience, from aspects of nursing care which in the practical situation had seemed to them to be essential to quality. Whilst the choice was a personal one and motivation was therefore maximised, a considerable amount of guidance was given in group discussions and by meetings with the Steering Committee. Only two of the six topics were those originally selected by the research assistants. One was helped to select one topic from many; one changed her topic of study after reflecting on whether she could sustain work on it for two years; another was advised to change her topic in view of her lack of background in a special aspect of nursing, and another was advised to change her topic because a great deal of research had already been carried out in her first topic of choice. The topics finally studied by the first group of six cover a wide range of types of nursing problems. This is an asset in terms of the objective of the total Project in that tools were developed for testing the quality of care in many aspects of nursing.

The significance of individual studies for the total project

Full accounts of the first six studies are to be published in separate reports. In this account only a brief description of the studies is given. An attempt to place all the studies in a common analytical framework is made. This includes:

1   The factor which was judged to be critical to the quality of nursing care.
2   The research design used.
3   The tools developed during the study.
4   The factors measured in each study.
5   An indication of possible categories of classification.

Those suggested are:

(i)	Categories of class of nursing care (following the definitions given by Goddard (1952))	basic, technical, administrative
(ii)	Categories of level of initiation of care	doctor initiated nurse initiated
(iii)	Categories of the direction of care	institutionalised personalised
(iv)	Categories of patient need	physical emotional and psychological social therapeutic
(v)	Categories of nurse performance factors	personality training knowledge perception skills – manual social

It is not suggested that these categories are final or exhaustive or that a satisfactory taxonomy of typology has been established. For the Project to accomplish its aims, the achievements of individual studies must be analysed and a synthesis made of their contribution to the total aim. This is necessarily an aspect of the study which will develop as succeeding studies are added to the store. A final synthesis will be the task of the

Steering Committee and the present Project Leader, Mrs. U. Inman. It is suggested, however, that some of the categories outlined above may be useful indicators of a more general application of the tools developed for a specific purpose.

The limitations of the studies

It is important to stress the limitations of the studies. They were undertaken by individuals with the minimum of help from observers, interviewers and mechanical analysis, i.e. within the restraints of finance. Hence, none of the studies was able to use random sampling techniques though care was taken to select a representative population from different types of hospital in London and the Regions where this was possible. From this it will be seen that it is impossible to generalise from these studies without testing them on a larger scale. Further, the studies were undertaken by a group of carefully selected nurses who none-the-less were in a learning situation. Additionally, the Project Leader was in a learning situation. So much learning took place during the two years that no member of the group would claim that the studies are without criticism.

The achievements of the studies

At the same time, it is useful to state what these pioneer studies have accomplished.

1   Individually, they have amassed a great deal of information about aspects of nursing care. Much of it may be known or sensed by experienced nurses, but within the limitations of the studies the facts have been placed on a more scientific basis. Because areas that are critical to the quality of care were studied some of the findings will give nurses with a care for standards cause for thought and, it may be, concern. If these are discussed and patient care improved then the individual studies will have accomplished a great deal.

2   More important than the individual findings in terms of the total project is the fact that a series of research tools has been developed. There is a wide range of type of tool-questionnaire, Q-sort, ranking and rating tools, observation schedules, etc., and a wide range of aspects of nursing has been studied as indicated by the categories of classification. It may be that with the second six studies presently being conducted the Project will have been so seminal in alternative approaches and over so wide a range that the tools could be tested as a battery before the six-year period is completed. It will be the task of the Steering Committee to reach a decision on this.

3   The objective of the Project that nurses should be involved in research has been achieved in large measure. Both nationally and internationally, the studies have received note and discussion. The Department at the Rcn has become a focus of enquiry, discussion and advice on nursing research and there has been a reciprocal benefit to the Research Discussion Group at the Rcn in the research assistants' association with it. In addition, there are longer-term benefits to the profession from this learning experience. One research assistant was granted a third year

of secondment to complete a Ph.D. and in that year was able to make a valuable contribution to the analysis of research for the Department of Health and Social Security. Another was appointed as a Research Fellow at the University of Wales and a third is working in medical research. Not only are research assistants returning to the clinical situation with new insights but some are making a continuing career in research.

SUMMARY OF THE STUDIES

1 Pre-operative starvation

(a) *The critical factor* in the quality of care was judged to be the period for which some patients were starved before operation. It was hypothesised that this was sometimes unnecessarily long.

(b) *The research design* was evolved to find by questionnaire:

    (i) the medical policy for pre-operative starvation, its purpose and the medical perception of how the policy was carried out in practice;

    (ii) the nurse's perception of medical policy, the reasons for it, and the organisation of care in practice.

The importance of the study is in developing a method for studying an area of technical nursing based on medical policy.

(c) *Tools developed*

    (i) Questionnaire to determine (i) above.

    (ii) Questionnaire to determine (ii) above.

(d) *Factors measured*

    Minimum fasting times (policy)

    Fasting times in practice

    Ward–theatre liaison

    Patient knowledge and reaction

    Hospital policies and differences

    Ward and individual anaesthetists' differences in policy

    Planning and organisation of fasting régime

    Interpretation of régimes

(e) *Possible categories of classification*

    Interpretation of régimes

(i) Class of nursing care	Technical, administrative especially communications
(ii) Level of initiation	Doctor initiated
(iii) Direction of care	Both institutionalised and personalised
(iv) Patient need	Physical, emotional and psychological; Therapeutic
(v) Nurse performance factors	Perception of policy; Interpretation of policy; Communication skills

2 The unpopular patient

(a) *The critical factor* was the difficulty nurses experienced in relating to and caring for 'difficult' patients. It was hypothesised that there are no factors other than personality which makes a patient unpopular.

(b) *The research design included:*
- (i) the identification of unpopular patients by Q-sort and rating methods;
- (ii) The reasons given for such ranking and rating;
- (iii) a questionnaire of factors other than personality which could contribute to unpopularity, e.g. diagnosis, nationality, social class, stigmata, deafness, language difficulty, length of stay in hospital.

This part of the study was followed (on advice from the Steering Committee) by a comparative analysis in ward situations in which an attempt was made to compare discriminating behaviour.

The contribution of this study is in the human relations aspect of nursing. It is a beginning in developing methods of investigating the way in which difficulties in relating to patients may affect the quality of care given.

(c) *Tools developed*
- (i) A tool for assessing the popularity and unpopularity of patients:
  - (a) a ranking scale
  - (b) a rating scale
- (ii) Questionnaires to assess:
  - (a) factors accounting for unpopularity (patient)
  - (b) nurses' attitudes to patients
- (iii) Card-sort role definition tool   The nurses' view of the patient's role.
- (iv) A comparative analysis technique for discriminating behaviours.

(d) *Factors measured*
Popularity of patients
Factors affecting unpopularity
Nurses' attitudes to patients
Nurses' view of patient's role
Discriminating behaviours

(e) *Possible categories of classification*
- (i) Class of nursing care
- (ii) Level of initiation – nurse initiated
- (iii) Direction of care – personalised
- (iv) Patient need – social, emotional and psychological
- (v) Nurse performance factors
  Perception of patient's role
  Communications skills
  Group norms

3 Admission to hospital

(a) *The critical factor* in this study was the anxiety created by hospital admission and the factors in nursing care which can reduce this anxiety. It is hypothesised that admission to hospital is an anxiety-creating incident and that anxiety is reduced by the amount of information given to the patient about his illness, his treatment and his environment.

(b) *The research design* included questionnaires to measure the amount of communication received, its content and source and timing. Anxiety was measured on admission and subsequently by Cattell's I.P.A.T. Scale (1963). The importance of the study is in developing a method to measure the effectiveness of nursing care in reducing anxiety, which is a frequent objective.

(c) *Tools developed or used*
   (i) Cattell's I.P.A.T. Scale (1963) for testing level of anxiety
   (ii) Questionnaire to test patient's knowledge of the provisions and limits of the hospital service and their source of information; and their opinion of nurses.
   (iii) Schedule for analysis of admission procedures.

(d) *Factors measured*
   Admission procedures.
   Anxiety levels (patient) on admission and subsequently; communication of information; content, source and timing.
   Patients' opinions of nurses.

(e) *Possible categories of classification*
   (i)   Class of care   Administrative, communications
   (ii) Level of initiation   Nurse initiated
   (iii) Direction of care   Both personalised and institutionalised
   (iv) Patient need   Social, emotional and psychological communications
   (v)   Nurse performance factors Communications skills

4 The teaching and practice of nursing procedures

(a) *The critical factor* in this study was the frequently remarked difference between procedures as taught and as practised.

(b) *The research design*
   A check list was developed of one basic procedure as taught (a dressing technique) in behavioural steps using a modified work study method. The check list was then used in the ward situation and an analysis made to see if the deviations recorded followed any pattern in respect of ward, year of training, or for trained staff. The deviations from taught procedure were further analysed for suspected dangerous practices.

   The study begins to develop a method of analysing nursing skills so that the effect of training on subsequent performance can be measured and its contribution to patient welfare (safety) estimated.

(c) *Tools developed or used*
   (i)   Check list analysis for nursing procedures
   (ii) Ward schedule for recording ward variables
   (iii) Nurse questionnaires giving demographic data, motivation on entering

nursing and opinions about nursing (developed from questionnaire by Mrs. R. Pomeranz).

(d) *Factors measured*
Non-conformity with taught procedure
Individual and ward scores of non-conformity
Personal data – nurses
Motivation on entering nursing
Opinions about nursing
Ward variables
Teaching method variables
Suspected dangerous practices

(e) *Possible categories of classification*

(i)	Class of care	Technical
(ii)	Level of initiation	Nurse initiated
(iii)	Direction of care	Institutionalised
(iv)	Patient need	Physical, therapeutic
(v)	Nurse performance factors	Training – learning of skills
		Group pressures
		Manual skill
		Personal factors

5 Care of patient's bowel function

(a) *The critical factor* was the frequency of worry and concern expressed by patients about their bowel habits. It was hypothesised that the quality of nursing care influences the worry and concern expressed.

(b) *The research design* established by questionnaire:
  (i) Alterations in bowel habit on hospitalisation;
  (ii) Related factors such as changes in diet and activity;
  (iii) Provision for nursing care – equipment, privacy, etc.;
  (iv) The organisation of nursing care, including giving of aperients;
  (v) The relationship of worry and concern to the above factors.

The importance of the study is in establishing a method of studying an area of basic nursing care, the needs, provisions and organisation of care. The method demonstrates whether care is individualised or institutionalised.

(c) *Tools developed*
  (i) Interview schedule (patient)
  (ii) Interview schedule (nurse)
  (iii) Schedule for calculating staffing ratios

(d) *Factors measured*
Home and hospital bowel habit
Worry about bowel habits
The use of aperients
Opinions on the use of bedpans, commodes, etc.
Home and hospital diet

Drugs being taken
Demographic factors
Reporting and recording of bowel action and use of aperients
Nursing practice of bowel care
Ward environmental features
Policies for bowel care
Staffing ratios

(e) *Possible categories of classification*

(i)	Class of care	Basic, administrative
(ii)	Level of initiation	Nurse initiated
(iii)	Direction of care	Institutionalised
(iv)	Patient need	Physical, psychological
(v)	Nurse performance factors	Practical skill, communications skill, perceptions, knowledge

6 Nursing care in paediatric units

(a) *The critical factor* in this study was the effect on the young child of separation from his mother during hospitalisation, and the emotional care given by nurses.

(b) *The research design* included:
  (i) an activity analysis of the nurses;
  (ii) a concurrent analysis of the emotional state of the child related to interaction with nurses, visitors, etc.
  (iii) a questionnaire to elicit the nurses' perception of their role in emotional care and their training and background to prepare them for such care;
  (iv) a questionnaire based on the recommendations of a report on *The Care of Children in Hospitals* (Platt Report).

  The importance of this study is in developing methods of studying the emotional care given to children in hospital.
  (i) in terms of other demands on time;
  (ii) in terms of role perception;
  (iii) in terms of attempts made to implement recommendations.

(c) *Tools developed*

(i)	Activity analysis schedule and categories	
(ii)	Analysis schedule for emotional state of child	
(iii)	Questionnaire	perception of role
		training for role
		demographic features
(iv)	Questionnaire	implementation of policy in Platt Report

(d) *Factors measured*
Nurse activities
Bed occupancy
Staffing ratios
Patient activity with special nursing needs, mobility and how time spent
Nurse contact with children and length of contact

Child contact with others
Emotional state of child
Demographic factors (nurses)
Nurses' understanding of children's emotional needs
Extent of implementation of recommendations of above report

(e) *Possible categories of classification*

(i)	Class of care	basic, technical, administrative
(ii)	Level of initiation	nurse initiated
(iii)	Direction of care	personalised
(iv)	Patient need	emotional and psychological
(v)	Nurse performance factors	perceptions, training, social skill

Members of the Steering Committee 1967–1969

Miss M. F. Carpenter, S.R.N., S.C.M., R.N.T., Dip. in Nursing (London)	Chairman Director of Education, Rcn
Dr. J. A. D. Anderson, M.A., M.D., D.P.H.	Department of Social Medicine, Guy's Hospital and London School of Hygiene and Tropical Medicine
Miss J. Cooper	Statistician, London School of Hygiene and Tropical Medicine
Mr. J. B. Cornish	Department of Health and Social Security
Miss J. K. McFarlane, B.Sc. (Soc.), S.R.N., S.C.M., H.V. Tutor's Certificate	Project Leader, Rcn
Miss M. Scott Wright, M.A., Ph.D.	Matron, Middlesex Hospital
Miss H. M. Simpson, B.A., S.R.N.	Nursing Officer (Research), Department of Health and Social Security
Miss J. Woodward, M.A. Ph.D.	Department of Industrial Sociology, Imperial College of Science and Technology

Members of the Project Committee 1967–1969

Dame Kathleen Raven, D.B.E., S.R.N., S.C.M.	Chairman Chief Nursing Officer, Department of Health and Social Security
Mrs. E. G. Croft	Department of Health and Social Security
Dr. Gillian Ford, M.A., B.M., B.Ch.	Department of Health and Social Security

Miss S. M. Collins, S.R.N., R.S.C.N., R.N.T.   Chairman of Rcn Council
Miss G. E. Watts, S.R.N., R.N.T.   Chairman of the General
                                                Nursing Council for England
                                                and Wales

With Members of the Steering Committee

Representatives of RCN Council on the Editing Committee

Miss L. Hockey, B.Sc. (Econ.), S.R.N.,   Research Officer, Queen's
    S.C.M., H.V. Tutor's Certificate, Q.N.   Institute of District Nursing
Miss P. Nuttall, S.R.N., M.C.S.P.   Editor, The Nursing Times
Miss M. B. Whittow, S.R.N.   Ward Sister, University
                                                College Hospital

The first team of research assistants

Mrs B. L. Franklin, B.Sc. (Nursing), University of Florida
Miss S. Hamilton-Smith, S.R.N., S.C.M. (Part 1)
Miss P. J. Hawthorne, S.R.N., S.C.M., Certificate in Social Science, Diploma in
Applied Social Studies
Miss J. Hunt, B.A., S.R.N.
Mrs F. Stockwell (née Bowker), O.N.C., S.R.N., R.M.N., R.N.T.
Miss L. A. Wright, S.R.N., D.N.

NOTES

* *The Study of Nursing Care Project Reports*, Series 1, Introduction. London, Royal College of
Nursing. pp. 10, 11–27, 6–7. Reprinted with permission of the Royal College of Nursing.

Chapter 2

The unpopular patient

FELICITY STOCKWELL

Introduction

The late 1960s and early 1970s were a landmark in the development of UK nursing research, as well as in British culture as a whole. The Briggs report was published in 1972 with its much quoted call for nursing to become a 'research-based profession' and the English Department of Health and Social Security funded a series of seminal research projects, 'The Study of Nursing Care'. Jimi Hendrix died, Deep Purple, Led Zeppelin and Eric Clapton's Cream were at the height of their powers, and some of us were wearing flares with no sense of irony.

One of the projects in the 'Study of Nursing Care' series was Felicity Stockwell's inquiry included here. Her research looked at the all-pervasive, yet easily overlooked issue of how nurses in general hospital wards enjoyed caring for some patients more than others, and asked whether this led to any differences in the quality of care that popular and unpopular patients received. Rather like listening to music from the early 1970s, reading Stockwell's report reminds us both of what was good about the products of that era and how much things have changed. One of the contributions to culture made by the 1960s and 1970s was a rejection of bureaucratic impersonality and a new concern with the individual and the individual's experiences and emotional fulfilment. Nurses also became more interested in the human interactions involved in their work and talk of holism and care came to the fore at about this time. Perhaps US psychologist Maslow's ideas about self-actualisation (mentioned by Stockwell) that seemed to articulate such feelings could only have developed out of a period of great economic growth and optimism that characterised the 1960s and the early part of the 1970s. (The middle and late 1970s saw the global rise in the price of oil and the election in Britain of Margaret Thatcher). As Maslow's theories claim, concern with these issues depends on more basic needs being largely fulfilled.

Stockwell's first question is whether popularity and unpopularity can be detected. She set about investigating this by asking nurses how much they either enjoyed or did not enjoy caring for particular patients, and devised a scoring scheme for their replies. With simple mathematics she could then derive average popularity scores for individual patients and average ratings made by each nurse. However, these average scores did not appear to reflect what she observed of the interactions within the ward, and this suggested an alternative, but equally simple approach of asking nurses to rank the most popular and unpopular patients that they were nursing. Stockwell preferred this approach because it enabled her to then ask nurses *how* they came to these judgements, which provided her with a new and interesting source of data. From a survey of behavioural literature and of the nursing literature that existed at the time – much of it from the US – she hypothesised that a number of patient characteristics were associated with unpopularity. These were largely confirmed by the nurses' own comments and included being a 'foreigner', having been in hospital for more than three months, having 'some kind of defect' and having a psychiatric disorder. Her conversations with nurses revealed considerable complexity and apparent contradiction in how nurses felt about individual patients with these characteristics. For example, she notes how one elderly woman with dementia who shouted noisily on the ward was accepted, while certain stroke patients who were aphasic or dysphasic and could also be noisy, were not.

Stockwell recorded a great amount of detailed observation about the atmosphere on her study wards and the flavour of the interaction between nurses and patients as well as among patients themselves. From these descriptions, nurses emerge as surprisingly uncritical of their attitudes and behaviour although they do not appear to be entirely unreflective. In fact, from our 30-year perspective, Stockwell's report is surprising in a number of ways. With such meticulous observation of nurses' behaviour and access to their own detailed accounts of their working experiences, she almost entirely ignores sociological literature on professional groups, and does not apply behavioural or other theory to the nurses' own roles and norms. Since then, of course, this work has been done with, among others, Joanna Latimer addressing the similar question of how nurses 'constitute' different classes of patient whose existence in the acute ward may support nurses' own professional project or be an affront to it (Latimer, J. 1997. 'Giving patients a future: the constituting of classes in an acute medical unit.' *Sociology of Health and Illness* 19: 160–185).

Stockwell's hope for her report was that:

> It should stimulate us to make greater efforts in the training of nurses so that emotional care of the patient is appreciated as a part of total patient care. It should help us to recognise that the study of behavioural sciences by nurses should be directed to an understanding of ourselves and our own human reactions to people as much as to an understanding of the patient. Leaders of professional teams such as ward sisters will recognise their part in creating a climate in which the human relations aspect of nursing will be recognised and maintained at a high standard.

Though her method may strike us now as rather unreflective and unsophisticated, proceeding as it does with a strong flavour of common sense and with instruments that are generally developed from scratch, Stockwell's meticulous approach and intelligence account for the interest and usefulness of this study today.

STOCKWELL, F. (1972)

The Unpopular Patient*

A STUDY OF INTERPERSONAL RELATIONSHIPS IN GENERAL WARDS

The original impetus for this study came from an interest in the care given to patients classified as 'difficult' by the nursing staff, and from a need to know more about the problems presented by such patients in order to help nurses understand and care for them.

The requirements of the project, of which this study forms part, were to devise some means of assessing the quality of nursing care in general wards.

It was hoped to combine these two facets by exploring the nature of popularity and unpopularity of patients with nursing staff and determining whether there was any measurable difference in the quality of nursing care they received.

The study has devised means of identifying popular and unpopular patients, explored possible reasons for patients being thus classified and examined the nurses' attitudes and behaviour towards them.

A quantitative approach was originally formulated and carried out but it was eventually felt that more information about interactions in the ward situation was needed and therefore a qualitative 'comparative analysis' was carried out to lay the foundations for more realistic measurements of nursing care in this area.

SUMMARY OF CONCLUSIONS

The chief aim of this study was to determine whether there were some patients whom the nursing team enjoyed caring for more than others and, if this proved to be so, to ascertain whether there was any measurable difference in the nursing care afforded to the most and least popular patients.

The first part of the work shows that it is possible for nurses to identify both popular and unpopular patients by means of the rating and ranking scales developed in the study. Of these, the ranking scale proved to be the more effective tool.

Reasons for patients' unpopularity were mostly related to personality factors and physical defects such as deafness but patients of foreign nationality and those whose present stay in hospital was longer than three months also proved to be significantly more unpopular than others.

In an attempt to gain more information about what might influence the nurses' enjoyment or lack of enjoyment in caring for particular patients, an attempt was made to define the nurses' view of the patient's role in the ward. In the process of a *comparative study* in four wards this was related to the patients the nurses stated they most enjoyed and least enjoyed caring for and to any variations in the amount and type of interaction that they had with them.

A quantitative evaluation of nurse/patient interaction was not attempted, but there were some observable differences in the ways in which nurses interacted with the most and the least popular patients.

In contrast with the findings of Viguers, R.T. (1959) this second part of the study showed that least attention was given to those mid-group bedfast patients who were neither particularly popular nor unpopular with the nursing staff. This finding was not anticipated.

On the whole, nurses felt that the carrying out of nursing tasks provided adequate opportunity for interaction with the patients while the patients expressed in varying degree that they did not have enough contact with, or information from, the nurses. Both nurses and patients felt, however, that stopping just for conversation was not part of the nursing task.

PROBLEMS, HYPOTHESES, QUESTIONS TO BE ANSWERED, AIMS AND METHOD OF STUDY

The problem

The basic problem underlying this study is to determine whether there is a difference in the quality of nursing care given to popular and unpopular patients and, if there is, to ascertain whether the difference is measurable as a criterion of the overall quality of nursing care given by a team of nurses to a group of patients.

The hypotheses

Arising out of the problem are two *hypotheses:*

1   That there are some patients whom nurses enjoy caring for and who are more popular than others with nursing staff.
2   That there are observable and measurable differences in the nursing care given to popular and unpopular patients.

In trying to formulate the means of testing these hypotheses, it became apparent that many questions arose which could not be answered by reference to existing theory or from the findings of relevant studies.

Questions

1   Is it possible to determine whether there are some patients who are more popular and some who are less popular than others?
2   If this is so – why?

3   If this is so, are there any reasons in common given for this?
4   Is there an 'ideal patient role' that makes a patient enjoyable to look after?
5   Do deviations from this role make the patient unpopular with the nurses?

Aims

1   To devise a means of identifying popular and unpopular patients in general wards.
2   To identify factors that might account for the popularity and unpopularity of patients.
3   To define the nurses' view of the patient's role.
4   To ascertain whether the degree of popularity influences any aspects of nursing care given to the patients.

Method of study

1   Rating and ranking techniques for identifying popular and unpopular patients.
2   Analysis of factors that might account for patient unpopularity.
3   Content analysis of the attitudes of nurses expressed about their patients.
4   Card sort technique for exploring the nurses' view of the patient's role.
5   A comparative study to gain further information about nurse/patient interaction.

FOUR WARDS COMPARED

Observations of the patients' role in the wards

In order to gain more information about the nurses' view of the patients' role in hospital wards, it was accepted by the researcher that people who conform to group norms will be more liked than those who do not, therefore the patients that the nurses most and least enjoyed caring for were identified and their behaviour observed. An attempt was made both through observation and questioning to ascertain what sanctions the nurses employed to reward conforming behaviour and to deter non-conforming behaviour; but subjective evaluation had, of necessity, to play a large part in this.

When nurses changed their opinion of how much they enjoyed looking after patients, an attempt was made to find out what influenced this change.

Finally the nurses' descriptions of their opinion of ideal and least ideal patients were examined and compared with the observations made in the ward by the author.

Behaviour of popular patients

In each of the wards there were one or more patients who were particularly able to communicate with nurses in passing, usually with some sort of cheering or light-hearted remark, and they all ranked high in the nurses' enjoyment of caring for them. In **Ash Ward** the patient most able to do this was a young woman who had been in and out of hospital a lot and on this occasion had been in for six weeks. She was confined to bed, but was situated nearest to the nurses' station. She knew the nurses by name and took an interest in their doings. She also had a small daughter who was brought to visit her every day and this helped to provide a focus of interest and an excuse for stopping at her bedside.

In **Elm Ward** the patient the nurses most enjoyed looking after was a man who had been very ill, but who was then up and about. His work had brought him into contact with hospitals and he liked to think he was familiar with the ways of ward life, but was fairly discreet in communicating this to the nurses. On occasion he would tell the junior nurses what to do and this detracted from his popularity with them. He was the centre of the up-patient group and was very helpful to the patients and the nurses would go to him to borrow a watch with a second hand if they were without one. Much of the interaction he initiated was in a bantering or jocular tone and this meant that his occasional expressions of anxiety were not taken seriously, but he circumvented this by arranging for his wife to see the consultant about his worries. Incidentally, this led to several patients doing the same thing.

The most popular patient in **Fir Ward** was a woman who was mobile and independent. She was only occasionally spontaneously talkative, but she always looked up in a friendly way as the nurses went by and laughed if they joked with her or nearby patients and she was willing to do small jobs if asked. Another patient who was very popular in this ward was an old lady who was very demented, very deaf and almost blind, but in her demented state she was perpetually having tea parties and the nurses were identified as friends from the past and invited to join her. They would play up to her delusions, pretending to be the duchess of this and that and they found her very amusing.

As **Oak Ward** was divided into two parts for nursing administration the nurses were ranking two different groups of patients, but there was one patient who had been placed in both areas and was known to all the nurses and they all enjoyed looking after him. He had been resuscitated following three episodes of cardiac arrest and, although he was somewhat apprehensive, this was appreciated by the nurses and was counterbalanced by his good sense of humour and great determination to get well again. In a quiet and undemanding way he always had a word for the nurses as they passed his bed.

Other patients whom the nurses indicated they enjoyed looking after shared these attributes of being able to facilitate communications and approach life in the ward with humour. The other things that these patients, apart from those in the geriatric ward, had in common was that they were all recovering from or showing remission during a fairly severe degree of illness and were able to express gratitude for this.

Summary

Patients the nurses enjoyed caring for:

- Were able to communicate readily with the nurses.
- Knew the nurses' names.
- Were able to joke and laugh with the nurses.
- Cooperated in being helped to get well and expressed determination to do so.

Behaviour of 'least' popular patients

The patients whom the nurses indicated they did not enjoy looking after fell into two main groups. There were those who indicated that they were not happy to be in the ward, or with what was being done for them, by grumbling and complaining or otherwise demanding attention. In the second group were those whom the nurses felt did not need to be in hospital, or should not be in that particular ward, and whose personalities did not outweigh this judgement.

Two of the patients in **Ash Ward** fitted into the 'grumbling' category: both were rather lonely widows and one of them was heard to say how embarrassing it was never having any visitors. Both were overtly self-pitying and found more than their present predicament and the ward to grumble about. One of them did not appear to be particularly miserable, although she had a reputation with most of the nurses for being a grumbler and moaner. On one occasion however, she indulged in some fairly aggressive teasing, as when she was being given her tablets she said to her neighbour 'I'm going to shoot this nurse!' and the nurse replied 'You can't get guns on the National Health', which elicited the response 'Well it will have to be poison then – slow poison'. Another patient whom the nurses did not enjoy looking after was a women very crippled with rheumatoid arthritis. She did not grumble, but she became very cross and sarcastic when frustrated either by being kept waiting for assistance or when a nurse was called away in the middle of doing something for her. She commented to the observer that she was always left until last by the nurses and quoted them as saying, when they eventually came to put her to bed 'We've come to do old nuisance now'.

Two patients whom the nurses did not enjoy looking after also fitted into the second group. One was a man, admitted in a semi-conscious state following an overdose of barbiturate, who was categorised as being 'psychy' and elicited quite a lot of positively expressed hostility from the nurses. He was extremely restless and antagonistic while semi-conscious and he was rather frightening. A seconded psychiatric nurse said she could not get near him 'because the other nurses make him so aggressive'. It was a fellow patient who stayed by him, calmed him and eventually persuaded him to drink. On regaining consciousness he was very apologetic and ingratiatingly docile, but, as one nurse said, 'I must admit, I haven't spoken to him since he came round and I don't want to. You don't know whether to pretend you don't expect him to hit you or to keep well clear in case'.

Another patient in the second group was a West Indian woman whom the nurses suspected of malingering. She had been admitted for investigation of possible hypertension, found to have nothing that warranted treatment and was discharged home. Within 24 hours she was back again, having fainted in the street. In the ward she lay unhappily in bed, resisting attempts to encourage her to sit up or get up. The 'encouragement' given by the nurses was rather half-hearted and she was described as 'a misery who is only homesick and won't help herself'.

In **Elm Ward** there was very little overt grumbling but this was the ward where the patients indulged in the most 'jocular grumbling' among themselves, mainly about the food, the cold (especially in the sitting room) and being disturbed by the nurses during their rest hour after lunch. Sometimes the nurses were intended to hear the exchanges, but they would take up the humour aspect, ignoring the underlying complaint. So, in this ward, the two patients whom the nurses least enjoyed caring for were in the group of those not needing to be in hospital. Both these patients had diabetes which was being controlled by diet and they both tested their own specimens and charted the results. The older of the two men was described by the nurses as being lazy and helpless because 'he just lies around on his bed all day'. On several occasions he complained of the cold to his neighbour but he did not communicate this to the nurses. The other patient did not think he should be in hospital and was reluctant either to test his urine specimens (sometimes guessing the results), or to keep to his diet, though the nurses did not seem to be aware of this. The fact that he continually expressed a desire to be away from the place and chivvied the doctors to discharge him seemed to make the nurses very disinterested in his welfare and progress.

The patients the nurses least enjoyed caring for in **Fir Ward** were two women, diagnosed since admission as having endogenous depression, both of whom were volitionally retarded, looked miserable and did not appear to be making any progress. There was also a woman with severe dementia who had contracture deformities and was very noisy and physically aggressive when the nurses attended her.

In **Oak Ward** the man the nurses most positively did not enjoy caring for did not have a stated diagnosis. He had been admitted previously with a duodenal ulcer and the nurses indicated that on this occasion he had only been admitted to give his wife a rest because he pretended to be so helpless and was such a worrier about his bowels. He was very able to demand the nurses' attentions, although they observably turned deaf ears to his calls and avoided the vicinity of his bed as far as possible.

There were also three patients recovering from strokes who aroused the antipathy (somewhat guiltily expressed) of the majority of the nurses, including the sister. All three patients were aphasic or dysphasic, but two of them were able to make quite a noise when more than usually frustrated. One of them had been in the ward for over a year and attempts to transfer him to other accommodation had proved unsuccessful. There was a feeling on the part of all the staff that such patients should not be in an acute medical ward and they were placed in an area away from the other patients during the day. Attitudes towards their treatment and the consequent behaviour of these three patients differed noticeably in comparison with those of two similar patients in **Elm Ward**. There the ward sister particularly favoured the older dependent men and this seemed to be communicated to the nurses, several of whom counted one or both of the 'stroke' patients among the ones they enjoyed caring for.

Summary

Patients the nurses least enjoyed caring for:

- Grumbled and complained.
- Communicated lack of enjoyment at being in hospital.
- Implied that they were suffering more than was believed by the nurses.
- Suffered from conditions the nurses felt could be better cared for in other wards of specialised hospitals.

Attitudes expressed by the nurses about patients they most enjoyed caring for

In the three medical wards, the most spontaneous and frequently given reasons for enjoyment in looking after patients related to the patients being fun or amusing, having a good sense of humour and being friendly and easy to get on with. In **Fir Ward** the majority of the nurses gave as their reason for enjoying caring for the most popular patient the fact that she was the most sensible. As one nurse said 'Obviously you like the most sensible'. It was the second most popular patient that the nurses found amusing and here the accent was placed on the fact that she was so entertaining and 'you could not help laughing *at* her'.

Sometimes a nurse would say that the person she most enjoyed looking after was a patient who did not rank high with any of the other nurses. In these instances the reason invariably given was that this was the patient they knew best, often explaining why this was so, such as the fact that they had 'specialled' him when ill, or had accompanied him to a lengthy investigation; on two occasions the nurses had met these patients before in a different ward.

In two of the wards, the sisters indicated that among the patients they most enjoyed caring for were those they knew best because they had been in and out of the ward several times over a long period. In one instance a patient so mentioned was a man whom the rest of the nursing team said they did not enjoy looking after. Very few nurses spoke of the enjoyment they obtained from the actual nursing as a criterion for ranking the patients.

Summary

The majority of the nurses included among the reasons given for choosing the patient for whom they most enjoyed caring, some reference to the patients being fun, having a good sense of humour, being easy to get on with and friendly.

Some individual preferences related to how well the nurses knew the patient.

Very few of the reasons given related to the nursing needs of the patients.

Attitudes expressed by the nurses about patients they least enjoyed caring for

Two main attitudes were expressed by the nurses about the patients they least enjoyed caring for, which linked with the two groups described under the behaviour of least liked patients. The first of these related mainly to the 'grumblers' and 'moaners' and the patients who demanded unnecessary attention, where the nurses described various feelings of frustration and impatience. For example, 'He tries my patience to the limit. He is so pre-occupied with minor things and demanding attention when others need it', and 'You can't get away from her'. In exploring such sentiments further, the nurses indicated that the best way of dealing with people who demanded attention was to ignore them as far as possible and to show them that other patients needed the nurses' attention more than they did. Nobody could recall an actual incident of 'being

caught' by a patient and not being able to get away. It appeared that they were express-
ing a fear that this might happen rather than describing the discomfort of a
remembered experience. If a nurse expressed this particular sentiment about a patient
and later in the interview, when discussing what the nurse did during slack periods in
the ward and the use of these for talking to or listening to the patients, the observer
asked whether such a patient could provide a good excuse for stopping to talk for a
while. This suggestion was mostly dismissed by indicating that if you gave in to such
people you just stored up trouble by making them worse and no one would thank you
for that.

The second attitude related to the patients whom the nurses felt did not need to be
in hospital or whose condition did not warrant their being in that particular ward. In
these instances the nurses expressed irritation that such patients wasted their time, to
which sometimes an afterthought was added that perhaps they could not help it. On
the whole they were dismissed as being nuisances or hypochondriacs, and in one
instance as being psychopathic. When asked how they knew when a patient was gen-
uinely suffering or 'putting on' symptoms, the answers were that 'you can just tell', or
sometimes because the doctor or sister had told them. In one ward the sister was heard
to explain during a reporting session that a patient's fainting attacks had been diagnosed as psychogenic; this did not mean that the nurses should ignore them, but just
not to make too much fuss about them, which showed that possibly she had an awareness of the nurses' natural inclinations. In another ward when the sister was talking
about a patient admitted for investigation of abdominal pain who was known to have
been treated previously for cancerphobia, she told the nurses not to take too much
notice of him as he was just a hypochondriac with probably nothing the matter.

With regard to the patients whose condition the nurses felt was not suitable for
their particular ward, the sentiments expressed implied a reluctance to provide the
necessary care even though it was within the team's capabilities. For example, the
three stroke patients in **Oak Ward** were grudged the amount of care they needed,
albeit somewhat guiltily when expressed to the observer. In another ward a patient
admitted in an unconscious state following a head injury elicited a lot of resentment
about the amount of care he needed, whereas unconscious patients admitted to the
same ward following cerebro-vascular accidents who needed the same amount of
care and observation were given it unstintingly.

Sometimes the nurses' antipathy towards patients arose or coincided with the fact
that they did not feel competent to provide the necessary care and this was particularly
the case with patients diagnosed as being in need of psychiatric treatment. In all the
wards extremely negative sentiments were expressed about such patients and sometimes the behaviour of the nurses seemed designed to exacerbate the patients'
symptoms. The most extreme example of this occurred in **Fir Ward**, where an elderly
woman was admitted with a diagnosis of agitated depression. The week before, a
patient with senile dementia had been admitted who was considerably more noisy,
restless and uncomprehending, but senile dementia was acceptable to the nursing staff
and although this patient was not popular, she was fitted into the ward routine with the
minimum of trouble. The woman with agitated depression was received and treated
quite differently and the sister and permanent staff seemed to be glad when she

proved 'unmanageable' and was transferred to a psychiatric hospital. In one of the medical wards a patient admitted for investigation of headaches was diagnosed by the houseman as being a hysteric, and the nurses laughed at the accounts of him groaning whenever he was aware of a member of staff was around. When a psychiatrist, who was asked to examine him, suggested he should have further investigations at another hospital as his symptoms were consistent with early cerebral tumour, he was totally disbelieved by doctors and nurses, but they arranged his transfer with such comments as 'they are welcome to him' and 'it won't take them long to see through him'. Thus rejection or ridicule was usually the lot of such patients and the nurses either saw them as too 'mad' for their care or else as playing up and not in need of hospitalisation.

Summary

Frustration and impatience were expressed about patients who grumble, moan or demand attention, also irritation about patients considered to be wasting their time. Psychiatric patients were overtly rejected or ridiculed.

Use of sanctions

Where rewards or deterrents are employed in a group situation they give some indication of which behaviours are approved and which disapproved, but it is an extremely elusive aspect to observe. When the nurses were asked how they might indicate approval to the patients they enjoyed caring for and disapproval to the patients they least enjoyed caring for they found it difficult to express. Several of them said they treated all the patients the same and three nurses ranked the patients only on the understanding that the order in which they placed the patients made no difference to the way in which they treated them.

When nurses did recognise that there was possibly some difference in their behaviour they were reluctant to verbalise what this might be, except in a very general way, such as 'well I suppose I would be willing to put myself out more for someone like Mr.—'. These observations are, therefore, subjective interpretations of observed behaviour relating to those patients known to be more and less popular with the nurses.

Sanctioning behaviour could operate in several areas. Where the nurse came into contact with a patient because of carrying out a nursing task she could vary the way in which she approached a patient, the length of time she spent with him and the degree to which she personalised the interaction. The observer found these variations most noticeable when watching the ward sisters doing their daily round of the patients but they were also noticeable during temperature and medicine rounds and the serving of meals.

Other discriminatory behaviour was observed, particularly in relation to food. A patient might ask for a second piece of cake as a tea trolley returned past his bed and one might be given some, another refused and yet another given some but with a sarcastic remark. The same pattern was observed if a patient missed coffee through being out of the ward, with one person being allowed to get some for themselves, of having it fetched by a nurse, or being refused it. An unpopular patient who had been starved all day for tests to be carried out was given a plate of macaroni cheese for supper, which he did not fancy. He asked if there was any alternative and was told 'No', but his neighbour asked another nurse for some ham and salad which was also one of the diet meals, instead of his macaroni, and when given some he exchanged his plate with that of the other patient.

Discrimination was especially observable in **Oak Ward** where rules for patients were most rigidly enforced, though some patients were allowed to smoke or have visitors out of hours without comment, while others were constantly chivvied and their relatives asked to leave.

The nurses seemed to think that ignoring patients was the most powerful deterrent to unacceptable behaviour and certainly some unpopular patients had requests ignored or forgotten. For example, when a staff nurse was doing a round of the patients a man asked if he could have his letters if the post had come as it was his birthday. She said she would look, then contacted the kitchen to order a special cake for his tea but appeared not to notice that the post was already on the desk. Over an hour and a half later the man asked a junior nurse and she went to ask the staff nurse who was sitting at the desk with the post in front of her. She picked the letters up, saying 'I hope Mr.— has got something as it's his birthday'.

Apart from 'forgettings' some other 'ignoring behaviours' were probably not used as sanctions but were possibly due to the nurses' inexperience and lack of supervision, as when an elderly patient was given meat for lunch, which he was unable to cut up and when a patient who was supposed to be having complete rest had his lunch left on his locker and had to prop himself on his elbow in order to eat it. Similarly, patients described feeling upset when nurses chatted to each other, excluding them from the conversation, while carrying out care for them, but this seemed to be the practice of some nurses irrespective of whom they were caring for, rather than happening to just one or two patients.

A few positive rewards were seen to be given to patients as when the nurses clubbed together to buy a present for a girl who was having her birthday in hospital, and when the sister in one ward went to a great deal of trouble to arrange for a man to visit his crippled wife at home before he went to a convalescent home. Possibly the largest area of rewarding behaviour on the part of the nurses was the way in which they accepted favours from the patients. For example, laughing at jokes made by popular patients, accepting compliments and such things as sweets, fruit and newspapers from them, while refusing such offers from unpopular patients, unless they were given as a farewell present on their departure.

Summary

Rewarding behaviour by the nurses:

- Willingness to give more time.
- Allowing a more personalised interaction.
- Willingness to accept gifts and favours.
- Allowing lapses in keeping the rules.

Deterrent behaviour by the nurses:

- Ignoring the patients.
- Forgetting patients' requests.
- Refusing gifts and favours.
- Enforcing rules.
- Using sarcasm.

Observations of nurse/patient interaction in the wards

Patterns of interaction

The most striking aspect of interaction patterns in all the wards was that they were almost entirely task initiated. Nurses did not approach patients unless they were going to carry out some treatment or provide some service or unless they had some specific information they wanted to collect, and on the whole patients did not approach the nurses unless they had a specific need. There were some exceptions to this general pattern. In **Ash Ward** there was a junior pupil nurse who was able to make comments to the patients in general and if anyone responded she would carry on further conversation with them. If other nurses were not busy, such as when waiting for the meal-trolley to arrive for lunch, they would then gather round and join in.

In **Elm Ward** there was a Malaysian student nurse who was also State Enrolled, she would leave her colleagues when, in a slack period they had gathered in the sluice or treatment room, and approach elderly and lonely patients to get them talking and cheer them up.

Apart from these exceptions, it held true that on the whole when nursing tasks were completed the nurses removed themselves from the patient areas. This might have been because the observer was present, but remarks made by the patients indicated that this was a usual pattern. Thus one patient said 'Sometimes there are so many nurses they are falling over each other to do things for you and then suddenly you can't get a nurse anyhow'. Certainly, episodes were observed in each of the wards where one patient suddenly needed help and the other patients rang their bells or called and the observer was unable to find a nurse. After one of these episodes when a patient had fainted and seven minutes had elapsed before a nurse answered the bells, a patient said: 'I don't know where they get to – it's all right for me because I am independent, but I see the old ladies leaving their tea because they don't know whether they'll be able to get a bed-pan when they need one'. This remark, made in a well-staffed ward, underlines another problem in nurse/patient interactions, which is the difficulty that some patients have in attracting a nurse's attention when there is one in the ward. Several of the nurses and some of the patients commented on the frustration and annoyance they felt when a nurse was interrupted in the middle of a task and it might be this that accounted for the singleness of purpose of some nurses while in the ward area that prevented them from hearing or seeing some patients' request for help or attention. On a few occasions patients were purposely ignored or told curtly that they would have to wait; as these were the people who were classified as demanding or unpopular in other ways this very observable behaviour possibly helped to deter other patients from making requests.

One of the factors that distinguished popular patients was that they were able to attract the nurses' attention and initiate conversation with them and this was also observed by other patients who sometimes asked them to act as intermediaries in making their requests or voicing their complaints. If such a patient was ambulant, a bed-ridden patient might ask him for a drink of water or a urinal rather than 'trouble' the nurses.

On the whole the patients seemed very well aware of each other's needs and were very alert to each other's conditions when the nurses were not in sight. However, in all the medical wards there seemed to be a tacit understanding among the patients as to who they could do things for and who needed to have a nurse's attention. Thus in **Elm Ward** a patient recovering from a stroke, but still very helpless, was wheeled by the nurses into the sitting-room. Shortly after, the other patients left the sitting-room and returned to the ward, whereupon the man started calling for a nurse. The other patients had some chat and laughter about the nurses expecting him to stay in the sitting-room in the cold and eventually one of them went to see what he wanted. He asked to be wheeled back to the ward but was told that a nurse would have to do this. The ambulant patient returned to his fellows without getting a nurse and the calls started again until the ward maid went and wheeled him back to his bedside. An elderly man in the same ward, who was almost as helpless, was felt by the nurses not to be as incapacitated as he seemed. On some occasions the ambulant patients provided almost all his nursing care, such as helping him out of his chair and accompanying him to the lavatory while encouraging him to walk on his own, or cutting up his meat and making sure he had biscuits with a cup of tea when he hadn't eaten any lunch. It seemed as if the nurses were unaware of this, but on one occasion a nurse said 'Mr. X will you try your charm on Pop? He won't take his tea for me'. A comparable situation occurred in **Oak Ward** where there was another patient who was very helpless following a stroke, with hemiplegia and aphasia. He had been a very independent man and tried to continue that way in the ward. He was given a tripod walking aid but found it almost impossible to get out of his chair and would fall on the floor; as he had to climb four steps to reach the lavatory it was impossible for him to get there unless someone lifted his paralysed leg up each step. It was nearly always an ambulant patient who helped him up the steps and usually a patient who went to his aid when he fell. A nurse sometimes had to be collected to assist because he was so heavy but they did not go of their own volition if the patients got there to help first.

It was noticeable in all the wards that there were some patients who had practically no verbal contact with the nurses or other patients for hours at a time. These would be patients who figured as neither popular nor unpopular and who were not acutely ill but were confined to bed. Routine tasks, such as temperature recording and serving of meals were carried out for them by nurse after nurse without a word being exchanged. For example, a patient in **Ash Ward** saw the nurse coming round to weigh everyone and when the scales were placed at the foot of her bed she got out of bed, stood on them, had her weight recorded and got back into bed without either of them saying a word. It is possible that such patients do not want to talk to anyone but it seems more likely that they could not take the initiative in starting conversation, since they talked with other patients when they were allowed up and could mix more freely, and did not rebuff any conversational openings offered to them.

Summary

Nurse/patient interactions were mainly task-initiated.

Nurses were not available in the patient areas when there were no tasks to be carried out.

Interactions with some patients were mainly non-verbal.

Joking, teasing and banter

Many of the interactions in the wards were conducted in a joking, teasing or bantering manner. There were a few patients and a few nurses who were particularly adept at initiating interactions of this sort, but other people would join in fairly readily.

Much of the conversation among groups of ambulant patients took the form of jocular banter and jocular grumbling. The subjects for the grumbling were for the main part of the food, the cold, noise and disturbed rest. There were innumerable examples in this area, fairly typical being exchanges such as:

'How's your lunch?'

'I never have gone much for seaweed.' (Referring to the cabbage.)

'They should take some of the stalks out.'

'Philip Harben wouldn't recognise it. They could make him feel useful here.'

or:

'It's cold this morning.'

'Trying to kill us off I expect – make room for the next blokes.'

'They should issue us with fur coats, but they would have to be long ones.'

Where the majority of patients were confined to bed there was noticeably less banter. Perhaps this was because it was impossible to obtain the necessary privacy. It also seems as if bed patients made more overt complaints than ambulant patients and, while this was only an impression, it was true that practically all the patients whom the nurses stated they did not enjoy caring for because they grumbled and complained were confined to bed.

While the amount of bantering conversation between ambulant patients seemed fairly constant in the three medical wards, there was quite a difference in the amount of teasing and joking between patients and nurses, most being in **Elm Ward** and least in **Oak Ward.** The observer was convinced however that, since it occurred frequently, it was an important facet of communication. In the geriatric ward there was a little teasing and banter between some of the nurses and patients, but because of the nature of the patients' conditions and the fact that this ward had the largest number of foreign-speaking nurses there was only a small amount of lighthearted interchange.

Sometimes patients tried unsuccessfully to make jokes and usually they were the ones who were not very popular with the nurses. For instance, when a rather isolated patient had been taken for the first bath he had had for some time, he said to the nurse:

'I feel a new man. That's my birthday bath' to which the nurse responded 'Is it your birthday then?' 'Yes' he said, 'I only bath on my birthday!' This was said with laughter, but the nurse solemnly wished him 'Many happy returns.' Other patients got the point and laughed at the nurse, but she chided them for not greeting him also.

On some occasions remarks made by patients that were intended seriously were taken as jokes or teasing by the nurse. One example of this was an enquiry by a young lad with diabetes as to whether he should return the protamine zinc insulin which he had at home and no longer needed. He said 'I've got fifteen bottles of "protein" zinc insulin at home. Do you want them?' The nurse replied 'Yes, I don't mind having some of *that*', and another patient joined in with 'If it goes well with gin I'll have some too!' There was laughter and the nurse went away leaving the query unanswered. Another incident concerned a patient who had been given breakfast when booked for an I.V.P. which had then had to be postponed to the following day. At tea time he approached the nurses taking the trolley round and asked if he was allowed to have supper because of the test or should he have something extra to eat now. The nurses as a group responded teasingly, saying he shouldn't be worrying about supper when it was only tea time; as he was so lazy and lay on his bed all day he should be eating less, not more and no one actually answered his question.

It was observable that teasing and banter could be used in a rewarding way and in a deterrent way. A popular patient in one ward whose wife had sent him a large bunch of red roses on their wedding anniversary was teased in a way that enhanced the value of the roses both to him and to other patients who could see them. In the same ward there was a young Malaysian patient who was not very ill, not very cooperative and who tried to be too familiar with the nurses, demanding their attention. He constantly boasted about how much money he earned and two nurses colluded in saying that he would need a lot of money when he got the bill for his stay in hospital. He did not know whether to believe them or not and, when they went on kidding him, the librarian joined in agreeing with the nurses. Eventually, he started coughing and asked for some cough medicine. One nurse went away to fetch some linctus and came back with it, saying 'It's only coloured water, but we'll make you pay for it'. The nurses left the ward and after a while the patient approached another man to enquire about who did have to pay for treatment in the ward.

It was not uncommon for the patients to tease the nurses and many patients expressed appreciation of nurses who could take a joke. However, quite a number of nurses said that being teased by patients was one of the displeasures of nursing and, as one nurse said, the patients she did not enjoy caring for were the ones who teased her. It was possible for teasing to incapacitate a nurse, as when the patients in one ward were teasing a junior student nurse about which side of an extra bed to put a locker where there was very little space. Each side she put it they made up reasons why it should go on the other side, until she left it at the foot of the bed and went away. Eventually another nurse put it in place without a comment from anyone.

The patients' banter and teasing of the nurses could be rewarding or deterrent and, while comments about the nursing staff were usually sympathetic and favourable, if there were nurses or nursing situations that upset the patients they would come in for very ribald banter treatment. A nurse in one ward was so unpopular that the patients joined with other nurses when imitating and joking about her; in another ward a small group of patients tried to get the nurses to join in their complaining banter about the ward sister.

Summary

Joking, teasing and bantering interchange was common in the three medical wards.

Jocular grumbling, which occurred most among ambulant patients, appeared to limit formal complaining.

Teasing and banter were used in different ways with popular and less popular patients.

Nurses' attitudes to interaction with patients

When asked about the pleasures and displeasures in nursing, many of the nurses said that the things they enjoyed were working with people and the fact that nursing was never boring, and the things they disliked were being too busy, being interrupted while doing a task and not being treated with enough consideration by senior members of the nursing staff. When the observer tried to discover what constituted being 'too busy' and when it had last occurred, it became apparent that this was an abstract fear rather than a reality frequently experienced; further discussion elicited the fact that all the nurses would rather be busy than not have enough to do. This held true in all the wards, but in **Fir Ward** the nurses felt they were kept busy most of the time, particularly the pupil nurses who were of the opinion that the work there was much too hard and physically exhausting and they thought they would become ill if they did not soon move to another ward.

In the medical wards the nurses described various feelings of distress and guilt they had experienced when there was not enough work to fill the time. They said it was possible to make some tasks, such as doing the medicine round, last a long time or else to find jobs to do outside the ward area. When asked how they viewed going into the ward and talking to or listening to a patient at such times, the consensus of opinion among the nurses was that your colleagues would consider you to be slacking if you did that and this made you feel guilty. On the whole they felt that the sisters in these wards would not mind, but in **Ash Ward** and **Oak Ward** they thought the sisters would check up extra well to make sure everything was done. If it was certain that all the necessary tasks had been done, it seemed to be more acceptable to read the patients' notes than to go and talk to them.

The nurses were asked with whom, at the present time, they would have a conversation if they were sure that nobody would mind and, with one exception, they said it would be one of the patients they enjoyed looking after. The one exception was a nurse who said she would talk to someone who did not have any visitors, but when asked who was in this category at the moment, said there was no one, although this was the ward where one of the unpopular patients had complained of the embarrassment of not having any visitors.

On the whole, the impression gained from the nurses was that they enjoyed talking to and learning about the patients as they carried out nursing tasks, but they did not feel there was any need for them to be more freely available for more of the patients and anyway there was no legitimate time for this. In **Ash Ward** to which student psychiatric nurses were seconded it was suggested by general student nurses that they talked to the patients too much, making them too dependent and unwilling to go home.

Summary

The nurses felt that they had enough conversation with patients while carrying out nursing tasks.

They felt guilty if they 'chatted' to patients because their colleagues would think they were slacking.

They felt uncomfortable during slack periods in the wards but did not feel that having conversation with patients constituted 'work' at such times.

If they stopped to talk to patients, nurses would choose the patients they most enjoyed caring for.

Patients' attitudes to interaction with nurses

Common to all the wards were comments from patients about how busy the nurses always were but how cheerful they managed to be in spite of this. If any omissions or mistakes were noticed, they were explained away and forgiven because the nurses had so much to do and so many things to think about. With this went a feeling that the nurses should not be bothered with trivial matters, and although some patients wished it was otherwise, it was a code that was strictly enforced by the patients among themselves, as well as being endorsed by the nurses. One patient who had been a nurse many years before was telling her neighbour about the discipline there used to be in the wards and how much easier it was when everyone knew 'what was what'. She said 'Now the nurses are running all over the place and there is no peace, but they are not doing anything for you and you don't know where you are' and it was accepted by them both that there was nothing to be done about it. Referring to changes in the amount of discipline in the ward, another patient said, 'It's the free and easy atmosphere that amazes me. You don't feel so in awe, but you need to know that things aren't going to slip – I don't think nurses notice things like they used to.'

Several patients expressed bewilderment or anxiety about the number of nurses belonging to the ward and not being able to work out who was going to be there. One woman who had been in hospital many times previously explained to a recently admitted neighbour that, when she first comes in she picks a nurse she feels she can depend on and then when she is around asks her anything she needs, but patients with less experience of hospital had difficulty in determining who it was legitimate to interrupt in order to ask for something. In the two wards where there were ward clerks it was noticeable that many patients were able to approach them when they felt they should not bother the nurses. Sometimes the shyer patients would ask other patients to make requests for them or would seek reassurance that it was all right to ask.

Many of the patients implied that their own worries and needs were not serious enough for the nurses to be concerned about and, when talking among themselves, they quite often commented on the excellence of the care given to very ill patients and expressed confidence that as soon as anything was seriously wrong with anyone the nurses noticed and did something about it quickly and you could not really expect more of a hospital ward. There was, however, an undertone of regret that more time was not available for their concerns and occasional frustrated outbursts about being kept waiting or having nursing attention interrupted indicated a felt lack of attention.

Summary

The patients felt the nurses were too busy to be bothered with trivial matters.

Patients would welcome more opportunity to voice worries and needs, but felt this could detract from nursing care given to the seriously ill.

SUMMARY OF PART II

By a process of selective observation in four wards an attempt was made to explore and record the behaviour of nurses and patients as they interacted with each other. Popular and unpopular patients were identified and special attention paid to any differences in the way the nurses behaved towards them.

Interviews with the nurses and talks with the patients explored some of the attitudes about roles in the ward situation and what constituted desirable and undesirable behaviour.

NOTES

The Study of Nursing Care Project Reports, Series 1, No 2. London, Royal College of Nursing. pp. 10, 11, 12–13, 45–61. Reprinted with permission of the Royal College of Nursing.

Chapter 3

Information

A prescription against pain

JACK HAYWARD

Introduction

Jack Hayward's chapter is one of the 12 pieces of research which formed the Study of Nursing Care project, funded by the UK Department of Health and Social Security, administered by the Royal College of Nursing, and carried out during the early 1970s. Like the other research from this landmark project which is included in this volume, Hayward's piece tackles an area of fundamental importance to nurses, the prevention of anxiety and the alleviation of pain by means of giving (relatively) simple information to patients. Also like the other studies, he approaches the issue with a direct simplicity.

Hayward's introduction reads as an uncannily contemporary statement, pointing out that professional judgement is an inadequate guide to efficacy of treatment and patient impact. What is needed, he argues, are 'objective indices of nursing care', not only because patient welfare is the ultimate criterion, but because patients are developing a 'consumer attitude to health care'. This is not because of the impact of Thatcherism and the New Right – still seven years in the future – but because of the maturing of the NHS itself: few patients now remembered the pre-Health Service 'charity bed'. A further reason for the promotion of research in nursing was that it could lead to increased job satisfaction because research which would identify a body of specifically nursing knowledge and expertise could contribute, along with more enlightened employment attitudes, to increased personal fulfilment on the part of the nurse. But one adjustment would need to be made before this was possible, and this was to more closely align nurse teaching and nursing research. Hayward argues that nursing was an unusual profession because of the way that these two functions were separated and that this led to long-term delays in feeding the findings of research into nurse teaching.

Hayward's research question was as simple as his research design. He carried out an experiment in which one group of surgical patients is given specific information about ward practices, procedures and the pain that they might expect postoperatively, while a matched control group is not. He measured the possibly different impacts of these strategies by assessing postoperative anxiety, use of analgesia and overall well-being. His conclusion was, perhaps not surprisingly, that information did appear to alleviate anxiety and lead to less drug use after surgery. He measured his outcomes with a combination of preexisting instruments, such as the S-R Inventory of Anxiousness, and newly developed tools, including the Patient Subjective Scale which included a pain 'thermometer' (a cardboard representation of pain levels) as well as simple, if probing questions, including 'What single thing contributed most to your comfort and well-being whilst recovering from your operation?'

Hayward and his assistant took turns at being 'informer' and 'observer'; the informer randomly allocating the first suitable patients into either the informed or control group and providing a schedule of information tailored for the operation that each 'informed' patient was expecting. On the morning of the informed group's operation, the informer visited and repeated the set of information. The observer, who was, for the most part, blind to the grouping, visited the patients for the first five postoperative days and recorded the relevant data. According to his report, the procedure worked well with 68 patients participating fully in the study in one hospital. Hayward repeated the experiment, with some modification, in a second hospital with a further 66 patients. The chapter of his report included here gives the results.

When discussing the implications of his findings, Hayward points to previous and contemporary research which had stressed patients' dissatisfaction with the paucity of the information they were given. He also highlights a Ministry of Health report from 1963 which had stated that, if doctors could not supply patients with the information they needed, then the responsibility fell on the nursing staff, and preferably upon the ward sister. Though the implications of this research seem straightforward, Hayward is aware that considerable reorganisation would need to occur if ward sisters were to spend what he estimates as the 30–40 minutes required with each newly admitted patient, particularly given the fact that such nurses appeared to spend only a very small proportion of their time in actual patient contact. Such a change would need support 'from the highest levels of nursing management'. He also suggests that paternalistic attitudes to health care are outmoded and recommends that patients' needs for information are taken seriously and that nurse educators play their part in making students aware of the undesirable effects on patients of high levels of anxiety. However, Hayward is reluctant to propose simplistic changes to ward structures and roles. He concludes his report with an acknowledgement of the complexity of health care organisation:

> . . . the ultimate aim of nursing research must be to examine the effects of various nursing procedures in terms of patient welfare. It is thus the *process* of nursing which requires detailed scrutiny, and this involves studying the ward as a social unit, no one part of which can be satisfactorily examined without considering the others. Quality of care is obviously a multifactorial process and, as so often occurs in complex situations, the interactions between factors may exert more significant influences than the major factors themselves.

HAYWARD, J. (1975)

Information – A Prescription Against Pain*

FORMULATION OF HYPOTHESIS AND RESEARCH DESIGN

The main experimental hypothesis was formulated as follows: patients who were given information appertaining to their illness and recovery would, when compared to an appropriate control group, report less anxiety and pain during the post-operative recovery period.

Adequate testing of this hypothesis required a suitably controlled situation. In planning the effects of treatment or experience on a group of patients it is usually necessary to observe a control group, the characteristics of which largely resemble those of the experimental group. As comparison may be influenced by a wide range of personal characteristics such as age, sex, and number of previous admissions, a process of 'matching' is frequently adopted. This involves the comparison of 'pairs' of subjects who share common characteristics including the operation type, e.g. two males, aged 31–40 years, with similar social and educational backgrounds, admitted for partial gastrectomy, one of whom would join the experimental group, the other the control group, i.e. a 'matched pairs' design.

There are, however, two varieties of possible matching (Billewicz, 1964). In the former, patients are matched pair for pair as described above. The second method, described by Billewicz as 'frequency matching', is where the identity of actual pairs is not preserved, but the composition of the experimental and control groups is so manipulated that the distribution of sampling between the matching categories is the same in each group. Therefore the experiment is performed on two comparable groups rather than on several comparable pairs. As really close matching of the type described is difficult in clinical research (it may be difficult to 'match' patients on more than two or three variables) frequency matching is a useful approach.

Before finishing the research design, the following underlying assumptions were isolated:

1   That pain is a combination of physical and psychological factors which, taken in their entirety, form the pain experience.
2   That pain and anxiety are closely related phenomena, i.e. as anxiety increases the awareness of pain increases.
3   That the reduction of uncertainty about future events is a viable way of reducing anxiety.
4   That considerable evidence exists to show that the reduction of excessive anxiety in surgical patients is desirable.
5   That nursing information is that information which a trained and experienced surgical nurse could reasonably be expected to possess and to pass on to patients at opportune times and in an appropriate manner.

The investigation commenced in the two surgical wards from which patients for the initial interviews were drawn, and involved two researchers who alternated in role between 'informer' and 'observer'. To help eliminate bias from the observations, or at least to balance inevitable bias, the following procedures were incorporated into the experimental design.

1   After considerable rehearsal of aims and objectives, the initial 'informer' was selected from the two researchers by the spin of a coin. This person was responsible for the selection of suitable patients and their random allocation to either informed or control groups *without communicating this information to the observer*, so that the subsequent post-operative data were collected by someone who was 'blind' as to whether the patient belonged to the informed or control category. After every 10 patients, the roles of informer and observer were reversed.

2   After perusal of past records and discussion with medical staff, appendicectomy was chosen as the 'least serious' operation for inclusion. The sample was drawn largely from patients whose operations were deemed of 'moderate severity', e.g. cholecystectomy; the upper limit was left open at this stage, but in fact tended to be determined by necessity for transfer to intensive care.

3   Male and female patients were included and it was hoped that possible observer bias due to sex differences would be nullified by having a male and female researcher.

4   Patients were seen by the informer as soon as possible after admission, an interview room was provided for this purpose. Their approval and cooperation was sought, after which the admission procedure (described later) took its course.

5   Following their operation, patients were visited thrice daily by the observer who recorded progress for the first five days of the recovery period.

MEASUREMENT TOOLS USED (DEPENDENT VARIABLES)

1 The S–R Inventory of Anxiousness – used on admission

As anxiety formed an important feature of this investigation, it was obviously desirable to incorporate some type of measure. The *S–R Inventory* (Endler *et al.*, 1962) attempts to measure anxiety-proneness of individuals in response to specified situations, e.g. during a visit to the dentist, or after accidentally cutting a finger. It is, therefore, an estimate of the way a person habitually responds, i.e. 'trait anxiety', and should not be particularly sensitive to short term fluctuations in anxiety state (Appendix C).

The inventory was originally devised by considering the relative contribution of situations and individual differences in the production of anxiety. Furthermore it allows the effects of specific situations to be separated from the modes of response which serve as reactions, e.g. one person's response to a visit to the dentist may emerge in the cardiovascular mode – 'my heart pounds' – whereas another may react by sweating.

The original inventory consisted of 11 situations thought to be familiar to college students. It included both social and non-social situations, which varied from innocuous to threatening. Choice of situations for inclusion was largely dependent upon the use to which the inventory was directed; therefore, in the present case, half of the situations chosen were relevant to the present research which were presented with half from the original inventory (Endler and Hunt, 1969).

The format consisted of 10 situations and nine modes of response, plus two supplementary questions. Each response was rated on a five-point scale, with a high score indicating high anxiety.

The *S–R Inventory* was thought suitable for this particular research as situations appropriate for the purpose could be specifically chosen, leaving modes of response virtually the same as in the original version. Some initial concern was felt about the number of responses required – a total of 110 – but these fears were not realised, perhaps owing to the repetitive nature of the layout.

In summary, the main objective in using a pre-operative measure of anxiousness was to test its ability to predict post-operative pain as measured by analgesic consumption and patients' verbal report. If this is the case, it should then be possible to establish this relationship statistically.

2   Patient Subjective State Scale (PSS)

This included a number of questions relating to patients' state of well-being which were documented by the observer three times a day. The response was rated on a five-point scale and entered on the data sheet. Considered in order of presentation the questions were:

i *The pain thermometer (a visual cardboard scale)*

Some of the difficulties of measuring pain are considered in Chapter 1. However, the pain thermometer was used by Joyce (1968) and Lasagna (1958) and received favourable mention from both:

> The researcher presents a pain thermometer to subjects, asking them to place at appropriate 'temperatures' the main points, very severe, severe, moderate and slight. By then calculating the number of degrees between pain levels, it was hoped that one would have some measure of the relative importance assigned to these levels by different people. (Lasagna, 1958)

In order to keep to a five-point scale the following 'temperatures' were used:

a   I have no pain at all
b   A little pain
c   Quite a lot of pain
d   A very bad pain
e   As much pain as I could possibly bear

The colloquial nature of these phrases reflect the comments of ward patients when replying to the question, 'How much pain have you?' Patients were shown the pain thermometer at the pre-operative interview and given an explanation of how it worked.

Question ii

Is your pain local, that is, just around the site of the operation, or is it wide-spread?

It is a common clinical observation that wound pain may sometimes be restricted to the immediate area, whereas at other times, or in other patients, it may be widespread. It is accepted that the origins of widespread pain may be diverse, e.g. 'wind', nevertheless the question was included on clinical evidence that widespread pain often appears to be reported by more anxious patients.

Question iii

How do you feel in yourself, by that I mean what sort of mood are you in and how is your morale?

It was hypothesised that less anxious patients would report higher morale; a major finding of Egbert *et al.* (1964). Clinically speaking, high morale should be characterised by alertness, increased level of overall activity and an interest in decision taking, all of which should expedite both biological and psychological recovery.

Question iv

Have you any feeling of sickness (nausea)?

For many years clinical evidence has suggested the existence of a positive relationship between level of anxiety and post-operative vomiting in surgical patients, a hypothesis tested by Dumas and Leonard (1963) and upheld following a well-controlled experiment. Anxious patients vomited in the recovery room significantly (the word *significantly* denotes statistical significance when used in this report) more than did less anxious ones.

These four questions were asked three times daily; the following three questions were asked only on the morning visit:

Question v

How did you sleep last night?

Causes of sleeplessness vary widely and include individual variations in sleep patterns, insomnia due to anxiety, noise in the ward, pain and the necessity for night-time treatments. Despite these variations it was decided to compare informed and control patients' ratings of this variable.

Question vi

How are you managing your food?

A general assessment of appetite.

Question vii

During the initial interviews with post-operative patients the following question was asked 'What single thing contributed most to your comfort and wellbeing whilst recovering from your operation?' Answers varied considerably but the six most frequently occurring were (in random order), visiting time, talking to other patients, tablets or injections, talking to your doctor, nursing attention, and talking to sister or nurses. These findings were subsequently assembled to form a multiple choice question which was printed on a card and shown to patients on the morning visit. The question 'Which of these, if any, have been the greatest source of comfort to you over the past twenty-four hours' was asked and the choice recorded. If none of these factors was relevant, patients' own feelings were noted.

It is important to recognise that recordings on the PSS are observers' ratings of patients' statements, which are, in effect, a translation of the patients' comments and run the risk of bias. In order to minimise the risk, pilot trials, during which both investigators visited a patient simultaneously and recorded reactions independently, were carried out. After a number of practice ratings, final trials on eight patients were recorded by both investigators and the agreement between them assessed statistically by means of Spearman's Rank Correlation. (A measure of association between two variables. See appendix note on Statistics.) The resultant figure of 0.88 indicated a high level of observer reliability.

3 Post-operative analgesic consumption

This has been widely used as an indirect index of pain and seems, at first sight, to offer an objective measure. Although requests for analgesics might reasonably be expected to reflect levels of pain, the issue is complicated by individual differences between patients, especially in their willingness, or otherwise to request drugs. The protocols reported in Chapter 4 indicate some of the uncertainties expressed by patients as to the procedures for requesting drugs and their fears about side effects. Hence, it is perhaps too optimistic to consider analgesic consumption as a truly accurate measure of pain, but, when considered with other measures, it forms useful and easily quantifiable data.

A record of all analgesic drugs given for the first five post-operative days, calculated from the time of operation, was therefore added to the patients' records. To compensate for differences in the type of analgesic used, e.g. omnopon or pethidine, the drug dosages were reduced to a 'morphine equivalent score'. This was achieved by establishing the dose of a given drug which was, according to the pharmacological literature, equal to 10 mgs of morphine sulphate, and calling this 10 units (Lasagna and Beecher, 1954; Egbert *et al.*, 1964), thus making comparison possible.

4 Post-operative vomiting

Incidence of vomiting was recorded by a small chart attached to the patients' chartboards. This was completed by nursing staff who entered each incidence of vomiting day and night, supplementary information being provided by Question 3 of the PSS.

5 Ward sisters' assessment

Sisters were asked to rate the post-operative progress of each patient on the basis of her own professional judgement on a five-point scale ranging from 'unusually well' to 'very slowly' (Appendix F). This served the important double functions of, firstly, involving the ward nursing staff in the research, and secondly, seeing if variations in other measures of post-operative progress would be paralleled by a rating based upon professional insight. The scale was completed on the sixth post-operative day.

6 Patients' discharge rating

This was an attempt to obtain patients' feelings about participating in the research, particularly the thrice-daily post-operative visits. Again, a five-point scale ranging from 'very helpful' to 'a nuisance' was used (Appendix G). The ratings were anonymous and patients were asked to seal the answers in the envelope provided, which would not be opened until the end of the trials. Although it was difficult to obtain unbiased statements under such conditions it was felt that these scales would provide some feed-back about the visits.

   The aim, therefore, was to provide a fairly extensive insight into the post-operative recovery of each individual patient by means of the above records.

PROCEDURE FOR PATIENTS' ADMISSIONS

Most patients' first encounter with hospital took place in the out-patients' department, usually following referral by their general practitioner and with the aim of seeking a consultant's opinion. If an operation was then required, the patient was usually informed at the time and then waited a length of time which varied according to factors such as the urgency of the medical condition, the length of waiting lists and whether treatment was being provided privately or under the National Health Service.

   Notification of the date and time of admission is sent about 10 to 14 days beforehand. A booklet providing information about the hospital was also sent at this time. After reporting to the ward at the given time, patients were allocated a bed, after which they undressed and gave their day clothes to accompanying relatives or friends, there being no storage facilities available.

Although a distinct procedure for 'booking in' patients existed, this was not the responsibility of any particular grade of staff, although it tended to fall to the most senior nurse present. The patient's name, diagnosis, age and religion were entered into the ward book. A label was attached to the right wrist. At this time it was customary for a 'consent to operation' form to be signed, by which patients gave formal consent to the administration of an anaesthetic and also acknowledged that it could not be assumed that the operation would be performed by a particular surgeon, a point which occasionally provoked reactions from patients who had assumed just this.

During the period of observation the investigator made an attempt to establish a 'pattern' of routine admission procedure, a ploy which brought success only in the more obvious things such as personal details. What sort of information, if any, passed between the nurses responsible for admissions and the patient being admitted, was almost impossible to isolate beyond the fact that some nurses were largely silent, at best answering direct questions, at worst adopting a discouraging demeanour. The majority of nurses attempted to allay fears by 'cheering up' rather than by giving information which may have been more effective. Most routine questions were answered readily, but more specific things were often referred either to the doctor or ward sister.

Perhaps the most striking thing to emerge was that no one person was designated for admitting patients. It depended upon who was available at the time, which meant that some patients were admitted by the ward sister, others by an enrolled nurse.

Occasionally, patients were admitted 48–72 hours before they were to undergo surgery, but usually it was one day before. Following the admission procedure, patients may or may not be confined to bed, and at some time during this pre-operative stage a routine medical examination was performed, followed by an anaesthetist's assessment. During this time, specific pre-operative instructions relating to diet, rest, or any restriction where the patient's co-operation is essential were given, but although questions about general post-operative procedures may be answered, little information of this sort was directly offered. It is obviously difficult to generalise where no specific data were recorded, but the contention of Cartwright (1964) that more information appears to be given to patients in the higher socio-economic groups, finds support from the present observations, largely it would seem, because of their greater articulateness and more questioning manner.

Experimental procedure

Following the cross-checks on observer reliability, the procedure was as follows:

Operation lists were obtained several days in advance of admission, so as to identify suitable patients, i.e. those admitted for appendicectomy or more severe operations. If doubts arose about suitability, medical staff opinion was sought.

The initial choice of informer/observer was determined by a coin-toss and subsequently followed in random order. The informer then randomly allocated the first group of patients to informed or control groups.

An example of the research admission procedure now follows:

Pre-operatively

1 Self-introduction to patient with brief description of what would be involved, followed by a request for co-operation.

> Good day Mr./Mrs. . . ., I am . . . and I am from the Royal College of Nursing. My colleague . . . and I are interested in the way people respond to coming into hospital and having an operation. To do this, we are asking the co-operation of patients having certain operations. This involves asking you some initial questions, followed by a short interview, and then we keep in touch with you during your stay. Would you care to participate?

2 If the patient agreed to co-operate, main personal details were recorded. Then,

> We are particularly interested in the sort of things that worry you. We have a scale here (produce scale) which asks you to grade some common situations.

The *S–R Inventory* was explained. To facilitate this, some examples of five-point scales were devised which patients completed under supervision until they were demonstrably competent.

3 'Informed group' patients then received the schedule of information based upon Appendix D but tailored to each type of operation. Again, if uncertainties existed with regard to individual patients, the doctor was consulted. Every effort was made to make the interview as informal and free from tension as possible and emphasis was laid on major issues in each category rather than giving a wealth of information.

Control group patients were engaged in conversation for an equivalent time. It would be naive to assume that this had no effects, but direct information-giving was avoided.

4 On the morning of the operation, a bedside visit was made to informed patients during which the informer reiterated the central points of information covered during the admission interview. Control patients were visited for an equivalent time and engaged in conversation.

Post-operatively

A morning visit was made by the informer for the first five post-operative days. A record of relevant data was collected by the observer on three separate visits; morning, midday and evening.

The research team were initially very concerned about the effectiveness, or otherwise, of the system of grouping patients and how successfully the observer could be kept 'blind' to this grouping when patients were being visited thrice daily. It was soon realised that the greatest threat would come from the patients themselves who could easily 'leak' some details of the pre-operative interviews and thus 'give the game away'. In view of these anxieties, patients' cooperation was sought. It was explained that different groups were being followed and it was important that the observer remained unaware of what transpired at the interview. Therefore, patients were asked to refrain from volunteering information relating to admission, a policy which was successfully followed in the majority of cases.

The first hospital – results and analysis

A total number of 92 patients were approached and invited to participate in the project. From this number complete data were obtained from 68 patients. Reasons for discarding the 26 others included:

1   Two patients preferred not to participate: one because she had not written anything for 20 years and was concerned at the idea of so doing, the second refusal gave no reason.
2   After being interviewed on the day of admission, a history of recent psychiatric illness was subsequently discovered in five patients. Data were collected as arranged and discarded.
3   Post-operative emotional instability developed in four patients which rendered data collection uncertain.
4   Seven patients developed post-operative complications which delayed, or rendered atypical, their recovery.
5   Eight patients went straight from the operating theatre to the intensive care unit. They were visited and the data discarded.

Table 3.1 gives the range of operations. Tables 3.2 and 3.3 show the sample characteristics of those patients for whom data were complete.

Table 3.1   The first hospital: operation types for sample patients

Number of patients	Operation
8	Pyeloplasty
18	Hysterectomy
4	Gastrectomy
4	Vagotomy and pyloroplasty
4	Nephrectomy
2	Resection of colon
2	Cholecystectomy
10	Appendicectomy
4	Haemorrhoidectomy
6	Herniorrhaphy
2	Partial thyroidectomy
4	Others
68	

Table 3.2   Sample characteristics of those for whom data were complete

Variable	Number	Sex	
		Male	Female
Sex			
Male	26		
Female	42		
Age			
16–29		8	14
30–44		5	14
45–59		5	12
60+		8	2
Socio-economic status			
Registrar	1	1	–
General's	2	4	4
Classification	3	10	13
	4	3	18
	5	8	7
Marital status			
Married		17	29
Single		8	11
Widow/er		1	–
Divorced		–	2

The outcome of this first experiment was obviously of great importance, firstly, to assess the feasibility of this type of research in hospital wards and secondly, to assess possible effects of information on pain and anxiety.

DATA COLLECTION

There were no apparent problems relating to the collection of operation lists and selection of sample patients proceeded as planned. The varied days and times of admissions necessitated both investigators working irregular hours, an unimportant factor for the first research assistant, but one which created problems for subsequent ones.

The research assistant in this type of project was much more than a relatively uninformed data collector. Owing to the 'crossover' nature of the study design, i.e. alternating between informer and observer, the assistant played an integral part in the organisation and day to day running of the project, a role calling for considerable commitment, therefore it was difficult for this role to be carried out by other than a full-time assistant.

A rather unexpected problem occurred with patients who were admitted on Saturdays or Sundays. Owing to the policy of virtually unlimited visiting, it was often difficult to interview patients without them having to leave relatives or friends waiting at the bedside. It was thought preferable to wait for visitors to depart before interviewing as it was thought that the alternative may cause patients to hurry their responses, not to mention inconveniencing visitors.

Table 3.3 Sample characteristics

(i) Total sample

Variable	Mean	Standard deviation	N
Age	40.02	15.46	68
Social class	3.60	0.98	68
Previous admissions	1.35	1.29	68
Birth order	3.57	2.30	68
Length of stay in days	11.45	6.52	68
Total analgesic units	69.41	44.34	68
Admission anxiety score	195.87	55.30	40

(ii) Experimental group

Variable	Mean	Standard deviation	N
Age	41.73	16.20	34
Social class	3.56	0.925	34
Previous admissions	1.33	1.28	34
Birth order	3.52	2.28	34
Length of stay in days	11.55	7.33	34
Total analgesic units	59.85	35.38	34
Admission anxiety score	200.04	54.74	26

(iii) Control group

Variable	Mean	Standard deviation	N
Age	38.85	14.56	34
Social class	3.61	1.08	34
Previous admissions	1.31	1.29	34
Birth order	3.40	2.26	34
Length of stay in days	11.35	5.69	34
Total analgesic units	78.97	50.50	34
Admission anxiety score	188.14	59.35	14

The procedure for pre-operative interviewing worked satisfactorily, a side-room offering suitable accommodation for this stage. No untoward difficulties arose over the giving of information, as this was preceded by careful preparation in line with the operation type and other relevant factors. The *S–R Anxiety Inventory* is one of the longer self-report scales and some concern was felt initially that patients may find its completion tedious. In fact, the average time for completion was 20 minutes, which, although long by some other test standards, seemed quite acceptable to these patients. To some extent this problem of length was helped by the similarity of scoring on each page, the only change being the situation described at the top.

The demonstration five-point scale was extremely useful. It ensured that no patient could start the anxiety inventory without firstly demonstrating competence.

Objectives in these first trials of the *S–R Inventory* were:

1   To ascertain whether variations in post-operative state, especially pain as assessed by analgesic consumption, could be predicted by the anxiety score on admission.
2   To gauge patients' reactions to the inventory.
3   By administering the inventory a second time, usually the day before discharge, it was hoped to gain insight into its test–retest reliability, i.e. would patients' second completion relate closely to their first? A total of 34 patients completed two inventories.

FINDINGS

1 To detect possible predictive validity, admission anxiety scores were completed with post-operative analgesic scores from the 40 patients who successfully completed this inventory. For this purpose, the statistical calculation of product-moment correlation (see Appendix note on correlation) was performed, a technique which allows the relationship between two variables to be expressed. The resultant figure of 0.264 signified a moderate positive relationship, which was subsequently shown to be significant at the 5% level (see Appendix note on test of significance). Thus, the implications are that the admission anxiety score acted as a moderately good predictor of post-operative analgesic consumption for this group of patients.

2 Similar correlations were calculated between admission anxiety and all other variables, but of these, only the 'length of stay' result was significant (1% level). This very interesting finding does not support the contention of Janis (1958) discussed in Chapter 3, who suggested that similar levels of pre-operative anxiety were experienced by all patients irrespective of severity of the impending operation. The present findings do not strengthen this viewpoint, for in this research the major factor in length of stay was operation type (patients who developed post-operative complications were excluded from this calculation) and, quite clearly, the higher levels of anxiety were recorded by patients undergoing operations of greater severity.

3 Correlations were calculated relating analgesic consumption to each of the 10 situations forming the anxiety inventory. From these comparisons the relative contribution of each situation can be examined and an 'hierarchy of relevance' established. Table 3.4 shows correlations between analgesics and each situation, calculated for informed and control patients. It may be seen that situations 7, 8 and 5 are significant contributors for informed patients, while situations 2, 3 and 6 appear to exert little influence.

An unfortunate error in data collection meant that only 14 control patients completed the inventory. Significant comparisons were rendered less probable because of low numbers, only situation seven reaching the 5% level. However, the overall pattern appears similar with situations 7 and 5 showing the highest and situations 2, 3 and 6 the least relationships with analgesic consumption.

An attempt was made to provide two separate categories of 'Threat' situations in the *S–R Inventory* designed for this project. Situations 4, 5, 6, 7 and 9 provided physical

Table 3.4   Correlations for S–R situations 1–10 and post-operative analgesics, informed and control group

	Analgesics	
Situations	Informed	Controls
1 (Crowded room)	0.23	−0.13
2 (Blackout)	0.01	0.08
3 (Visiting the ill)	0.03	0.07
4 (Opened letter)	0.26	−0.09
5 (Dentist)	0.35 *	0.37
6 (Standing on ledge)	0.11	0.05
7 (Operation necessary)	0.47 †	0.46 *
8 (Medical examination)	0.39 †	0.12
9 (Cut finger)	0.22	0.23
10 (Crowded train)	0.31	0.22
	N = 26	N = 14

* Significant at 5% level
† Significant at 1% level

threat whilst situations 1, 2, 3, 8 and 9 represented psycho-social threat. In order to assess possible relationships between these two categories and analgesic consumption the correlations shown in Table 3.5 were calculated for both informed and control groups. Means and standard deviations are also shown.

For both groups the mean scores for physical threat situations were higher than the corresponding scores for psycho-social threat situations while for the informed group a significant positive correlation between physical threat and analgesics emerged. The psycho-social threat correlation for the same group failed to reach significance. A similar pattern was found for the control group, although neither correlation reached significance.

Although not exposing great differences, in response to physical and psycho-social threat situations, these results indicate that higher anxiety was recorded for those situations concerned with direct physical threat.

4 Thirty-four patients completed an *S–R Inventory* on admission and then again before discharge from the wards. The second test was to gain insight into the test–retest reliability of the inventory, using correlations between the admission and discharge scores to examine this. The total included 21 informed group and 13 control group patients and the correlations were 0.88 and 0.83 respectively. These results imply that the inventory is robust in the test–retest sense. It must also be remembered that the patients concerned underwent surgery involving varying degrees of trauma during the intervening period, a fact which supports the contention that the *S–R Inventory* measures anxiety-proneness rather than 'state' or transient anxiety.

The above findings indicated that this particular method of measuring anxiety had advantages such as ease of completion and relevance to hospital situations. Additionally the results showed that the inventory possessed reasonable predictive validity for post-operative pain as assessed by analgesic consumption. Further testing of this measure was thus indicated.

Table 3.5   Type of threat situations compared with analgesics informed group

Variable		Mean	St. deviation	N
Analgesics		59.86	35.39	34
Admission	Physical	105.65	30.64	26
Inventory	P/S	94.38	25.42	26
Discharge	Physical	93.19	32.63	21
Inventory	P/S	83.57	33.14	21

Pearson Product-Moment Correlations

Variable	Analgesics	Adm. P.	P/S	Dis. P
Analgesics				
Admission P	0.364*			
Admission P/S	0.2890 n.s.	0.836		
Discharge P	0.336*	0.938	0.792	
Discharge P/S	0.332*	0.879	0.852	0.912

*Significance level of $p < 0.05$ (1 tailed)
P = Physical threat
P/S = Psycho-social threat

Control group

Variable		Mean	St. deviation	N
Analgesics		78.97	50.51	34
Admission	Physical	99.14	32.82	14
Inventory	P/S	89.00	29.07	14
Discharge	Physical	83.62	23.77	13
Inventory	P/S	80.00	28.29	13

Type of threat situations compared with analgesics

Pearson Product-Moment Correlations

Variable	Analgesics	Adm. P.	P/S	Dis. P
Analgesics				
Admission P	0.251 n.s.			
Admission P/S	0.099 n.s.	0.839		
Discharge P	0.436 n.s.	0.864	0.719	
Discharge P/S	0.209 n.s.	0.700	0.924	0.817

P = Physical threat
P/S = Psycho-social threat
n.s. = not significant at $p < 0.05$

POST-OPERATIVE DATA – PATIENTS' SUBJECTIVE STATUS SCALE

The pain thermometer

Patients reported few problems in understanding and using this device and data collection was straightforward. It was hypothesised that informed patients would record lower ratings than control patients, and scores for each of the five post-operative days were compared between 34 informed and 34 control patients. Although these scores were rated on a five-point scale, it was felt that they were not a truly 'equal interval' measurement (a scale where the distances between any two numbers on the scale are of known size). For this reason the Mann-Whitney test (Siegel, 1956) (see Appendix note) was used to detect possible significant differences between informed and control patients. In spite of the informed groups' consistently lower scores, the only significant differences were for Day 5, which was the final day of data collection, when informed patients were significantly recording less pain. In other words, informed patients seemed to be reaching a relatively pain-free state more rapidly than the patients in the control group, a finding which provides support for the anxiety-reduction hypothesis.

Pain: local or general

This question proved rather difficult for the observers to rate satisfactorily, as patients' answers tended to be rather non-specific. It is also possible that sources of pain other than from the wound made accurate delineation a matter of guesswork for some patients. However, data were recorded for all 68 cases, but subsequent statistical analysis failed to reveal significant differences between the two groups.

Morale

Observers reported that this question presented few difficulties to patients who seemed able to differentiate their answers clearly and without ambiguity. Following data analysis the hypothesis that informed patients would report higher morale than controls was supported on Day 4 (2% level), Day 5 (5% level), with Day 2 narrowly missing significance (6%).

This was an encouraging result as other workers have reported an increased sense of wellbeing in patients who are well informed. When the data from Questions 4 (Nausea) Question 5 (Sleep) and Question 6 (Appetite) were compared, analysis failed to show significant differences.

COMFORT AND REASSURANCE

This was the multiple-choice question where patients were asked to rate, randomly, the presented six sources derived from initial interviews or, alternatively, to add their

Table 3.6   Patient State Scale, Question 7, 5th day following operation: Patients' first choice as percentages

Sources	%
Other patients	19.4
Visiting time	14.6
Talking to sister or nurses	10.4
Tablets or injections	11.8
Talking to your Doctor	10.3
Nursing attention	33.4
Total	100.0

Table 3.7   Ward Sister's assessment of patient progress

Statement	Informed	Controls	Total
Unusually well	5	2	7
Better than usual	8	7	15
About average	13	15	28
Not as well as usual	4	5	9
Very slowly/not well at all	4	5	9
Totals	34	34	68

own comments. Table 3.6 gives the percentages of items given a rank of one, i.e. those considered most important.

WARD SISTERS' ASSESSMENTS

Sisters completed this scale on the sixth post-operative day. Results are shown in Table 3.7.

Although the ratings tended to classify the informed group as making better progress than controls, the scores did not differ significantly. Thus patients' own ratings of their level of morale (Question 3) were not reflected in the Ward Sisters' ratings of progress.

POST-OPERATIVE ANALGESICS

The procedure for analgesic administration was similar for the male and female wards, and, as house officers were responsible for patients in both wards it was possible for analgesics to be standardised (unless medically contra-indicated). By far the most commonly prescribed analgesic was Omnopon (Papaveretum), usually in 20 milligram doses given by injection. The main supporting analgesic was Fortral (Pentazocine) given either by injection or tablets. The manufacturers state that 40 milligrams of Pentazocine are equivalent in analgesic effects to 10 milligrams of morphine sulphate.

Following the doctor's prescription, the major responsibilities as to when patients 'needed' analgesics fell upon the nurses. The actual time that elapsed between patients' request and the administration of the drug varied considerably, due largely to administrative problems, e.g. unless a registered nurse was on duty the drug had to be taken from the cupboard and checked by a registered nurse from another ward, or by a nursing officer. This process was often further complicated by factors such as staff shortages, meal times and the general availability of trained staff. Patients reported these problems as being especially pressing at night.

For purposes of analysis the time of operation was noted for each patient and Day 1 was the 24 hours after this, right through to Day 5, thus analysis was for 'patient days' rather than for orthodox time. The procedure followed by nurses when recording analgesics was standard throughout; the date, time and dosage of each drug being entered on a medicine chart kept at the foot of the bed. This made data collection very straightforward.

The method envisaged of matching informed and control patients by operation type and as closely as possible on other variables was so that a 'matched-pairs' type of analysis could be used. However, in some pairings the ages were rather disparate, and as the sample contained a preponderance of females the 'frequency-matching' approach, considered earlier, was used.

The hypothesis under test was that due to decreased post-operative anxiety, informed patients would request significantly fewer analgesics than control patients. The mean dosage for informed patients was 59.86 units, whilst for controls the mean dosage was 78.97. When the 34 pairs of scores were compared statistically using a 't' test (see Appendix A note on statistics used) the result was significant at the 2.5% level. Figure 3.1 shows these differences in graphic form.

The influence of age

It was hypothesised that an inverse relationship would emerge between these two variables based upon the following assumptions:

1   Older patients tend to complain less.
2   Pain tolerance increases with age as a function of learning.
3   The age disparity between nurses and elderly patients may hinder communication of distress.

This hypothesis received statistical support for the entire sample at the 5% level of significance, for the control group at the 2.5% level, while the informed group failed to reach significance. This latter finding is of particular interest as it is possible that informing patients of all ages how to request pain relieving drugs partly nullified the effects of age which are seen clearly in control patients' data.

It is clear from these results that younger patients tended to receive more analgesics, especially in the control or non-informed group. This finding was supported by

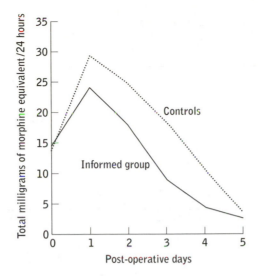

Figure 3.1   The first hospital: post-operative analgesics

considerable observational evidence as it was the experience of all concerned that younger patients complained strongly if they were not warned to expect severe pain. The pain came as an unpleasant shock. A moment's reflection will, however, reveal that it is quite possible for a young adult in present-day society never to have suffered the experience of severe pain, in fact a type of learning deficit. In view of the major aims of the experiment it is interesting to note that Table 3.8 shows correlations for both the age and social class variables as being lower for informed than for control patients. Therefore it seems a reasonable suggestion that informing patients of all ages and classes will reduce the differentials usually found in analgesic requests.

The influence of social class

The relevant literature often suggests that social class plays a part in analgesic requests, it being considered that the greater articulateness and social competence of the higher social groups allows a more rapid formation of communication links with medical and nursing staff. Such patients are likely more often to adopt a 'consumer' view of medical care and are frequently better informed about citizens' rights. In view of these factors it was not surprising to find a positive statistical correlation between social class and analgesics for both informed (2.5%) and control (1%) patients. The reduction mentioned above, in the effects of age found for informed patients, seems reflected in the social class findings, in that the influence of class was much more pronounced for control patients than for informed. This is entirely reasonable as the effects would operate as though under ordinary conditions.

Table 3.8   Correlates of age and social class

Informed group

Variable	Mean	Std. deviation	N
Social class	3.59	0.93	34
Age	41.74	16.19	34
Analgesics	59.85	35.39	34
Anxiety	200.04	53.74	26

Pearson correlations

	Social class	Age	Analgesics
Social class			
Age	−0.22		
Analgesics	0.35 *	−0.27	
Anxiety	0.09	0.11	0.34

Control group

Variable	Mean	Std. deviation	N
Social class	3.62	1.07	34
Age	38.85	14.60	34
Analgesics	78.97	50.51	34
Anxiety	199.14	59.35	14

Pearson correlations

	Social class	Age	Analgesics
Social class			
Age	−0.35		
Analgesics	0.43 †	−0.37	
Anxiety	0.71	−0.22	0.188

* Significant at 5% level
† Significant at 1% level

Post-operative vomiting

The collection of these data presented unforeseen problems, particularly for night duty, during which time nurses were unable to record with accuracy. As a result this part of the investigation was abandoned. A further complication was that nausea and vomiting are associated with certain analgesic and other drugs, thus confounding the situation further.

DISCUSSION

Any discussion of the actual findings must be preceded by a consideration of two crucial factors: firstly, the reactions and views of those patients who participated in the research, and secondly, the reactions of ward staff. As a direct indication of what patients felt about being visited by the research team the results of Patients' Discharge Ratings are shown in Table 3.9.

Table 3.9   Patients' statements regarding research visits

Statement	%
1 Very helpful	19.3
2 Slightly helpful	35.3
3 No effect	35.3
4 Unhelpful	8.8
5 A nuisance	1.3

These statements show a preponderance of favourable responses, which, although the conditions under which these ratings were collected may allow room for bias, nevertheless provide a direct statement. In addition to discharge comments, the very high response rate was a favourable index. All patients were told that participation was voluntary and that they could ask to withdraw from the project at any time. In fact, only three patients out of almost 100 preferred not to collaborate, and of those who consented, only two asked to withdraw during the course of data collection. Several favourable letters were received after patients had gone home.

Co-operation of doctors and nurses from both wards was excellent. Considerable interest in the project was shown by a wide range of staff and it was especially encouraging that junior nurses were among the most avid questioners. To a certain extent the study design hampered a free exchange of information between researchers and staff, because involving nurses too closely would have increased the bias risk.

A less satisfactory aspect of data collection was an imbalance between numbers of patients admitted, resulting in a preponderance of females. This was due primarily to lack of demand. At the time there seemed few indications that these numbers would balance, therefore data were collected in spite of the relative lack of males.

A disadvantage arising from male and female patients being nursed in separate wards was that sex differences tended to be confounded by differences in ward staffs. For some areas of research this may not be important, but where analgesics are concerned the differences are crucial. It is true that the prescription of analgesics was as standardised as circumstances allowed, but prescription forms only a small part in the chain of processes which decide whether or not a patient receives the drug. As the investigation progressed it became quite clear that the major responsibility for these decisions fell on the nurses and that discernible differences in approach existed between the male and female wards.

The male ward tended to use a 'routine' method of analgesic administration, based largely on assumptions that certain operations required certain dosages of analgesics. Some male patients did not obtain relief from pain following the 'routine' drug dosage and consequently requested more. This departure from normal practice led some nurses to express slight resentment when referring to those patients who persistently requested analgesics over and above the 'recognised quantity' for their particular operation. Conversely, female patients were encouraged to request analgesics rather than 'suffer in silence', therefore the total dosage received was determined more by individual demand than by ward routine.

Of course, an important variable to consider is that both male and female patients are nursed mainly by female nurses, and that this may, in itself, lead to variations in the decision-taking that precedes the giving of drugs, a factor noted by Bond and Pilowsky (1966) in a discussion of analgesic administration by nursing staff:

> Comparison of the average pain scores of those patients (who had not communicated pain) with those of patients who requested or received drugs indicates a more satisfactory therapeutic relationship between women patients and nursing staff than between male patients and nursing staff.

The authors develop this further by suggesting that female nurses identify more easily with their own sex than with male patients, and consequently are able to recognise need more quickly and easily in women; they continue,

> The greater need for males to communicate distress may be linked with the popular conception that women tolerate pain better than men, and that complaints made by women were more readily accepted as an indication of genuine discomfort.

The point which plainly emerges from the above discussion is that the doctor's prescription which legitimises the giving of analgesics, is, when compared with the nursing contribution, a relatively minor influence as to whether or not a patient ever receives the drug.

In spite of the equal distribution of 'contact time' between informed and control patients significant differences emerged in analgesic consumption and level of morale. Additionally informed patients reported significantly less pain than controls on Day 5. These findings indicate that just 'talking to the patients' is less effective in reducing anxiety (as measured by the indices used) and pain than 'informed talking'. That social interaction may play an important part in relieving fear and anxiety would not be denied but, from the present evidence, social interaction plus information is still better.

The *S–R Inventory of Anxiety* gave encouragement to the view that this type of test could be especially useful in identifying sources of anxiety in patients. There were few problems associated with completing the scale and the high test–retest reliability showed that patients were consistent in response. Furthermore, the significant (5%) positive correlation between admission anxiety and analgesics showed that the inventory could claim a certain predictive validity for this purpose. The contention receives further support when the mean admission anxiety scores for the informed and control patients are compared with analgesics received.

This comparison must obviously be considered when evaluating the correlations involving prediction, for if the mean anxiety score of control patients was substantially higher than that of informed patients interpretation problems would arise. Table 3.10 shows that the reverse occurred, i.e. that admission anxiety was higher for informed

Table 3.10 Means of admission anxiety and analgesics compared for informed and control groups

Group	Mean admission anxiety score	Mean post-operative analgesic drugs
Informed	200.03	59.86
Control	188.14	78.97

than for controls.

It was apparent that some of the situations used for the *S–R Inventory* were more relevant than others, a point which would need discussion if further use were contemplated.

Patients' answers to the wide range of questions used for the PSS were each recorded on a five-point rating scale. With the exception of the pain thermometer and morale sections, the scale generally failed to reveal major differences between the groups. This leaves the possibility that differences in patients' condition were restricted to these two areas, or that the scale was insensitive to subtle differences in condition. The fundamental nature of rating scales may account for some of these problems, for, although useful for many purposes where standardisation and reliability are involved, by their very nature they tend to be insensitive to material that cannot easily be categorised. However, it was difficult to visualise a reasonable alternative in view of the clinical constraints on data collecting which operate under hospital ward circumstances.

Again, although the pain thermometer only detected significant differences on Day 5, it is problematic whether replacement of this device by another form of pain 'measure' would be entirely advantageous. The ease and simplicity of this method makes it ideally suitable for post-operative use, where any lengthy or complicated process is obviously undesirable.

The significant differences in morale between informed and control groups were an encouraging findings. When morale is high, patients tend to be more alert and active and require fewer analgesics. This increased mobility is especially important in the prevention of complications such as deep-venous thrombosis and chest complications: additionally, the improved circulatory rate provides more satisfactory healing of wounds. The desirability of high morale for a patient's own state of well-being scarcely requires mention (Revans, 1964).

It is interesting to consider the answers to Question 7 relating to sources of comfort. These tended to be answered fairly consistently from day to day, with the 'Tablets or Injections' response more prominent in the first three days than in the last two, although these differences were not significant. Table 3.6 (page 59) shows all patients' first choice as percentages on Day 5. No significant differences emerged between informed and control groups.

The relative importance to 'Nursing attention', 'Visiting', and 'Other patients' is roughly comparable with other survey findings, although the high rating given to 'Other patients' deserves mention. Talking to Sister or Nurses was included to compare its position with 'Nursing attention' and it is seen that to these patients talking, whether by doctors or nurses is not a magical panacea. Without question, a large part of nursing attention involves what Argyle (1973) has called non-verbal communication. This author presents the findings of many experiments involving human communication and finds non-verbal communication far more effective than language in the understanding of attitudes, feelings and emotions. As so much of nursing attention is concerned with these particular aspects of behaviour it is hardly surprising that the 'mere word' falls far short of what is required by patients in distress.

It is encouraging to find that the Ward Sisters' ratings of patients' progress followed the research findings. Although differences were not statistically significant, they rated the informed patients as making better progress than the controls on the basis of professional judgement. One sister felt that there was a tendency to rate the progress of all patients as slightly better than would be the case if a completely objective answer were given, largely because unfavourable ratings may be taken as a reflection on standards of care.

The significant relationship (5%) between length of stay and admission anxiety, coupled with the higher average scores for the 'physical threat' situations on the S–R Inventory indicates that patients in this sample showed higher anxiety for the more serious operations. This is quite different to the findings of Janis (1958) who considered that severity of operation made little contribution to pre-operative anxiety, but a major contribution to post-operative anxiety.

Although not a main feature of this investigation, an attempt was made to note excessive emotional or physical reactions of patients who either scored very low on admission anxiety or who strongly denied anxiety during the pre-operative interview, i.e. exhibiting the psychological mechanism of denial. Janis (1958) found that these patients tended to show severe emotional upset during the post-operative phase, sometimes to such an extent that recovery was retarded. Similar cases did occur during the present investigation, but infrequently. However, it is an interesting aspect of anxiety in patients and one in which further study is merited.

The information schedule as used in this first experiment was rather an unrefined instrument. For individual patients the items included almost certainly formed a hierarchy of relevance, in which some items were more important than others in reducing anxiety, but as this obviously varied according to individual needs and requirements, the data allowed little insight into these differences. One of the more interesting issues concerned the type of information provided and the possibility of its being obtained from alternative sources. Therefore, it is quite possible that routine information about everyday procedures on the ward could come from a variety of sources, but that this may be less so for information considered as 'technical or professional'. Further trials could usefully determine if the anxiety-reducing effect would still be found if the 'schedule' were restricted in this way. Furthermore, the reduced length would allow patients to concentrate upon central issues without being swamped by minutiae.

The 'open' or 'Nightingale' wards in which the investigation was carried out provided a 'social' environment in which many patients derived comfort and reassurance from contact with their neighbours. At the same time, many patients who participated in this research echoed the findings of surveys (e.g. Cartwright, 1964) in that most open wards are noisy, sometimes unpleasant, and make few concessions to privacy: e.g. in response to the question 'How did you sleep last night?' a patient replied archly that this was decided by the noise level of the ward rather than by any differences in his condition. Additionally, the open ward system possessed serious drawbacks when trying to examine relative differences in analgesic consumption between male and female patients; any such variations could be also accounted for by differences in policy between male and female ward staffs, i.e. the effect would be 'confounded'. (A statistical term denoting an uncontrolled variable which could also account for the findings.) One way out of the predicament would be to find a ward in which male and female patients are nursed by the same staff. In newer hospitals containing small wards or cubicles this seemed a feasible proposition and so attention was turned to this type of ward for the next phase of the project.

NOTES

The Study of Nursing Care Project Reports, Series 2, No. 5. London, Royal College of Nursing. pp. 67–93. Reprinted with permission of the Royal College of Nursing.

REFERENCES

Argyle, M. (1973). *Social Interaction.* Methuen, London.

Billewicz, W. Z. (1964). Matched samples in medical investigation. *British Journal of Social and Preventive Medicine, 18,* 167–173.

Bond, M. R. and Pilowsky, I. (1966). Subjective assessment of pain and its relationship to the administration of analgesics in patients with advanced cancer. *Psychosomatic Research, 10,* 203–208.

Cartwright, A. (1964). *Human Relations and Hospital Care.* Routledge and Kegan Paul, London.

Dumas, Rhetaugh, G. and Leonard, R. C. (1963). Effect of nursing on the incidence of postoperative vomiting: a clinical experiment. *Nursing Research, 12,* 12–15.

Egbert, L. D., Battit, G. E., Welch, C. E. and Bartlett, M. K. (1964). Reduction of postoperative pain by encouragement and instruction of patients. A study of doctor–patient rapport. *New England Journal of Medicine, 270,* 825–827.

Endler, N. S., Hunt, J. McV. and Rosenstein, A. J. (1962). An S–R inventory of anxiousness. *Psychological Monographs,* 76, 16 (Whole No. 536), 1–33.

Endler, N. S. and Hunt, J. McV. (1969). Generalisability of contributions from sources of variance in the S–R inventories of anxiousness. *Journal of Personality, 37,* 1–24.

Janis, I. L. (1958). *Psychological Stress.* Wiley, New York.

Joyce, C. R. B. (ed.) (1968). *Psychopharmocology: Dimensions and Perspectives.* Tavistock Publications, Lippincott, London.

Lasagna, L. (1958). The clinical measurement of pain. *Annals of the New York Academy of Science, 13,* 28–37.

Lasagna, L. and Beecher, H. K. (1954). Analgesic effectiveness of codeine and meperadine (Demeral). *Journal of Pharmacology and Experimental Therapeutics, 112,* 306–311.

Revans, R. W. (1966). *Standards for Morale.* Oxford University Press, London.

Siegel, S. (1956). Nonparametric statistics for the *Behavioural Sciences.* McGraw-Hill, New York.

Chapter 4

An investigation of geriatric nursing problems

DOREEN NORTON, RHODA MCLAREN, A.N. EXTON-SMITH

Introduction

When one thinks of nursing research the subject of pressure sores is often the first to come to mind. Pressure sores have almost become synonymous with nursing research, partly on account of the unique role they have played in the history of research. But more than that 'Pressure sores have long been regarded as the emblem of bad nursing'. They may generate a sense of guilt which sometimes leads to denial or minimising of a problem. As such their importance is symbolic and scientific as well as historical. Fewer subjects have occupied the attention of researchers with so little apparent reward. Not only were they one of the earliest problems to be tackled, but notwithstanding their association with certain diseases such as paraplegia, they were considered *par excellence* a nursing problem. This attention was also born out of a more activist approach towards rehabilitation and a growing scepticism surrounding bed rest.

A pioneering study of its kind, the work of Norton, McLaren and Exton-Smith aimed at identifying the factors which predisposed the elderly to pressure sores, and the prophylactic and therapeutic measures that may be employed to prevent them. The study was part of a wider collection intended to use research in a practical way to shed light on and help to resolve health care problems of the elderly. Written at a time when geriatrics was becoming a speciality in its own right, it was part of a wider effort to attract talented and dynamic practitioners into the field. This required nothing short of a cultural revolution – to turn a backwater and professional *cul-de-sac* into a specialism of prestige. One of the authors was a leading light in this reform movement, A.N. Exton-Smith, Professor of Geriatric Medicine at University College, London. Research would play an important role in destigmatising the sector, with its connotations of Poor Law and chronic sick.

The growth in the sector was remarkable. By the early 1960s some 250 departments of geriatrics had been established in the UK. A comprehensive approach to the

delivery of care required teamwork and that collaborative spirit that animates the collection. The depth and breadth of the studies is impressive. The unifying theme was that
of design; ranging from the pattern of the in-patient day and its diurnal rhythm of care
to ergonomics and equipment. Much of the research focused upon surveying and
observing activities of daily living and designing different modes of service delivery and
technical aids for patient care. Others focused on the spatial environment and
ergonomics, the design of furniture, equipment, aids and adjuncts to care and rehabilitation. Thus, sterilisation techniques, materials science, the properties and uses of
plastics, foams, commentaries on incontinence and even art therapy formed part of the
panoply of care. No detail or aspect of design was left untouched, the design of clothing, dressing gowns, night dresses and bed jackets all found a place in this remarkable
volume. The latter in particular were perhaps the most novel and neglected. The impact
of costume and dress codes in care, and their capacity to confer dignity as a defence
against institutionalisation were ultimately to prove of practical as well as sociological significance.

It is the sensitivity and subtlety with which problems are articulated that is so
impressive. We are swept along by the self-evident logic of the case for reform.
Nevertheless, there is a quiet evangelism at work in that there is a confessional quality to the work. So much so that the stimulus to much of it was the negative experience
of one member of the team, Doreen Norton, then a student nurse. Ms Norton tells us
she has the unfortunate experience of causing a disabled elderly patient to suffer pain
when trying to dress her in a hospital nightgown. Her question 'why don't they make
things the right shape and save all this trouble?' prompted a number of the questions
which formed the basis for many of the studies. Research in this instance seems to have
begun as a form of repentance. But what was Ms Norton to do with her question?
There was no tradition of research by a nurse, 'no machinery by which funds and facilities can be made available to a nurse for practical nursing research'. Yet what was
produced by these pioneers was probably the first programme of research in nursing.
Remarkably, in 1959 a geriatric nursing research unit was established in the
Whittington Hospital. Its sponsors, the Governors of the National Corporation for the
Care of Old People, the Archway Group Management Committee and the Matron of
the Whittington Hospital formed a consortium of funders. It was also the first opportunity for a nursing research team to join forces with what was then known as geriatric
medicine in investigating practical nursing problems in the care of the elderly in
hospital.

Many of the problems were found to be more complex than formerly supposed.
Indeed, some were shown to require special study in themselves. 'It was, we discovered,
not only a question of practicalities – the design of a nightgown – this or that type of
chair for this or that type of patient – but of principles; the principles of assessing and
meeting the needs of individual patients'.

It was fortuitous perhaps that this initiative coincided with the adoption of a more
activist agenda in rehabilitation and elderly care. The subjects chosen for research
lacked the lustre and glamour of high-tech bioscience, but they spoke of the everyday
problems facing nurses and patients. It is their very familiarity that makes them vulnerable to dismissal and neglect, as they take on the stigma of their subjects. Research

has played an important role in de-stigmatising and changing attitudes towards elderly care, and this is a model collection in this regard.

But what Norton is much better known for is her production of a classification system with which to assess the risk of patients developing sores. Her research began here and was to become one of the touchstones of nursing in this area. The eponymous scale made Norton a household name in clinical nursing care. In all, three studies were conducted: a survey of nursing regimes used to 'treat' pressure sores (e.g. local applications such as spirit, soap, Witch Hazel, zinc cream), a trial involving 218 patients and 4 applications (a zinc cream, 2 types of silicone cream and cleansing the skin with an antibacterial agent, PHisohex), and finally a trial of 100 female patients involving the relief of pressure by frequent turning. In each case, consecutive patients admitted without pressure sores were observed. Only sores which showed a break in the skin surface of the 'pressure area' or blisters occurring over the heels were considered to be pressure sores. One of the main findings from the survey was the linear relationship between the scale assessing risk and development of sores. Another point of interest was the plethora of potions used to treat pressure sores. Fourteen such preparations and different ways of applying them, such as tar paste, a number of which subsequently turned out to be damaging. Certain preparations, such as Witch Hazel were regarded as harmful, only zinc cream remaining as of potential benefit. Further controlled trials would be needed to confirm this. The interpretation of findings was confounded by length of stay and therefore period of risk.

The second and third studies were trials testing different types of preparation and the effect of turning patients on the development of sores. The second trial concluded that no benefit could be derived from such local applications, even when combined with an active management policy of early ambulation. Indeed, what was identified was the harmful effect of some treatments, such as spirit and frequent application of soap. The third confirmed that patients at risk derived benefit from frequent turning: 'Relief of sustained pressure by 2–3 hourly turning is effective in preventing pressure sores in the majority of cases even when the general condition of the patient is extremely poor'. Attention was drawn within the study to understanding the aetiological principles, especially the physiology of tissue damage. In this regard, the authors applied lessons learned from the care of paraplegic patients and the fallacy of erythema as an indicator of superficial tissue damage. The most striking lesson and principle learned is that, contrary to convention, the more dangerous deep sores began with necrosis of subcutaneous tissue – muscle and fascia escaping detection until breakout on the surface. The prevention of deep pressure sores can occur only by preventing compression. One of the silent and underplayed findings from the study was the comparable incidence of pressures sores between bedfast and chair-bound patients at risk. This was a finding that was to form the basis of further research and it is to that that we now turn.

NORTON, D., R. MCLAREN AND A.N. EXTON-SMITH (1975)

Introduction; and A study of factors concerned in the production of pressure sores and their prevention*

INTRODUCTION

Geriatric nursing has long been recognised as being largely routine work of a particularly heavy nature. So accustomed have nurses become to its difficulties that many now accept them as an inevitable part of the nursing care of old people. This attitude is understandable, and indeed praiseworthy, but it does not meet the needs of present day conditions and those of modern geriatric medicine.

AIMS AND PROPOSALS

The aims of this investigation were threefold: (1) to improve nursing techniques in the management and care of the elderly sick; (2) to provide greater comfort for the patient and increase his independence; (3) to reduce the work of nurses both in time and effort. To this end, a number of observational studies and practical experiments were envisaged.

The original proposals for research were drawn up under five headings: Incontinence, Pressure Sores, Clothing, Furniture and Equipment and Nursing Techniques. These five headings alone, however, gave little indication of the issues involved. The proposals were therefore accompanied by 'explanatory notes', from which the following extracts are taken.

> It is believed, and can only be proved by experiments, that nurses in their anxiety to get things done quickly, tend to do more for elderly patients than perhaps is really necessary, and so create work for themselves while at the same time depriving old people of any initiative they possess.
>
> It is also believed that an over-indulgence of nursing care in hospital (prompted by the custom of having ward routines completed by a given time) tends to make the elderly patient dependent upon the nurse, and that many geriatric nursing problems and hospital after-care difficulties are created as a result.
>
> A fundamental purpose governing these proposals for research is to establish a new approach to the nursing care of the elderly patient in hospital.
>
> If these patients are to help themselves, material things must be adapted to their needs and capabilities, therefore the design of beds, chairs and clothing will be examined.
>
> Continuing further the principle of trying to help elderly patients to help themselves, consideration must be given to the instruction needed by nurses in the care of the elderly sick.

As yet there is no universally known and accepted methods and techniques laid down for nurses in the care of old people as there are, for example, for the nursing care of infants.

The 'paediatric' nurse receives instruction in every aspect of the infant's care – diet and correct method of feeding, bathing and dressing, and the way to hold and support a child when learning to walk. She is also taught elementary child psychology and is made aware of the importance of environmental factors. The 'geriatric' nurse, on the other hand, must work without special instruction to guide her. The demand for a comprehensive textbook of geriatric nursing indicates that there is now a great need for geriatric nursing procedures to be developed and established.

The practical experiments undertaken in this research would aim to develop geriatric nursing procedures which would be universally accepted as being in the best interests of the elderly patient.

Only one long-term study of a statistical nature is planned. This will consist of conducted trials of various methods in the prevention and treatment of pressure sores.

All the geriatric nursing problems described as being in need of investigation are likely to exist in the care of a single patient, and each problem the cause or effect of another. Only by considering the nursing care of elderly patients over a long period is there any likelihood of solving or alleviating any specific nursing problem.

(Extracts: 'Explanatory Notes', March, 1959)

THE HOSPITAL SETTING

The hospital in which the nursing research unit was established has 1,100 beds and serves a large and diverse community of North London. It is a nurse-training school for State Registration and State Enrolment. It is divided into three wings which, before the National Health Services Act came into force in 1948, were three separate hospitals.

When the study began, all five geriatric wards, accommodating 120 patients, were in the same wing of the hospital. Three wards, one for men and two for women, each with 28 beds, were in the same block; two smaller wards, one with 20 beds for women and one subdivided with eight beds each for men and women, were in the next block. The wing was built in 1869 and Florence Nightingale was concerned in the appointment of its first Matron.

The geriatric wards are staffed by full and part-time State Registered Nurses, State Enrolled Nurses and pupil nurses.

The aims and functions of the geriatric department and details of the patients are discussed in Section 2.

ESTABLISHING THE RESEARCH UNIT

The first member of the nursing research team took up her appointment on 1st July, 1959. The second, a ward sister of the hospital, was not appointed until three months later (owing to the printing strike which delayed advertising the post). This delay had its advantages as it allowed a settling-in period during which the unit itself and personal relations in the hospital were established.

A room attached to one of the geriatric wards had been set aside as an office; this was equipped by the third week. In establishing the unit itself many problems were encountered, some anticipated, some unforeseen. One time-absorbing factor was to fit the unit into the framework of the hospital administration while at the same time retaining its individuality. Senior officers of all departments assisted in every possible way. Owing to the size of the hospital, however, and the need for discussion with many officers in various departments, some time had to be spent in identifying these people and in explanations before specific matters could be dealt with.

Settlement of the terms of appointment of the nursing team required negotiation. This was to be expected as the employment of nurses for an independently financed research project within a hospital had hitherto been unknown. Selection of uniform may appear to be a trivial matter but had, in fact, to be seriously considered; the team needed to be dressed in a manner which would make them acceptable to patients and nursing staff yet not associated with any particular authority. Although it was the wish of the hospital to reduce the number of people wearing white coats there was no alternative but to adopt them.

Both members of the team were non-resident, but had the privilege of dining with the ward sisters and charge nurses and sharing their sitting room.

The importance of establishing good relationships with the staff of the geriatric wards was realised from the outset, but this presented no problems whatever. The following letter was sent to all nurses working in the wards.

July, 1959

Dear Nurse . . . ,

I had hoped that it would be possible to tell you personally of the Geriatric Nursing Research which is to take place in this hospital during the next two years, but as this has proved too difficult to arrange I take this opportunity of writing to you so that you may know what is happening.

Perhaps I should first explain that I am a nurse, and, like yourself, experienced in the care of old people. I am, therefore, very aware of the problems which face you in the geriatric wards. It is because of these problems that this research is being undertaken, and it is our earnest hope that between us we can find a solution to them.

Before we can find the answer to any of the problems like incontinence, pressure sores, heavy lifting, difficulty in dressing and feeding helpless patients, etc., we have to collect all the facts about them. These facts alone may be startling to a great many people. Perhaps you yourself will be surprised to learn how many soiled sheets you have to change in the course of a week. Collecting these facts will be the most tedious part of this research, and will mean extra work for you at times, but I am sure you will realise that the results of it could make all the difference to your work in the future. There will be occasions when an observer will be in your ward making notes of the nursing care given to patients, and I would like to stress that the observer is not there to criticise your work, but merely to record facts of the nursing problems with which you are dealing.

As we try different experiments we will again need your help, and although you may be convinced that a particular thing you are asked to do will not be satisfactory, it is only by carrying it out faithfully that it can be proved.

In the course of your work you have no doubt had ideas as to how certain problems can be overcome, and this research is a golden opportunity to present them. The Geriatric Nursing Research Office is on Ward . . and you are welcome to come at any time to discuss them.

In conclusion I would like to say that I deem it a privilege to work amongst you, and I am confident that the research team will receive your full co-operation.

Yours sincerely,
D.N.

Contacts with manufacturers of hospital furniture and equipment were also established in the early stages. A letter was sent to twelve companies which resulted in ten offering to lend products for trials.

By the first week of October, 1959, the research team was ready to begin its work in the wards.

SCOPE OF THE REPORT

This being the first attempt to study the basic nursing care of old people in hospital, it has been necessary to describe its problems in great detail and to try to show how they arise. Much of this report, therefore, will be familiar to those experienced in geriatric nursing. And where we have failed to suggest a possible solution to a particular problem at least some satisfaction may be derived from seeing it recognised and presented.

From this it will be anticipated that many of the problems were found to be more complex than formerly supposed. Indeed, some were shown to require a special study in themselves. As a result some modification of the original plan has been inevitable. It was, we discovered, not only a question of practicalities – the design of a nightgown – this or that type of chair for this or that type of patient – but of principles; the principles of assessing and meeting the needs of individual patients.

A study of factors concerned in the production of pressure sores and their prevention

The complications which may arise when the elderly are confined to bed on account of illness are becoming more widely known. In geriatric medicine it is now recognised that the patient should spend the minimum time in bed and independent activity must be restored as quickly as possible. Nevertheless, even with modern methods of medical treatment, the problem of pressure sores – usually regarded as primarily a nursing problem – remains. Sometimes, the development of a sore becomes as great, or even greater, a hindrance to recovery as the illness for which the patient is being treated.

In certain diseases, notably in paraplegia, the risk of development of pressure sores and their dangers are so great they have formed the basis of special studies.[1] But so far as the aged sick are concerned no comprehensive investigation has been undertaken. A variety of prophylactic and therapeutic measures are employed and no clear assessment has been made of their relative value.

DEFINITION

Two forms of pressure sore have been distinguished by Groth (1942).[2] The first is superficial and begins in the skin surface with maceration of devitalised skin; if allowed to progress it may form an infected shallow ulcer which is often painful. The second type is a deep sore which arises in those tissues overlying bony prominences and later extends to the surface. In this form, the progress of the tissue damage is from within outwards and considerable necrosis of muscle, fascia and subcutaneous tissue may have occurred even at a stage when the skin shows only erythema. Later the gangrenous lesion extends through the skin and in many cases down to the underlying bone. In practice it is usually possible to distinguish clinically between the two types of sore.

In the present study only those patients who showed a break in the skin surface of the 'pressure areas' or blisters occurring over the heels were considered to have pressure sores. Thus, patients showing skin erythema alone, without further evidence of tissue damage and which did not progress to actual ulceration, were not classified as having sores.

CLASSIFICATION OF POSSIBLE FACTORS

It is likely that many factors are involved in the production of pressure sores and for the purpose of studying their significance they may be grouped under two headings:-

(i) **Clinical condition of the patient**. His physical and mental state and particular aspects of his condition largely dependent on the nature of the illness.

(ii) **Nursing care**. The frequency and standard of nursing attention, the measures employed for the relief of pressure, the local applications to the pressure areas, the manner of nursing the patient (in bed or in a chair) and such external factors as the material of the mattress, mackintosh and drawsheet.

Clinical experience shows that the general condition of the patient is of great importance in determining whether or not a pressure sore will develop. It is essential, therefore, to have some method of assessing this.

METHOD OF ASSESSMENT

A method of assessing the patient's general condition by means of a simple scoring system was devised. (See Nursing Investigation (Pressure Sores) Form.) The scores range from a maximum of 20 for the patient who is in physically good condition, mentally alert, ambulant, capable of full mobility and not incontinent, to a minimum of 5 for a patient who is in very bad physical state, stuporose, confined to bed, immobile and doubly incontinent. It can be argued that mental states such as 'apathetic' and 'confused' are not strictly comparable on the basis of a quantitative score, but our classification was found to have the advantage that the state could be readily interpreted by nurses and closely similar scores could be obtained by different observers. To eliminate possible error, however, recordings were made by the same observer on every patient at weekly intervals. In this way changes in the patient's condition during his stay in hospital were assessed.

THE INVESTIGATIONS

Three investigations are described:-

I   A survey of 250 patients (Series I) in Hospital A, the nursing regimes already in existence being allowed to continue at the discretion of the ward sisters (i.e. the use of a variety of local applications including spirit, soap massaged into the skin, witchhazel, zinc cream, and a zinc cream preparation).

II   A trial, carried out on 218 patients (Series II) in Hospital A, of four local applications (a zinc cream preparation, two types of silicone cream and the cleansing of the skin with Phisohex).

III   A trial carried out on 100 female patients (Series III) in Hospital B, the main prophylactic measure being the relief of pressure by frequent turning of the patient.

In each investigation consecutive patients admitted without pressure sores were observed. All the patients were under the care of the same consultant physician and similar methods of management and treatment were practised in the various wards of both hospitals. Therapy aimed at the early restoration of independence by rehabilitation and nursing patients out of bed as soon as possible.

NURSING INVESTIGATION (PRESSURE SORES)

NAME _____ M/F ____ Age _____

Ward _____
No. _____

Diagnosis 1 _____
2 _____
3 _____

Date { Admitted _____
       Transferred _____
Discharged _____
Died _____

In bed _____

Obese _____
Average _____
Emaciated _____
Weight _____

A. Gen. Phys. Cond.
4. Good
3. Fair
2. Poor
1. Very Bad

B. Ment. State
4. Alert
3. Apathetic
2. Confused
1. Stupor

C. Activity
4. Ambulant
3. Walks/help
2. Chairbound
1. Bed

D. Mobility
4. Full
3. Sl. limited
2. V. limited
1. Immobile

E. Incontinence
4. Not
3. Occasional
2. Usually/urine
1. Doubly

F. Site/Pres. Sores
Sacrum
Hips (L or R)
Heels (L or R)
Knees   "
Elbows
Other

G. Type
Erythema
Blister
Superfic
Deep
Gangrene

H. Size

I. Change in Sore
1. Healed
2. Improved
3. Static
4. Worse

Date	A	B	C	D	E	F	G	H	I	Prevent. meas.	No. 24 hrs	Treat. meas.	No. 24 hrs	Appetite Good-Poor	No. 24 hrs	Drugs	Comments

Figure 4.1

I – Survey of 250 patients being nursed under existing ward routines

Earlier observations showed that a variety of local applications were being used during the routine prevention of pressure sores, none of which had been objectively assessed as superior to the others. In fact, ward sisters had individual preferences. It was decided that until such an assessment was made, there should be no change in the established ward routines and that we should investigate the incidence of pressure sores under existing conditions with the use of traditional procedures. As will be seen we obtained no evidence that the use of the various local applications had any great effect on the incidence of pressure sores, and therefore the analysis which follows can be taken as giving, within broad limits, a picture of the aetiological factors involved.

THE PATIENTS

The investigation is based on a series of 250 patients admitted to the geriatric unit of Hospital A. All patients have been included except those who had pressure sores at the time of their admission.

Age and sex

There were 102 men and 148 women; their age distribution is shown in Table 4.1.

The mean age of the 250 patients was 79.9 years, 25% being under 75 and 23% over 85. The women were, on the average, slightly older than the men.

Table 4.1   Age and sex distribution

	Total	Died	Discharged
Males			
Less than 75 years	33	8	25
75–84	47	17	30
85 and over	22	9	13
Total	102	34	68
Females			
Less than 75 years	29	8	21
75–84	84	22	62
85 and over	35	10	25
Total	148	40	108

Length of stay

The length of stay of the patients in hospital is shown in Table 4.2. It will be seen that most of the deaths occurred soon after admission; 63% within the first three weeks and that more patients died in the first week than in any subsequent week. 53% of the discharges occurred within three weeks. Only 5.6% died or were discharged after a hospital stay of eight weeks or longer.

As might be expected, of the patients who were discharged, the better their general condition on admission the shorter the time they tended to stay in hospital; whereas most of the early deaths tended to occur in those whose general condition on admission was poor. The relationship between the initial score (i.e. the assessment score on admission to hospital), the mortality and the lengths of stay of those patients who were discharged is shown in Table 4.3.

Table 4.3 shows that the mortality decreased as the initial score increased; of patients with a score of less than 12, i.e. patients who generally speaking were in poor general condition, immobile and incontinent, almost three-quarters died, whilst at the other end of the scale patients with maximal or almost maximal scores of 18 to 20 suffered only an 8% mortality. Correspondingly the patients who survived were in hospital longer when they had lower initial scores.

Table 4.2   Deaths and discharges grouped according to the length of stay

Length of stay	Total	Died	Discharged
Less than 1 week	33	18	15
1 week–	50	14	36
2 weeks–	57	15	42
3 weeks–	33	11	22
4 weeks–	22	3	19
5 weeks–	16	5	11
6 weeks–	16	3	13
7 weeks–	9	2	7
8 weeks or more	14	3	11
Total	250	74	176

Table 4.3   Mortality and length of stay related to initial score

Initial score	Total	Died		Discharged				
				Total	under 2 wks.	2 wks. +	4 wks. +	8 wks. +
Less than 12	42	30	72%	12	1	6	4	1
12–14	53	22	42%	31	5	11	12	3
15–17	92	17	18%	75	19	27	24	5
18–20	63	5	8%	58	26	20	10	2
Total	250	74	30%	176	51	64	50	11

INCIDENCE OF PRESSURE SORES

Of 250 patients admitted to hospital without pressure sores, 59 (24%) developed pressure sores at some time during their stay. The incidence was considerably higher among those who died (54%) than among those who were discharged (11%).

Although 70% of all the pressure sores developed within 2 weeks and 34% within one week, patients who died or who were discharged shortly after admission clearly ran less risk of developing them; the incidence of pressure sores in patients who were in hospital for at least two weeks was 74% among patients who died and 14% among those who were discharged. The relationship between the incidence of pressure sores and the initial score is shown in Fig. 4.2.

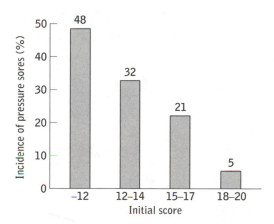

Figure 4.2   Relation between pressure sores and initial score.

   This shows an almost linear relationship between the initial score and the incidence of pressure sores: the proportion of patients developing pressure sores being almost 50% for scores less than 12 compared with 5% for scores of 18–20. The trend would doubtless have been even steeper had not many of those with lowest scores died within a few days of admission. The average initial score of all patients developing pressure sores was 12.9 (compared with 15.7 for those who did not). By the time these 59 patients actually developed pressure sores their average scores had decreased slightly to 12.3.

   There was, as might be expected, a large difference in this respect between the patients who died and those who were discharged. For the former the average score at the time of development was 11.0 compared with 14.9 for those discharged from hospital. These latter patients had treatable diseases and their pressure sores healed as their general condition improved.

   Three examples of the occurrence of pressure sores in relation to changes in score are shown in Figures 4.3, 4.4 and 4.5.

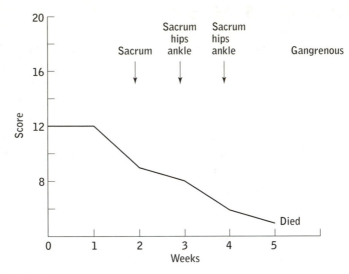

Figure 4.3   Mr. G. D.

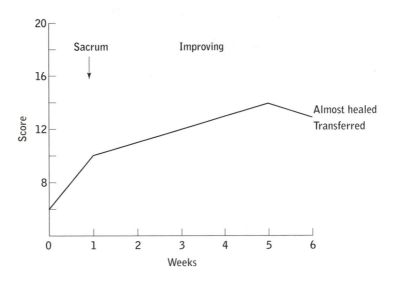

Figure 4.4   Mr. P. F.

Mr. G. D., aged 77, suffering from hemiplegia (Fig. 4.3) developed a pressure sore towards the end of the second week as the score fell to 9 from the initial level of 12; his condition continued to deteriorate and by the fifth week multiple gangrenous sores were present.

Mr. P. F., aged 72, suffering from hemiplegia and peripheral arterial disease (Fig. 4.4) developed a pressure sore within the first week after

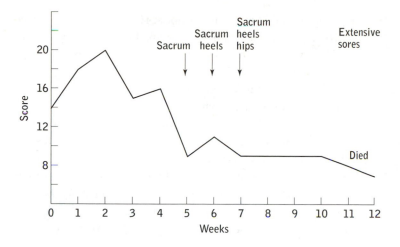

Figure 4.5   Mrs. A. J.

admission. Initially his general condition was very poor but as he improved the sore gradually healed.

Mrs. A. J., aged 80, suffering from Parkinsonism and congestive cardiac failure (Fig. 4.5). After an initial improvement in her condition she gradually deteriorated and a pressure sore of the sacrum developed when the score had fallen to 11. There was further very gradual deterioration in the next 7 weeks and she died with extensive pressure sores.

EARLY PRESSURE SORES

Important questions we wish to answer from the present data are – Which patients are likely to get pressure sores? Can the incidence of pressure sores be related to age, sex, the initial score and its components or the clinical diagnosis?

The main difficulty in answering these questions is that the stay in hospital varies considerably and therefore the time the patients are at risk varies. Moreover, many patients with low scores on admission died so soon after admission that there was insufficient time for pressure sores to develop. This difficulty can be partly overcome by re-phrasing the first question – Who gets pressure sores in the first two weeks? (these will be called early pressure sores – E.P.S.). As has been seen 70% of pressure sores developed in this period.

The 250 patients may be grouped as follows:-

Group A:	All patients who developed pressure sores within 2 weeks	41
Group B:	Other patients – still in hospital at 2 weeks	137
Group C:	Other patients – discharged within 2 weeks	49
Group D:	Other patients – died within 2 weeks	23

Patients within groups C and D were clearly not at risk for the whole 2 weeks but we can make an approximation to the truth by regarding them on the average as at risk for half the period. Thus we can define the early pressure sore ratio for any group of patients as the number of patients in group A expressed as a percentage of the total groups A and B, together with half C and D. Accepting this definition the Early Pressure Sore Ratio (E.P.S. ratio) for the whole series was 19%.

Table 4.4 shows how the early pressure sore ratio varies according to the age, sex and the initial score of the patients. The most striking feature is the very steep increase in the E.P.S. ratio as the initial score decreases, the ratio being 51% for patients with scores under 12 and only 4% when it is 18–20. Three-quarters of the patients who develop early pressure sores have initial scores within the lower range (less than 15) although only 38% of all the patients have scores within the same range. A lesser increase is apparent as the age increases, but there appeared to be no appreciable difference between the sexes.

Table 4.4   Variation of the E.P.S. ratio with the age, sex and initial score

	No. of patients	E.P.S. ratio
Total	250	19%
Male	102	18%
Female	148	20%
Age		
Less than 75	62	14%
75–84	131	19%
85 and over	57	25%
Initial score		
Less than 12	42	51%
12–14	53	25%
15–17	92	11%
18–20	63	4%

Components of score

Fig. 4.6 shows that all the individual components of the initial score are associated in quite high degree with the E.P.S. ratio. There is certainly a high correlation between these components and it is probably academic to attempt to ascertain which individual aspect is the most important. Assessment under the heading 'Incontinence' is probably the most useful single indication of the risk of developing early pressure sores; not only is there a sharper increase of the E.P.S. ratio for this component than for any of the others but it is largely independent of the method of management of the patient or of subjective judgments.

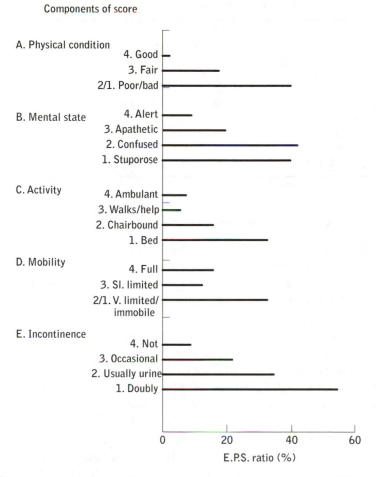

Figure 4.6   Relationship with individual component of Initial Score and the EPS ratio.

Diagnosis

In Table 4.5, the patients have been classified according to the nature of their illness.

It will be noticed that for the patients suffering from cerebrovascular disease, heart disease, respiratory disease and malignant conditions the E.P.S. ratio is similar to the overall figure of 19%. There is a higher than average ratio in patients with Parkinsonism, paraplegia and other neurological disorders and it is also worthy of mention that 3 of the 4 patients with peripheral vascular disease (included in miscellaneous) developed early pressure sores. The very low ratio seen in patients suffering from skeletal disorders (arthritis, osteoporosis, and deformities resulting from old fractures) can almost certainly be attributed to relatively high scores in this group of patients. For the most part their general condition was good, they were mentally alert and not incontinent.

Table 4.5 E.P.S. ratio related to the principal pathological condition

	Total cases	E.P.S. ratio
Cerebrovascular disease	65	20%
Parkinsonism and other neurological diseases	19	35%
Heart disease	39	20%
Respiratory disease (exc. Carcinoma)	47	20%
Alimentary disease (exc. Carcinoma)	12	20%
Malignant disease	16	22%
Skeletal disease	32	3%
Miscellaneous conditions	20	22%

Local applications to pressure areas

Earlier studies showed that no less than 14 different preparations or combinations of preparations were employed in the wards of the geriatric unit. The application of spirit or zinc cream after washing the area with soap and water were popular procedures. Many nurses had been taught to apply soap to the pressure areas and to massage it into the skin with the palm of the hand. In Table 4.6, the patients have been grouped according to the local application with which their pressure areas were treated. It has been necessary to exclude all those cases in which the type of local application was changed, those in which special preparations such as tar paste, thovaline, etc., were applied, and those who did not receive any form of local application.

Table 4.6 shows that, with the possible exceptions of witchhazel, and the Zinc Cream preparation†, none of these procedures had any striking effect on the E.P.S. ratio. After 23 patients had been treated with witchhazel, this application was discontinued since it was clearly not beneficial. The clinical states of the patients in the groups were considered to be comparable as shown by the close similarity in their mean ages and in their mean initial scores.

Table 4.6 Method of prophylaxis

Local application	No. of patients	Mean age	Mean initial score	Total with P.S. (%)	E.P.S. ratio
*S.W. (Soap massaged in)	68	79.3	14.1	23%	21%
S.W. Witchhazel	23	79.6	14.9	39%	30%
S.W. Zinc Cream	64	78.5	15.1	26%	18%
S.W. Spirit	23	81.4	15.8	26%	20%
Zinc Cream preparation†	27	81.4	15.5	15%	12%
Total	205			25%	19%

*Soap and Water.
† Formula – See Investigation II.

Any differences revealed by this table are certainly not large enough to vitiate the foregoing analysis of aetiological factors. The analysis suggests, however, that witch-hazel may be harmful and the zinc cream preparation may be beneficial. Only a controlled trail would confirm this.

THE INFLUENCE OF EARLY PRESSURE SORES

A question of some interest is – How does the occurrence of pressure sores influence the outcome? It is almost impossible to provide an answer because we cannot always distinguish between cause and effect; some patients get pressure sores simply because they are moribund whilst in others the development of pressure sores may occasionally be a cause of death. Even if patients in these extreme categories could be identified there are many cases in which cause and effect are inextricably interwoven.

Thirty of the patients with early pressure sores were still in hospital at two weeks; by this time 15 of them had scores in the lowest range (less than 12) compared with 12 in this range when they were admitted. No less than 17 of these patients were doubly incontinent at two weeks compared with only 10 on admission. By contrast the 137 patients who had remained free from pressure sores for two weeks in hospital had very much better scores at the end of the two weeks than when they came in: 81 of them (59%) had improved to scores of 18–20, only 35 (25%) of them had this score initially; only 2 patients had scores of less than 12 after two weeks compared with 11 on admission.

The prognosis of the two groups can be assessed according to their mortality and the length of stay in hospital of the survivors. The relevant figures are shown in Table 4.7.

It will be seen that the mortality was nearly 5 times as great in the group with early pressure sores than in the group without pressure sores. Of those patients who were discharged, 6 out of 8 with early pressure sores were in hospital for more than 6 weeks compared with less than one-quarter (25/117) of the patients with no pressure sores.

Thus the development of early pressure sores is associated with a very grave prognosis both in regard to the chances of the patient's recovery and the speed of recovery,

Table 4.7   Mortality and the length of stay in hospital of those who were discharged

Patients in hospital at two weeks	Total	Died No.	%	Discharged Total	3–4 wks	4–5 wks	6 wks +
With early pressure sores	30	22	73	8	1	1	6
Without pressure sores in two weeks	137	20	15	117	63	29	25

but the figures given do not indicate that the pressure sores themselves are responsible for these results since we know that the group with early pressure sores were in a less favourable condition when they were admitted.

LATE PRESSURE SORES

Of the 137 patients who were free from pressure sores at two weeks, 18 subsequently developed them (late pressure sores). Bearing in mind the small numbers, a limited comparison of the patients with early and late sores can be made and in respect of the initial scores, the figures are given in Table 4.8.

Table 4.8   Initial scores of patients with early, late and no pressure sores

Initial score	All patients with pressure sores		Patients without pressure sores
	Early	Late	
Less than 12	18	2	22
12–14	12	5	36
15–17	9	10	73
18–20	2	1	60
Total	41	18	191

If we compare the 18 patients who developed late pressure sores with the early pressure sore group, on the one hand, and on the other with patients who never acquired pressure sores it may be seen that as far as their initial scores were concerned they fell midway between the two groups. Only two of them had scores of less than 12 (compared with almost half in the early pressure sore group) but only one had a maximal score of 18–20 compared with about one-third in the group of patients who remained free from pressure sores.

SUPERFICIAL AND DEEP PRESSURE SORES

It is possible that some of the differences observed between the two groups of patients with early and late pressure sores might be due to differences in the type of sore. In Table 4.9 the 59 patients have been classified according to the type of their pressure sores.

Eighteen patients had deep, gangrenous or extensive sores and 14 of these occurred within the first two weeks. All but one of the patients with deep sores died. Superficial sores occurred relatively more often after two weeks; 23 of the 41 patients with this type of sore died.

On examining the scores of the patients recorded at the time the deep pressure

Table 4.9   Relationship between type of pressure sore (superficial or deep), the time of its development and the mortality

| Type of sore | Total | Time of development of pressure sore | | | | No. of deaths |
		under 2 wks	2 wks+	4 wks+	6 wks+	
Superficial	41	27	11	2	1	23
Deep	18	14	2	2	0	17

Table 4.10   Initial scores and scores at the time of development of pressure sores related to type of sore

| | Initial score | | Breakdown score | |
	Superficial	Deep	Superficial	Deep
Score				
Less than 12	13	7	18	9
12–14	13	4	5	6
15–17	12	7	14	3
18–20	3	–	4	–

sores occurred (breakdown score) we find that only 3 out of 18 (17%) had scores of 15 or more. On the other hand, for patients with superficial sores 18 out of 41 (44%) had scores of 15 and above; moreover, when the superficial sores occurred after two weeks eight patients had scores in the higher range (15 and above) compared with 6 whose scores were less than 15.

Thus, although deep sores still occur after two weeks, superficial sores are relatively more common at this stage of the patient's illness. Also in the present series late superficial sores developed slightly more often in those patients whose general condition was comparatively good. Since the general condition of the patient has a less direct influence in the causation of this type of late superficial sore it is here that the best prospects will be found for the prevention of pressure sores by improved nursing skills and techniques.

II – Trial of four local applications

The application of a zinc cream preparation may be of value since it replaces fat lost from the superficial layers of the skin by frequent washing with the use of soap. Moreover, for incontinent patients it may exert some protection from the contact of the skin with urine and fæces. The silicone creams are also reputed to be of value in this respect and a low incidence of pressure sores has been claimed with their use.

Special preparations

Trials of the following preparations were conducted:

1   A zinc cream preparation.[3]
2   A 20% silicone cream (Vasogen).
3   A 20% silicone cream with antiseptic (Conotrane).
4   Phisohex.

The techniques employed for their application are described below.[4]

The trials were carried out on 218 patients in the four wards of the geriatric unit of Hospital A. Each regime was allocated to one ward and in order to minimise any bias from difference in nursing standards between the wards a changeover of applications was made after three months.

RESULTS

The 218 patients were classified in four groups according to the application and the results are given in Table 4.11. The age composition and the mean initial score of the patients in the four groups are approximately the same. The incidence of pressure sores in the four groups may therefore be compared.

Table 4.11   Trial of special applications

Local application	No. of patients	Mean age	Mean initial score	Breakdown score	Total P.S.	E.P.S. ratio
Zinc cream preparation	39	81.5	14.8	13.4	8 (20%)	13%
Vasogen	66	80.2	16.4	12.7	17 (26%)	21%
Conotrane	69	82.0	15.6	15.3	16 (23%)	20%
Phisohex	44	80.0	16.5	15.4	10 (23%)	17%
Total	218					18%

The E.P.S. ratio in this second investigation was 18% and was therefore very close to that found in the first investigation under existing ward routine care of pressure areas. No striking benefit could be ascribed to the use of silicone preparations in the prevention of pressure sores. (It was noted that in the group treated with Conotrane the sores were all superficial and that many later healed or showed improvement; the high incidence in those treated with Vasogen is probably attributable to the low breakdown score and the high mortality of patients in this group.) The lower than average E.P.S. ratio for the group treated with zinc cream preparation indicates that this preparation affords some protection, and to a lesser degree so may the use of Phisohex instead of soap.

III – Trial of pressure sore prevention by turning

The first investigation revealed a relationship between the patient's clinical state and the incidence of pressure sores. It was shown that his general condition, particular aspects of his condition and, in some cases, the nature of his illness exert considerable influence in determining whether or not pressure sores will develop. Important though these clinical aspects may be, they are not the only factors concerned in the production of pressure sores: indeed, if they were there would be no prophylactic measures available to us other than those resulting from the treatment of the patient's illness and the improvement in his general condition.

The results of both the first and second investigation showed that in the prevention of pressure sores little reliance could be placed on the use of local applications. The purpose of this third investigation was to ascertain if the incidence of pressure sores could be reduced by quite a different nursing routine, namely, the relief of sustained pressure by frequent turning of all those patients considered to be especially at risk on the basis of their assessment score.

METHOD

The practice of routines involving frequent turning of patients requires an adequate number of nurses and their very close supervision. It was therefore considered desirable that the third investigation should be carried out in a small ward with a relatively high nurse/patient ratio. At the time the investigation was being planned the two small wards in the geriatric unit of Hospital A, owing to reorganisation, were about to be transferred to other wings of the hospital and their function changed. A preliminary investigation in one of these wards before the move took place, however, indicated that promising results might be obtained; the incidence of pressure sores in a series of 51 patients was reduced to 10%. A longer trial of this method of prophylaxis using frequent turning of patients was considered to be essential. The ward chosen was a geriatric ward in Hospital B accommodating 20 female patients. Apart from relatively larger numbers of nurses[5] there were two differences between the wards in Hospitals A and B which must be mentioned – in Hospital B, plastic instead of rubber waterproof sheets were used and indwelling catheters were commonly employed in the management of patients who were persistently incontinent of urine.

The 100 female patients studied were all newly admitted and were free from pressure sores on admission. Their illnesses were similar to those in Hospital A (see Table 4.12) and the selection of patients for either hospital was based only on the availability of beds at the time of admission and the geographical situation of their homes. The patients in the geriatric wards of the two hospitals were under the care of the same consultant physician and the same policy of medical management was practised (namely, early ambulation and the early restoration of independent activity by rehabilitation and the nursing of as many patients out of bed as possible during the daytime). As to the prevention of pressure sores, the application of soap was restricted to a minimum and there was no special application as a routine to the pressure areas.

Table 4.12   Diagnosis: comparison of Series I (148 female patients) with Series III (100 female patients)

	Series I %	Series III %
Cerebrovascular disease	25	33
Parkinsonism and other neurological disorders	8	5
Heart disease	18	20
Respiratory disease	15	11
Alimentary disease	6	6
Malignant disease	3	8
Skeletal disorders	17	11
Miscellaneous conditions	8	6
	100	100

But the position of patients was changed frequently during the time they spent in bed and in some cases as often as 12 times in the 24 hours.

RESULTS AND COMPARISONS OF INVESTIGATIONS I AND III

The main results of the third investigation are best shown by comparing the findings in Series I and III. As all the patients in Series III were women the corresponding results for the 148 female patients in Series I are presented. It will be seen from Table 4.12 that the patients in the two series suffered from similar illnesses, and when classified according to the site of their principal disease, there are roughly the same number of patients in each group.

Table 4.13 shows that the mortality in the two series was also similar. The length of stay was rather longer for patients in Series III probably because they were in a less favourable condition on admission (58% had initial scores of less than 15 compared with 37% in Series I). Both the longer stay and the poorer general condition would tend to increase the incidence of pressure sores.

The striking feature, however, is the remarkably low incidence of pressure sores in Series III compared with Series I. Because of age difference in the two series separate rates for early pressure sores are calculated for each age group: the marked differences between the results in Investigations I and III persist.

In Investigation III very few of the patients with low ratings for the individual aspects of their general condition developed early pressure sores. Only 2 of the 29 (7%) persistently incontinent patients in Series III developed early pressure sores compared with 11 of the 23 (48%) female patients in Series I. It is difficult to assess the influence of incontinence, however, because of its management in Investigation III – the patients considered at risk, by reason of being turned frequently, were changed more often and therefore exposed to a soiled condition for a much shorter period; urinary incontinence was also controlled in a few instances by catheter drainage.

Table 4.13   Comparison of the results of Investigations I and III

	Series I	Series III
No. of patients (females)	148	100
Age		
Less than 75 years	20%	26%
75–84	57%	57%
85 and over	23%	17%
Initial score		
Less than 12	15%	26%
12–14	22%	32%
15–17	28%	26%
18–20	25%	16%
Died	27%	28%
Discharged		
Less than 2 weeks	19%	8%
2 weeks –	25%	19%
4 weeks –	24%	32%
8 weeks–	5%	13%
E.P.S. ratio	20%	4%
E.P.S. ratio by age		
Less than 75 years	16%	4%
75–84	17%	4%
85 and over	32%	6%
Total pressure sores	26%	9%

Frequency of turning of patients

In the third investigation the aim was to prevent pressure sores by frequent turning of the patients, particular attention being paid to those who were considered to be especially at risk after assessment of their general condition had been made on the basis of the scoring system. In Table 4.14 patients have been classified in groups according to the number of times they were turned. It will be seen that 32 patients out of the 100 were turned 2–3 hourly (that is up to 12 times in the 24 hours) in some period of their stay in hospital. This was not always from the time of their admission, but 2–3 hourly turning was instituted when the general condition of the patient declined.

The mean initial score of the group of patients who were turned 2–3 hourly was significantly lower than that of the patients in the other groups who were turned less frequently; half of them had scores of less than 12. All 32 were being nursed in bed, 13 because they were quite immobile, but in the case of another 14 because their medical condition necessitated strict bed rest, although they were capable of greater activity.

Sixty-eight patients had their positions changed when they were washed, that is 4-hourly or less frequently. The majority were nursed out of bed during the day. None of these patients was classified as 'immobile' as each was capable of changing her own

Table 4.14   Frequency of nursing attention (i.e. 2–3 hourly turning with washing as necessary or washing up to 4 hourly with change of position of the patient)

Turning	No. of patients	Mean initial score
2–3 hourly	32	11
4 hourly	27	13
Routine attention, 2, 3 or 4 times daily	41	18

bodily position to a varying degree, and the nurses altered the position in bed during toilet rounds.

Relief of sustained pressure by 2–3 hourly turning is effective in preventing pressure sores in the majority of cases even when the general condition of the patient is extremely poor. As an example the following case may be mentioned –

> Mrs. H. a frail lady of 93 with chronic bronchitis and emphysema, osteoporosis of the spine and osteoarthritis. She died after 18 weeks in hospital. Her general condition remained fairly good until the 11th week after which it gradually declined. By the 12th week she was confined to bed, confused, and doubly incontinent and 2–3 hourly turning was instituted. She remained free from pressure sores (see Fig. 4.6).

Patients who developed pressure sores

Pressure sores developed in nine patients in spite of frequent turning (see Table 4.15). But all the sores were superficial and in those patients who recovered the sores healed

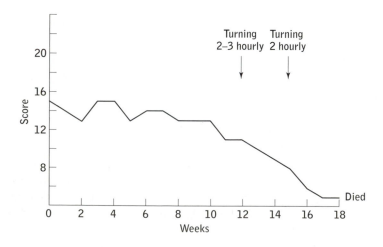

Figure 4.6   Mrs. H. The effectiveness of 2–3 hourly turning for preventing pressure sores in a patient whose general condition became extremely poor.

Table 4.15 Patients who developed pressure sores (Series III) (showing frequency of turning, initial scores, site and extent of pressure sores and outcome)

Case No.	Turning	Initial score	Site and size of pressure sore	Outcome	Change in sore
1	3 hrly	10	Sacrum, hip, knee all superfic.	Discharged	Healed in 4 wks
2	2 hrly	13	Sacrum, superfic. 1/2"	Discharged	Healed in 1 wk
3	2 hrly	8	Both heels, blisters	Discharged	Healed in 3 wks
4	(see text)	13	Hip, superfic. 1"	Discharged	Healed in 3 wks
5	(see text)	16	Hip, superfic. 1"	Discharged	Healed in 3 wks
6	4 hrly	15	Sacrum, superfic. 1"	Discharged	Improved
7	2–3 hrly	12	Sacrum, superfic 2"	Died	Improved
8	2 hrly	5	Hip, superfic. 2"	Died	Static
9	2 hrly	6	Sacrum, superfic. 1"	Died	Static

comparatively quickly (in less than 5 weeks) when the frequency of turning was increased to 12 times in the 24 hours.

Two cases are worth particular comment. In Case No. 4 the patient was ambulant and because the development of pressure sores was not anticipated no special prophylactic measures were practised. She was, however, very confused and the small superficial sore developed at the site of damage caused by scratching. In Case No. 5, the patient, who suffered from Parkinsonism, was also ambulant. She fractured her femur in the ward and following an open reduction with the insertion of a pin and plate she immediately developed a pressure sore of the right hip. This healed completely when two hourly turning was practised for the next four weeks.

DISCUSSION

In the first and second investigations no particular attention was given to the relief of pressure on those areas where pressure sores are likely to develop. Main reliance on prophylaxis was placed on local applications and on nursing patients out of bed as much as possible. A policy of management which aims at early ambulation and the early restoration of independent activity by rehabilitation may be only partially effective in reducing the time during which pressure is sustained by limited areas of the body. There are three noteworthy circumstances in which long periods of unrelieved pressure are likely to occur:

(a) In those cases where rehabilitation procedures fail or cannot be practised because the patient is too ill.

(b) In those patients who are 'chairbound' and may not be included in the normal routine of nursing attention for patients in bed. (See Individual Patient Studies.) Reference to Fig. 4.6 shows that in Series I the E.P.S. ratio for the patients nursed in chairs was 16%, that is, only slightly less than that for the series as a whole (19%).

(c) During the twelve hours or more when all patients are nursed in bed at night.

In all these circumstances particular areas of the body will be subjected to sustained pressures unless the patient is capable of changing his position himself or unless his position is changed either mechanically or by frequent turning by the nurses.

In certain units, especially spinal centres treating traumatic paraplegia, the importance of relief of pressure by 2-hourly turning of the patient has long been recognised (Guttman 1955)[6] and the value of these nursing procedures has been well proven. In fact when the dangers of immobility have been pointed out to them, nurses have been ready to practise these techniques in centres treating paralysed patients who are all at risk in regard to the development of pressure sores. But in geriatric wards, and indeed in general medical and surgical wards, where the number of patients at risk is relatively smaller (because many are capable of changing their own position in bed) the importance of these measures which aim at relief of pressure, either by frequent turning or by other means, has not been wholly appreciated.

The results of the first two investigations show that no reliance can be placed on the use of local applications to pressure areas in the prevention of pressure sores even when these nursing procedures are combined with an active policy of medical management which aims at early ambulation and the early restoration of independent activity. But the incidence of pressure sores can be strikingly reduced by instituting a nursing regime of changing the patient's position so that prolonged periods of unrelieved pressure are avoided. There is no doubt that in Investigation I, although many patients were nursed out of bed during their waking hours, most of the damage to their pressure areas occurred while they were in bed at night.

In standard teaching of nursing methods, considerable attention is paid to the toilet of pressure areas and to the use of local applications. These procedures are important and add much to the comfort of those patients who must spend long periods lying in bed. Some applications (e.g. witchhazel) have been shown to be harmful and others, such as the use of spirit and the frequent application of soap, may also be injurious and are certainly ineffective in the prevention of pressure sores. As skin toilet care is necessary and frequent attention is essential to incontinent patients, we recommend the use of the minimum amount of soap which should be rinsed off with adequate quantities of water before a bland emollient such as a zinc cream preparation is applied to the pressure areas.

Bettley (1960)[7] has drawn attention to the harmful effects to the skin of prolonged contact with soap and water, and as the toilet care of the pressure areas must be carried out several times a day and over a period of many months in some patients, the use of a soap-substitute seems worth considering. A detergent-antiseptic such as Phisohex appears satisfactory and the nurses find it pleasant to handle. But before it can be said to be free from injurious actions longer periods of trial are necessary.

Nursing procedures will only be sound if they are based on a knowledge of the aetiology of pressure sores. Local applications can, at best, only influence the incidence of superficial sores, and their use is based on the view that pressure sores start in the skin. As Groth[8] has shown, these superficial sores are the *least serious* form of pressure sore; the much more dangerous deep sore starts with necrosis of subcutaneous tissue, muscle and fascia which cannot be detected until it reaches the skin surface. Husain (1953)[9] has demonstrated in experiments on animals that skin is comparatively resistant to pressure and it may show only erythema at a stage when the underlying tissues have been irreparably damaged. Thus, on theoretical grounds, it is apparent that the prophylaxis of *deep* pressure sores can only be achieved by preventing compression of the tissues which support the body weight. These theoretical considerations find support in the results of the present investigation.

SUMMARY AND CONCLUSIONS

Three investigations were carried out: the first was a survey of 250 patients and in the analysis particular attention was paid to factors in the general condition of patients and in the nature of their illnesses which are believed to be of importance in the production of pressure sores; the second investigation assessed the relative value of special preparations applied to pressure areas in a further series of 218 patients; the third investigation carried out on 100 patients was designed to determine the effectiveness of frequent turning of the patients in order to prevent the action of sustained pressure on localised areas of the body.

A Clinical Aspects

1   In the first survey of 250 patients 59 (24%) developed pressure sores after admission. The incidence was 54% in the 74 patients who died and 11% in the 176 who were discharged.

2   Using a simple scoring system to assess the patient's condition an almost linear relationship was found between the score and the incidence of pressure sores. 5% of the patients in good general condition (scores 18–20) developed pressure sores compared with 48% of those whose general condition was poor (scores of less than 12). In general the development of pressure sores is associated with a falling score.

3   To overcome the difficulty of a variable period at risk (due to differences in length of stay in hospital) comparison was made between patients who developed pressure sores within the first two weeks (early pressure sores) and those who remained free from pressure sores within the same period. 70% of the pressure sores developed within the first two weeks and the risk of developing early pressure sores was 19%.

4   The average age of patients in the series was 79.9 years; nearly twice as many patients over 85 got pressure sores compared with those under the age of 75. There was no significant difference in the incidence between men and women.

5   A significant difference was found between the initial scores of the patients who developed early pressure sores and those who were free from sores at two weeks. Moreover, the individual components of the total score (based on ratings for physical condition, mental state, activity, mobility and incontinence) were all associated in high degree with the incidence of early pressure sores. Incontinence was found to be a sensitive index: of the 150 patients who were never incontinent 7% developed pressure sores, whereas for those who were persistently incontinent (of urine and/or fæces) 39% developed pressure sores.

6   A much lower than average incidence of pressure sores was noted in patients with skeletal disorders and a much higher than average in patients suffering from certain neurological disorders (Parkinsonism and paraplegia). There was little difference in the incidence of pressure sores in other groups of patients classified according to the nature of their illness.

7   Mortality was five times as great and the duration of hospital stay of the patients who were discharged was much longer in those with early pressure sores compared with the group without pressure sores at two weeks. This is not to say that pressure sores in themselves are responsible for these effects since the condition of the group of patients who developed early pressure sores was altogether less favourable from the time of their admission.

8   In general, patients who developed late pressure sores (after two weeks) had initial scores midway between those of the early pressure sore group and those of patients who never got pressure sores.

9   Eighteen of the 59 patients had deep, gangrenous or extensive pressure sores and 14 occurred within the first two weeks. All but one of the patients with deep sores died. Fifteen (83%) had low scores (of 14 or less) at the time of development of pressure sores.

10 Superficial sores were associated with a much less serious prognosis and *relatively* they occurred more often after two weeks. Eighteen of the 41 patients with superficial sores were in comparatively good condition, i.e. with scores of 15 or more at the time of the occurrence of the pressure sore.

B Nursing Aspects

1   The classification of the 250 patients in the first investigation according to the local application to their pressure areas showed that the type of application had little influence on the incidence of pressure sores, except that witchhazel was considered to be harmful. The frequent use of soap and the drying of the skin with spirit were of no value in the prevention of pressure sores.

2   In further trials on 218 patients (Investigation II) using special applications (a zinc cream preparation, silicone creams – Vasogen and Conotrane – and the use of Phisohex instead of soap for cleaning the skin) the overall incidence of early pressure sores was the same as in Investigation I. Phisohex appeared to be a satisfactory cleansing agent and in many ways seemed preferable to soap. It was considered that a zinc cream preparation may be beneficial.

3   From the results of these first two investigations it is concluded that local applications cannot be relied on to prevent pressure sores even when combined with a policy of medical management which aims at early ambulation and the early restoration of independent activity.

4   In a third investigation of a series of 100 patients the value of frequent turning of patients to relieve sustained pressure was assessed. By such routines it was found possible to achieve a striking reduction in the incidence of pressure sores. Only four patients developed early pressure sores and five patients developed sores later. All the pressure sores were superficial and five subsequently healed

completely when the frequency of turning these patients was increased to as many as 12 times in the 24 hours.

Of the 100 patients 32 were turned 2–3 hourly during some period while they were in hospital.

5   Equally remarkable in the third investigation was the absence of deep, gangrenous sores caused by the damaging effects of compression of muscle, fascia and subcutaneous tissues.

6   It is concluded that frequent turning to relieve pressure is an effective prophylactic measure even for very ill patients in poor general condition.

NOTES

An Investigation of Geriatric Nursing Problems in Hospital. Edinburgh: Churchill Livingstone. pp. 8–11, 194–223. Reprinted with permission of Churchill Livingstone.

1   Gutman, L. The Problem of Treatment of Pressure Sores in Spinal Paraplegics. Brit. J. Plast. Surg. 8, 196, 1955. Yeoman, M. P. & Hardy, A. G. Pathology of Pressure Sores in Paraplegics. Brit. J. Plast. Surg. 7, 179, 1954. Munro, D. Bedsores in Spinal Cord Injuries. New Eng. J. Med. 223, 391, 1940.

2   Groth, K. E. Experimental Study of Decubital Ulcers. Acta. Chirurg. Scand. 87, Sup. 76, 1942.

3   Zinc cream ¾: Vaseline / Olive Oil } ¼ (equal parts): Tinc. Benz. Co. (few drops).

4   Zinc cream preparation: Pressure areas washed with soap and water which was then rinsed off, area dried and cream applied every time attended.
    Silicone creams: A little cream gently massaged into the skin.
       Continent patients   –   Applied once daily.
       Incontinent   –   Area washed with warm water, dried and cream applied every time attended.
    Phisohex: Area washed and left wet; blob of Phisohex (about the size of little finger nail) lathered over area. Rinsed off and dried. A little dusting powder could afterwards be used.
       Continent patients   –   Applied once daily.
       Incontinent   –   Every time attended.
    In trials Nos. 2, 3 and 4 soap was not used except for washing when fæcal soiling occurred. Spirit was eliminated in all trials.

5   Nurse/patient ratio: Hospital A, 1 to 2.3. (See Sect. 2. Ward States.)
                            Hospital B, 1 to 1.4.

6   Gutman, L., The Problem of Treatment of Pressure Sores in Spinal Paraplegics. Brit. J. Plastic Surg. 8.196.1955.

7   Bettley, F. R., Effects of Soap on the Skin. Brit. med. J., i, 1675, 1960.

8   Groth, K. E., Experimental Study of Decubital Ulcers. Acta. Chirurg. Scand. 87, Sup. 76, 1942.

9   Husain, T., Experimental Study of Pressure Effects on Tissues. J. Path. Bact. 66, 347, 1953.

Chapter 5

Pressure sores

M.O. CLARK, J.C. BARBANEL, M.M. JORDAN, S.M. NICOL

Introduction

Pressure sores have a long-standing and anguished history within nursing research. This paper reports the findings from a survey undertaken in Glasgow to determine the incidence of pressure sores in the patient community of Greater Glasgow Health Board. Published before it was common to include research reports within mainstream journals in nursing, it bears the hallmarks of that time. It is not only diffident, but defensive about troubling the reader with such details as methods and results. The abstract is short and elliptical. The paper on the other hand is written with a clarity and narrative quality that is non-threatening to the reader, making it very easy to follow the decision trail. In this sense it has a certain home-spun charm, but could also be regarded as a potential model for finding more reader-friendly formats for presenting research.

The value of the paper lies in reminding us just how intractable a problem pressure sores have been within nursing, and the effort invested in identifying imaginative solutions. Looking back one is struck by the ingenuity of researchers, the ease and excitement they must have felt operating within a multi-disciplinary environment. The paper is multi-authored, the product of collaboration between an assistant nursing officer, computing officer and nursing academics, a health board equipment research committee and bioengineering unit at local university. The model of co-funding was enlightened too, even by contemporary standards. Rarely do managers or officials of health boards collaborate so closely with researchers. Much lip service is often paid to involving such parties as stake-holding partners. But here was a model operating spontaneously without the rhetoric of government behind it. This is instructive, for one of the criticisms levelled at nursing research has been its insularity. The paradox of nursing's success has been that it has since shed the early research partners upon which it relied for success. This is not necessarily the result of a robust self-sufficiency, but the product of the expansion of postgraduate research, often on a part-time basis which has not benefited from funding or the peer review processes associated with that.

The paper laments the lack of a solution to the problem of pressure sores, in spite of the high level of interest it generated. Interestingly, early research seems to have focused on practical or technical solutions in the absence of an epidemiological evidence base. Bioengineering in particular appeared particularly promising as a source of technical solution. Economics was also an important driver of research. But beneath these concerns lay the epidemiological, estimating the size of the problem and acquiring baseline data from which any change could be measured.

The aim of the study was to identify the incidence and severity of pressure sores in patients in the care of Greater Glasgow Health Board. The question then arose of how best to sample the population to provide a representative perspective on the problem. So many variables had to be taken into account, creating a complex model for analysis. In the end it was decided to undertake a census of all patients in care on a given day. Clear definitions of 'in care' were given; all hospital in-patients and all patients receiving a home visit from a district nursing sister on the day of the survey. Maternity wards, psychiatric and so-called mental handicap units, where patients were mobile, were excluded since pressure sores were believed to be rare in such areas. It was recognised that the data collection instrument needed to be simple to complete and easy to administer. Data on patients' age, sex, diagnosis, continence status, mobility, paralysis, level of consciousness and whether they had received a general anaesthetic in the two weeks prior to the survey were collected. Any pressure sores that the patient had, number, site and severity were also identified. Assessment, it was realised, could not rely upon a value judgement with wildly varying standards, so a severity guide was devised to assist in providing some consistency in measurement. Reliability checks were provided in the form of 'spot checks' in a random sample of 5% of all wards included in the survey and any discrepancy noted.

What is impressive is the scale of the project and the effort that was invested in gaining access, briefing, preparing and gaining the consent and co-operation of staff. Efforts were co-ordinated across five districts for which liaison officers were nominated to mediate between the project co-ordinator and ward staff. Liaison officers also acted as the delivery point for distribution of the survey instrument to wards and district nurses. Pilot testing estimated the timings for completion of the questionnaire.

The total number of patients involved in the study was 10 751 of which over 8000 were hospital and just over 2000 were district nurse patients distributed over some 45 hospitals and 34 specialities. We are not told what the total sample size was so it is difficult to estimate return rate and representativeness. The scores from the lowest grade in the scale for pressure sore severity provided reliability testing. The sheer logistics of conducting a survey of this kind are impressive.

What of the key findings? These suggested that the incidence of pressure sores rose with age. The most common site was the sacrum. The incidence of Grade 2 sores decreases, and that of Grade 3 increases with the number of sores per patient, and was statistically significant. The more sores the patient has the more severe they are likely to be. Severity of incontinence was also associated with severity – double incontinence having the greatest effect. Mobility scores were calculated according to patient dependency scores of Scottish Health Services Studies No. 9, and indicated that chairfast patients with a similar level of dependency to bedfast patients tended to have a slightly higher incidence of pressure sores, although these were not statistically significant. It was this latter finding, that it is pressure, irrespective of its origin, that is damaging, which was the most important insight generated by the study. And the warnings were clear. Unless preventive solutions were sought, the size and scale of the problem would only increase. As with many papers, it ends with the plea for more research. But interestingly, in the summary of the paper the authors make a point of stating they are presenting findings without interpretation. This suggests either that they believe the facts speak for themselves or feel they have to overcome the suspicion of the reader about the claims made by researchers. Either way, the approach has a freshness and its own virtues. Although the tone of the article is apologetic about research, ironically it may have given greater credence to its audience than researchers sometimes do today.

CLARK, M.O., J.C. BARBANEL, M.M. JORDAN AND S.M. NICOL (1978)

Pressure sores*

The problem of pressure sores is not a new one; indeed it can lay claim to antiquity since there was evidence of their presence in the mummified body of an Egyptian priestess (Thompson, 1961).

Continued awareness of and interest in the subject of pressure sores can be assumed by the number of articles which have appeared in the nursing press over recent years. We seem, however, to be no nearer a solution to the problem, and pressure sores still exist. But the number of people with pressure sores is not known, therefore, we cannot say whether the situation is improving, worsening or remaining static.

Doreen Norton is well known for her contribution to the subject of pressure sores particularly in relation to the development of a scale for identification of patients 'at risk'. While development of some pressure sores may be deemed 'inevitable', equally there may be others which are 'preventable' if some form of assessment is implemented as a routine measure in planning the nursing care of each patient.

BACKGROUND

Work began at the Bioengineering Unit of Strathclyde University in 1971 to investigate the mechanical causes of pressure sores. As part of this project it was estimated that the prevention and treatment of pressure sores cost the National Health Service approximately £60m a year (Fernie, 1973).

Following this, in 1974 the chief scientist of Scotland's Equipment Research Committee funded the project at the Bioengineering Unit of Strathclyde University to investigate mattresses and their coverings in relation to the part which they play in the production of pressure sores. In addition to the bioengineers, the research group contained a nurse whose role was predominantly concerned with patient contact when trials were being undertaken.

Further financial support was made available to the researchers in 1975 with the request that the newly appointed nursing research officer at the Scottish Home and Health Department should be the liaison officer to the project. A further nursing input was to be provided by an area nursing officer at the Greater Glasgow Health Board.

Doreen Norton was invited to speak at a symposium attended by nurses involved in the project, the bioengineering staff and students and the chief scientist's working party. Miss Norton spoke about previous research in which she investigated the problem of pressure sores on patients in geriatric hospitals. She demonstrated the scale which she used for identification of those 'at risk' of developing pressure sores (Norton et at., 1975). This scale entails nurses' professional judgement of the patient's physical and mental conditions, activity, mobility and incontinence.

Miss Norton contended that pressure should be relieved at a time interval according to the degree of risk to which the patient was exposed.

The bioengineers demonstrated the instruments which they had developed for scientific measurement of temperature, humidity and pressure at various points of contact between person and mattress and also for measuring the mattress properties. At the end of the day, it had to be admitted that there were still gaps in our knowledge which needed to be filled and that it was not yet possible to use these instruments in the day to day identification of those 'at risk'.

Many opinions are offered about the causes of pressure sores and the optimum preventive régimes which may be applied but there seems to be little evidence of any attempts to evaluate critically the different methods.

There seem to be three main components with regard to the prevention and treatment of pressure sores: the patient, nursing practice, and equipment such as mattresses, sheets. The interaction of each group with the others is not known and is further complicated by the many variables attached to each group. Even the size of the problem, that is, the number of patients affected, is not known because of the absence of any large scale epidemiological information in Britain.

In an attempt to remedy this situation, in part at least, a decision was taken that the Greater Glasgow Health Board, the Equipment Research Committee and the Bioengineering Unit of Strathclyde University, would jointly finance an investigation into the incidence of pressure sores in a given population of patients.

AIMS OF THE STUDY AND METHODS EMPLOYED

The aim of the study was to identify the incidence and severity of pressure sores in patients in the care of Greater Glasgow Health Board.

Considerable discussion took place to try to ascertain whether or not sampling of the population would give a truly representative picture of the problem and it was finally agreed that so many variables existed that sampling would be difficult. The decision was therefore reached that a census would be taken of all patients in care on a given day. 'In care' was defined as all hospital in-patients and all persons receiving a home visit from a district nursing sister on the day of the survey. The only exceptions to this would be maternity wards, psychiatric wards where patients were mobile, and wards which catered for patients who were mentally handicapped but fully mobile. These wards were omitted after discussion with nurse managers in the specialities, who considered that it was not reasonable to ask staff to become involved in a fairly time-consuming exercise when pressure sores occurred so rarely in these areas.

It was recognised from the outset of the study that because of the size much apparently relevant information about nursing practice, patient and equipment variables, could not be included and that detailed information on these counts would only be obtained in an in-depth study of a smaller sample.

A simple questionnaire was therefore designed and completed in respect of each patient in care on January 21, 1976. This questionnaire provided information about the patient's age, sex and diagnosis; his status in relation to continence, mobility, paralysis, level of consciousness and whether or not he had had a general anaesthetic at any time during the two weeks before the survey.

Information was also sought regarding any pressure sores the patient had in relation to their number, site and severity. Design of the section to collect this information proved difficult as great care had to be taken to remove, as far as possible, any value judgement about a pressure sore being 'bad', 'deep', 'large', 'small', and so on; at the same time it was not practical to implement any system which would accurately remove subjectivity. A new classification was therefore devised for the purposes of this study. Grade 1 – skin discoloration; Grade 2 – superficial pressure sore; Grade 3 – destruction of skin – no cavity; Grade 4 – destruction of skin – a cavity.

In order to assess accuracy and/or deviation of the responses, spot checks were undertaken in a random selection of 5% of all wards included in the survey. No spot checks were undertaken in the community because of the practical difficulties involved. The spot check related only to the findings reported about pressure sores and any deviation was recorded.

The district nursing officers were informed at an early stage of the proposal to conduct the study and they willingly agreed that the nursing staff should participate in this exercise.

There are five Districts in Glasgow and liaison officers were nominated to co-ordinate the survey between the project co-ordinator and the ward staff. Meetings were held with these officers when the purpose of the survey and the questionnaire were explained.

The liaison officers submitted lists of wards, bed complements and specialties and from this a master index was compiled for use of the project co-ordinator throughout the survey. It was also possible with this information to pre-code the questionnaires and deliver them to the liaison officers for distribution to the wards and district nurses.

A pilot study was carried out to test the questionnaire and to assess the amount of time which would be required to complete the questionnaire for a ward.

FINDINGS

The Greater Glasgow Health Board has a total bed complement of approximately 15,000 beds which are spread throughout 45 hospitals and encompass all the major clinical specialties. The district nursing staff provide home nursing services for a population of 1,105,645 (Scottish Health Statistics, 1975).

With the specialties omitted as previously outlined, the total number of patients involved in the survey was 10,751 of which 8,685 were receiving care in hospital and 2,030 had a visit from a district nurse on the day of the survey. The location of 36 people could not be identified due to irretrievable coding omissions. The hospital patients were being cared for in a total of 34 different clinical specialties.

The result of the spot check in 5% of the wards surveyed to assess the reliability of the data indicated that confusion had arisen over the interpretation of Grade 1 sores with the result that little reliance could be placed on these particular findings. Grades 2, 3 and 4, were acceptable, therefore it was decided that the analysis would be conducted on these grades only and that Grade 1 results would be totally excluded.

Tables 5.1 and 5.2 identify the sex and age distribution of the patients together with the incidence of pressure sores of Grades 2, 3 and 4 in these categories. Some totals are slightly less than 10,751 due to omissions in completion of questionnaires.

There were almost twice as many females as males in the survey and, as can be seen in Table 5.1, the females tended to have a slightly higher incidence of pressure sores than the males but this was not statistically significant.

It can be seen from Table 5.2 that the incidence of pressure sores tends to increase with age though in the 10–19 years group this shows an out of sequence figure. The patients in this group who had pressure sores – 12 patients – had diagnoses recorded as follows: five had congenital abnormalities (four of which were spina bifida); two had malignant neoplasms; two had cerebral paralysis; three were in hospital as the result of some accident.

The increasing survival rate of patients with congenital abnormalities such as spina bifida is seen as being a feature of the past 20 years and may be an explanation of the 10–19 year 'bulge' in pressure sores incidence shown on Table 5.2.

Table 5.1 Incidence of males and females with different grades of sores (expressed as percentage of patients in each group)

Sex	Percentage of patients with pressure sores (all grades)	Percentage with worst sores			No. of patients in each group
		Grade 2	Grade 3	Grade 4	
Male	8.0	4.5	2.1	1.4	3,896
Female	9.2	5.4	2.2	1.6	6,826
Total	8.7 (940)*	5.0 (544)*	2.2 (232)*	1.5 (164)*	10,722

*These numbers represent the actual number of patients.

Table 5.2   Incidence of patients in each age group with different grades of sores (expressed as percentage of patients in each group)

Age	Percentage of patients with pressure sores (all grades)	Percentage with worst sores Grade 2	Grade 3	Grade 4	No. of patients in each group
1–9	0.9	0.3	0.3	0.3	347
10–19	3.5	1.7	0.6	1.2	345
20–29	1.1	0.8	0.3	0.0	368
30–39	2.4	1.0	0.0	1.4	420
40–49	4.7	2.2	1.1	1.4	649
50–59	6.3	3.4	1.7	1.2	1,024
60–69	9.4	5.7	2.1	1.6	1.960
70–79	11.4	6.4	3.2	1.8	2,842
80–89	11.7	7.0	2.6	2.1	2,157
90+	13.2	7.9	3.7	1.6	378
Total	8.9 (932)*	5.1 (537)*	2.2 (230)*	1.6 (165)*	10,490

*These numbers represent the actual number of patients.
Note that children under one year are not included in this table.

Table 5.3   Incidence of patients with pressure sores by ward designation in specialties with more than 100 patients

Ward designation	Percentage of patients with pressure sores (all grades)	Percentage with worst sores Grade 2	Grade 3	Grade 4	No. of patients in specialty
Chest – inc. Tb	8.3	5.7	1.4	1.2	424
Dermatology	4.3	1.7	0	2.6	115
ENT	2.4	0.8	1.6	0	123
Geriatric assessment	20.6	14.1	2.8	3.7	320
Geriatric long-stay	10.7	6.0	2.7	2.0	2,042
Gynaecology	1.7	1.4	0.3	0	366
Medicine	10.7	6.6	3.2	0.9	1,017
Mental deficiency	2.4	1.9	0	0.5	212
Opthalmology	1.2	0.6	0	0.6	157
Orthopaedic	11.9	6.3	3.7	1.9	520
Paediatric	1.9	0.8	0.3	0.8	374
Psychogeriatric	9.2	6.4	1.6	1.2	1,046
Radiotherapy	10.9	5.4	4.7	0.8	129
Surgery	8.1	4.5	2.6	1.0	782
Urology	6.3	2.1	2.1	2.1	143
Young chronic sick	7.9	4.2	0.5	3.2	189
Community	8.7	4.6	2.3	1.8	2,030

Of the 35 specialties including community in which the patients were nursed, 17 had more than 100 patients being cared for within them and the incidence of patients with pressure sores by ward designation can be seen in Table 5.3.

The incidence of pressure sores has been shown to increase with age (Table 5.2) and the influence of people aged 70 years and over on the incidence within the different specialities as detailed in Table 5.3 is demonstrated in Table 5.4.

It is relevant to reiterate that 50% of the patients in the survey were aged 70 years or over and that the incidence of patients with pressure sores in this group was 11.6%, compared with an incidence of 6% in those who were 69 years of age or less.

The most common site of pressure sores was the sacrum followed by ischial tuberosities, hips, heels, ankles, elbows and knees. Some patients had more than one sore, and Table 5.5 represents the number of sores at particular sites and not the number of patients.

The majority of patients who had been reported as having pressure sores had a sore on one side only while 2.7% of the population had multiple sores ranging from two to the worst reported case (one patient) with 14 sores.

The incidence of Grade 2 sores decreases and that of Grade 3 increases with the number of sores per patient and this finding is statistically significant.

It can therefore be stated that the more sores a patient has, the more severe will be the sores.

Table 5.4 Incidence of patients with pressure sores by ward designation in specialties with more than 100 patients – a comparison of patients under 70 with those 70 years and over

Ward designation	Under 70 years		70 years and over	
	% of patients with pressure sores (all grades)	No. of patients in specialty	% of patients with pressure sores (all grades)	No. of patients in specialty
Chest – inc. Tb	5.5	273	13.7	139
Dermatology	2.2	93	13.6	22
ENT	0.9	107	12.5	16
Geriatric assessment	20.4	49	20.8	271
Geriatric long-stay	10.9	312	10.7	1,719
Gynaecology	1.0	303	7.7	26
Medicine	8.0	634	15.1	365
Mental deficiency	2.5	157	1.8	55
Opthalmology	0.9	114	2.3	43
Orthopaedic	7.1	354	22.6	164
Paediatric	1.9	367	–	–
Psychogeriatric	8.0	250	9.6	785
Radiotherapy	8.8	91	16.2	37
Surgery	4.7	596	18.9	180
Urology	4.7	85	8.8	57
Young chronic sick	5.3	170	31.6	19
Community	8.1	695	9.5	1,322

Table 5.5   Number of pressure sores at different sites

Site		Grade of sore 2	3	4
Sacrum		275	113	63
Ischial tuberosities	Left	89	28	15
	Right	90	24	15
Hips	Left	47	24	17
	Right	41	23	16
Heels	Left	46	40	25
	Right	44	41	26
Ankles	Left	22	12	6
	Right	34	8	13
Elbows	Left	17	4	4
	Right	18	6	3
Knees	Left	9	3	1
	Right	7	1	1
Other		63	41	14

The diagnoses of each patient were recorded and classified according to the International Classification of Disease Code (World Health Organisation 1967) and Table 5.6 shows the incidence of patients with pressure sores in diagnostic groups where the incidence was above the survey incidence of 8.8%.

A total of 61.8% of the patients were reported as being fully continent, a further 15.2% had 'occasional accidents', while 23% were incontinent of urine and/or fæces. The corresponding incidence of pressure sores in these three groups was 3.7%, 12.3% and 20.7% respectively.

When checking on the mobility of the patients, the classification used was that used in the patient dependency studies as per Scottish Health Services Studies No. 9 (1969), and Table 5.7 gives the details of pressure sore incidence related to these mobility classifications.

These results indicate that chairfast patients of the same general degree of helplessness as bedfast patients tend to have a slightly higher incidence of pressure sores though these results are not statistically significant.

Information about paralysis was sought and this revealed that 86.1% of the total population of patients had no paralysis, 10% were reported as having hemiplegia, 2.6% with paraplegia and 1.3% with tetraplegia; the incidence of patients with pressure sores recorded for these groups was 7.4%, 15.1%, 21.6% and 23.1% respectively.

The difference in overall sore incidence between hemiplegia and both para- and tetraplegia patients is statistically significant.

Table 5.6   Recorded diagnosis of patients with pressure sores together with severity of worst sore

| Diagnoses | % of patients with pressure sores (all grades) | Percentage with worst sores | | | No. of patients with diagnosis |
		Grade 2	Grade 3	Grade 4	
Multiple sclerosis	17.8	8.2	2.3	7.3	219
Paralysis agitans	17.0	9.5	4.7	2.8	212
Cerebral paralysis	14.8	7.6	3.5	3.7	512
Arthritis and rheumatism	13.8	8.5	2.7	2.6	732
Malignant neoplasms	12.3	6.4	4.2	1.7	692
Diseases of skin and subcutaneous tissues	11.8	4.0	2.5	5.3	323
Diseases of circulatory system	11.3	6.8	2.7	1.8	2,914
Diabetes mellitus	9.4	5.3	2.5	1.6	437

Table 5.7   Mobility related to patients with pressure sores expressed as percentage of patients in each group

| Mobility | % of patients with pressure sores (all grades) | Percentage with worst sores | | | No. of patients in each group |
		Grade 2	Grade 3	Grade 4	
Bedfast –					
totally helpless	18.6	8.9	5.9	3.8	650
partially helpless	17.5	9.7	4.3	3.5	514
not helpless	8.4	6.7	1.0	0.7	583
Chairfast –					
totally helpless	24.8	14.4	6.4	4.0	547
partially helpless	18.4	10.5	4.4	3.5	1,243
not helpless	10.6	6.1	2.2	2.3	784
Semi-ambulant	7.1	4.3	1.7	1.1	2,446
Totally ambulant	1.6	0.9	0.4	0.3	3,696
Total					10,736

SUMMARY

The objective of the survey was to identify the incidence of pressure sores in a given population on a given day. There is no indication that the particular day chosen was in any way atypical, therefore from the finding that 8.8% ($\pm$ 0.5%) of the population surveyed had a pressure sore on that day, it could be assumed that the objective of the survey was met and that valuable baseline data have been obtained.

The findings in relation to particular aspects, such as diagnoses and mobility, are presented without interpretation as further multivariate analysis will be conducted on the data available. Further in-depth study is also required to examine in greater detail the influence and/or interaction of the three main components in the prevention of pressure sores, that is, the patient, the equipment used, and the nursing care.

The one positive fact which emerges very clearly from the survey is the high incidence of pressure sores in the elderly. With the number of elderly people in the community likely to rise, with a probable increase in the number for whom care will have to be provided, it would be feasible to suggest that unless some suitable prophylactic measures are taken, the incidence of pressure sores will rise.

We should like to express our gratitude to the ward sisters, charge nurses and community nurses in the Greater Glasgow Health Board Area, without whose co-operation this study could not have been undertaken. We also appreciate the support given by senior nurse managers, Miss N. Roper, nursing officer at the Scottish Home and Health Department and Professor R. M. Kenedi of the Bioengineering Unit of Strathclyde University.

NOTES

Nursing Times 74 (9): 363–366. Reprinted by permission of *Nursing Times*.

REFERENCES

Fernie, G. R. (1973). *Biochemical Aspects of the Aetiology of Decubitus Ulcers on Human Patients*. Unpublished PhD thesis. University of Strathclyde, Glasgow.

Norton, D., McLaren, R., Exton-Smith, A. N. (1975). *An Investigation of Geriatric Nursing Problems in Hospital*, Churchill Livingstone.

Scottish Health Service Studies No. 9 (1969). *Nursing Workload per Patient as a Basis for Staffing*, SHHD, p. 41.

Scottish Health Statistics 1975, (1977). HMSO, Edinburgh

Thompson, Rowling, J. (1961). *Proc. R. Soc. Med.* 54, 409.

Chapter 6

A case study of the functioning of social systems as a defence against anxiety

ISABEL MENZIES

Introduction

Isabel Menzies has come to be a household name in nursing research. Her study 'social systems' stands out as a classic in the nursing canon. It continues to impress with its prescience and ability to speak to successive generations of nurses. Menzies' association with the Tavistock Institute and its applied psychoanalytic methods have left a lasting impression on the psyche of nursing. The central premise of much of Menzies' work is that change involves venturing into the unknown, provoking doubt and anxiety, often of a primitive and intense kind. The paper attempts to account for the high levels of stress and anxiety among nurses. Social organisations respond to such pressures by developing defence mechanisms by collusion, often unconscious, among members as an expression of externalised psychic defence mechanisms. Social organisations in turn are influenced by a number of interacting elements; their primary purpose, the social pressures and relationships within them, the processes for performing the task and the needs of members for satisfaction and support.

Hospitals are dramatic environments, evoking strong and powerful emotions. Menzies focuses on nursing and addresses the structure, culture and mode of operation of defence mechanisms to shield and protect nurses from emotionally distressing contact with patients. The study was commissioned by enlightened senior nursing staff of a general teaching hospital in London. Senior staff were worried by the high attrition rate of student nurses and the impact this had on the quality of patient care. Staffing crises resulted from the mismatch between changing patient needs and the shifts in the character of training provision. The erratic and unpredictable nature of these crises impacted negatively not only on students' training experience, but on patterns of patient care. Indeed some senior staff feared complete implosion of the allocation system under such pressure. The nursing service had adapted to this precarious situation through the development of a series of elaborate defence mechanisms. Defence mechanisms in this context make perfect sense where staffing patterns depend on a transient student workforce moulded to move around and adapt to sudden and frequent fluctuations in workload. Accordingly a 'good nurse doesn't mind moving . . . from ward to ward at a moment's notice'.

Menzies is best remembered for her insights into the splitting of the nurse–patient relationship. Illness and exposure to suffering create psychological stresses and physical demands that provoke fear, guilt and anxiety. The intimacy of patient care draws the nurse into a position that can be angst ridden. Splitting that contact up into a small series of tasks for a large number of patients prevents the nurse from concentrated encounters with the whole patient, and this brings with it anxiety. Defence mechanisms then create distance between the nurse and the patient. Such defences involve a complex choreography of evasion, involving emotional detachment of the nurse from the patient, denial of the nurse's feelings and the individuality of the patient by depersonalisation, and the constant redistribution of responsibility to avoid accountability. Each part of this edifice tends towards maintaining stability of the organisation in the face of turbulence and uncertainty.

It is difficult to do justice to the wealth of insight and richness of observation that the paper contains. Many readings of the paper are possible. The regime that Menzies describes can in some cases be considered a relic of a bygone age when nursing's rigid, ritualistic and repressive regime demanded a stiff upper lip, and patients were referred to as 'the appendix in bed six'. We now would regard this as a caricature of care, consigned to the realms of nursing mythology. But much of the study has itself become the subject of mythology in its retelling. The legacy of the study has tended to focus on the 'wastage' or work organisation, i.e. task allocation aspects, to the exclusion of the many other subtle and sophisticated analyses and arguments it contains. It is also admirably self-aware (as one might expect) as a research study, in the sense of its scepticism of 'surface' and its capacity to draw in qualifying distinctions and contradictions from private, or casual comments along the way. Unlike research papers today however, it is remarkably silent on methods and methodology. Large numbers of in-depth interviews were held, combined with observation, but little further light is shed upon processes of data collection. Today we would tend to think of a study of this kind as ethnography.

The impression one is left with is a sense of wonder that the system had not buckled under pressure from such a bleak, barren and at times brutal regime. The lack of support for all staff and the under-provision of care for a profession with a mandate to care seems staggering. Or does it? Some of you may perceive some traces of *déjà vu*. Menzies' critique is even more piercing when she argues that not only does the social defence system fail to alleviate anxiety, it can even create secondary anxiety. The consequence is that the nurse is severely limited in the capacity to 'master' anxiety and hence change. The debilitating effects of the defence system interferes with judgement, creating a self-perpetuating sense of deficiency and denial of the opportunity for self-development. In this, the nursing service fails its members. Menzies suggests that it was the more mature students who found the conflict between their own and the hospital defence system most intense. Anecdotally, it seemed that the students who did not complete training were, by and large, more mature, capable of intellectual, professional and personal development. Some who left were often spoken of as 'very good nurses'. If this were so then the driving out of students with greatest potential denudes the profession of talent and significant contributions to the theory and practice of the discipline. This vicious circle maintains the status quo by depriving the profession of its would-be reformers.

Illness provokes fear and stress for patients and their carers. Closeness and intimacy evokes a mixture of emotions which touches the vulnerabilities of all concerned. While Menzies acknowledges that the nurse is at risk of experiencing intense anxiety, this factor alone cannot account for elevated levels in nurses. Other factors within the nursing service need to be taken into account.

Menzies' key conclusion is that the nurses' task was not enough to account for the level of anxiety, and that the social defence system, while helping to avoid anxiety, did little to modify or reduce it. The picture painted is of an organisation afflicted by social pathology and the indictment was damning. Such changes as were introduced seemed to reinforce existing practices. While crisis seemed the key catalyst for action, the fundamental flaw remained of a failure to appreciate the real causes of the problem. The Cassandra-like quality of the conclusion was depressing, but should have been a jolt to a system under-performing and under-providing for its members, for which all shouldered some responsibility. At the time the paper stimulated 'antibodies' from within nursing, and indeed additional defence mechanisms in response to its criticisms. And, as far as methodology was concerned, this was to some extent justified. The paper was light on methodology. It is a tribute to the power of the paper and arguably the diligence and commitment of the nurses who responded that such a debate and dialogue took place, for such encounters were (and still are) rare in nursing. But Menzies' paper made an immediate impact, and has been cited in almost every paper on the organisation of nursing work and - practice since. It even contained the seeds of many reforms attempted since – patient allocation, team and primary nursing, clinical supervision, mentoring, reflective practice and support systems. It stands out as a beacon of insight and influence to which few can lay claim.

MENZIES, I.E.P. (1960)

A case-study in the functioning of social systems as a defence against anxiety*

INTRODUCTION

The study was initiated by the hospital, which sought help in developing new methods of carrying out a task in nursing organisation. The research data were, therefore, collected within a socio-therapeutic relationship in which the aim was to facilitate desired social change.[1]

The hospital is a general teaching hospital in London. This implies that, in addition to the normal task of patient-care, the hospital teaches undergraduate medical students. Like all British hospitals of its type, it is also a nurse-training school. The hospital has about 700 beds for in-patients and provides a number of out-patient services. Although referred to as 'the hospital', it is, in fact, a group of hospitals, which, at the time of the study, included a general hospital of 500 beds, three small specialist hospitals, and a convalescent home. The group of hospitals has an integrated nursing service run by a matron located in the main hospital. Nursing staff and students are interchangeable between hospitals.

The nursing personnel of the hospital number about 700. Of these, about 150 are fully trained staff and the remainder are students. The nurse-training course lasts four years. For the first three years, the student nurse is an 'undergraduate'. At the end of the third year she takes the examination which leads to 'state-registration', effectively her nursing qualification and licence to practise. In the fourth year, she is a postgraduate student.

The trained nursing staff are entirely deployed in administrative, teaching, and supervisory roles, although those who are deployed in operational units working with patients also carry out a certain amount of direct patient-care. Student nurses are, in effect, the nursing staff of the hospital at the operational level with patients, and carry out most of the relevant tasks. From this point of view, it is necessary that student nurses be deployed so as to meet the nurse-staffing requirements of the hospital. The student nurse spends comparatively little time undergoing formal instruction. She spends three months in the Preliminary Training School before she starts nursing practice, and six weeks in the nursing school in each of the second and third years of training. For the rest of the time, she is in 'practical training', i.e. acquiring and practising nursing skills by carrying out full-time nursing duties within the limits of her competence. The practical training must be so arranged that the student has the minimal experience of different types of nursing prescribed by the General Nursing Council.[2] The hospital offers, and likes nurses to have, certain additional experience available in specialist units in the hospital. The hospital's training policy is that the student nurse has approximately three months' continuous duty in each of the different types of nursing. Each student nurse must be deployed in a way that fulfils these training requirements. The possibilities of conflict in this situation are many. The nursing establishment of the hospital is not primarily determined by training needs, which take second place to patient-centred needs and the needs of the medical school. For some considerable time before the start of the study, the senior nursing staff had been finding it increasingly difficult to reconcile effectively staffing needs and training needs. Pressures from patient-care demanded that priority be given to staffing, and constant training crises developed. The policy of three-months training tours had in effect been abandoned and many tours were very short;[3] some nurses came almost to the end of their training without having had all the necessary experience, and others had a serious imbalance owing to too much of the same kind of practice. These crises created the more acute distress because senior staff wished to give increasing priority to training and to raise the status of the nurse as a student.

The senior staff began to feel that there was a danger of complete breakdown in the system of allocation to practical work and sought our help in revising their methods. My purpose in writing this paper is not, however, to follow the ramifications of this problem. I will make some reference to it at relevant points, and will consider later why the existing method persisted so long without effective modification in spite of its inefficiency.

The therapeutic relationship with the hospital was to some extent based on the belief that we would be wise to regard the problem of student-nurse allocation as a 'presenting symptom' and to reserve judgement on the real nature of the difficulties and the best form of treatment until we had done further diagnostic work. We began, therefore, with a fairly intensive interviewing programme. We held formal interviews with about 70 nurses, individually and in small groups, and with senior medical and lay staff; we carried out some observational studies of operational units; and we had many informal contacts with nurses and other staff. Respondents knew the problem we were formally studying, but were invited to raise in interview any other issues that they considered central to their occupational experience. Much further research material was collected in the later meetings with senior staff as we worked together on the findings from the interviewing programme.[4]

As our diagnostic work went on, our attention was repeatedly drawn to the high level of tension, distress, and anxiety among the nurses. We found it hard to understand how nurses could tolerate so much anxiety, and, indeed, we found much evidence that they could not. In one form or another, withdrawal from duty was common. About one-third of student nurses did not complete their training. The majority of these left at their own request, and not because of failure in examinations or practical training. Senior staff changed their jobs appreciably more frequently than workers at similar levels in other professions and were unusually prone to seek post-graduate training. Sickness rates were high, especially for minor illnesses requiring only a few days' absence from duty.[5]

As the study proceeded we came to attach increasing importance to understanding the nature of the anxiety and the reasons for its intensity. The relief of the anxiety seemed to us an important therapeutic task and, moreover, proved to have a close connection with the development of more effective techniques of student-nurse allocation. The remainder of this paper is concerned to consider the causes and the effects of the anxiety level in the hospital.

NATURE OF THE ANXIETY

A hospital accepts and cares for ill people who cannot be cared for in their own homes. This is the task the hospital is created to perform, its 'primary task'. The major responsibility for the performance of that primary task lies with the nursing service, which must provide continuous care for patients, day and night, all the year round.[6] The nursing service, therefore, bears the full, immediate, and concentrated impact of stresses arising from patient-care.

The situations likely to evoke stress in nurses are familiar. Nurses are in constant contact with people who are physically ill or injured, often seriously. The recovery of patients is not certain and will not always be complete. Nursing patients who have incurable diseases is one of the nurse's most distressing tasks. Nurses are confronted with the threat and the reality of suffering and death as few lay people are. Their work involves carrying out tasks which, by ordinary standards, are distasteful, disgusting, and frightening. Intimate physical contact with patients arouses strong libidinal and erotic wishes and impulses that may be difficult to control. The work situation arouses very strong and mixed feelings in the nurse: pity, compassion, and love; guilt and anxiety; hatred and resentment of the patients who arouse these strong feelings; envy of the care given to the patient.

The objective situation confronting the nurse bears a striking resemblance to the phantasy[7] situations that exist in every individual in the deepest and most primitive levels of the mind. The intensity and complexity of the nurse's anxieties are to be attributed primarily to the peculiar capacity of the objective features of her work situation to stimulate afresh these early situations and their accompanying emotions. I will comment briefly on the main relevant features of these phantasy situations.[8]

The elements of these phantasies may be traced back to earliest infancy. The infant experiences two opposing sets of feelings and impulses, libidinal and aggressive. These stem from instinctual sources and are described by the constructs of the life-instinct and the death-instinct. The infant feels omnipotent and attributes dynamic reality to these feelings and impulses. He believes that the libidinal impulses are literally life-giving and the aggressive impulses death-dealing. The infant attributes similar feelings, impulses, and powers to other people and to important parts of people. The objects and the instruments of the libidinal and aggressive impulses are felt to be the infant's own and other people's bodies and bodily products. Physical and psychic experiences are very intimately interwoven at this time. The infant's psychic experience of objective reality is greatly influenced by his own feelings and phantasies, moods and wishes.

Through his psychic experience the infant builds up an inner world peopled by himself and the objects of his feelings and impulses.[9] In the inner world, they exist in a form and condition largely determined by his phantasies. Because of the operation of aggressive forces, the inner world contains many damaged, injured, or dead objects. The atmosphere is charged with death and destruction. This gives rise to great anxiety. The infant fears for the effect of aggressive forces on the people he loves and on himself. He grieves and mourns over their suffering and experiences depression and despair about his inadequate ability to put right their wrongs. He fears the demands that will be made on him for reparation and the punishment and revenge that may fall on him. He fears that his libidinal impulses and those of other people cannot control the aggressive impulses sufficiently to prevent utter chaos and destruction. The poignancy of the situation is increased because love and longing themselves are felt to be so close to aggression. Greed, frustration, and envy so easily replace a loving relationship. This phantasy world is characterised by a violence and intensity of feeling quite foreign to the emotional life of the normal adult.

The direct impact on the nurse of physical illness is intensified by her task of meeting and dealing with psychological stress in other people, including her own colleagues. It is by no means easy to tolerate such stress even if one is not under similar stress oneself. Quite short conversations with patients or relatives showed that their conscious concept of illness and treatment is a rich intermixture of objective knowledge, logical deduction, and fantasy.[10] The degree of stress is heavily conditioned by the fantasy, which is, in turn, conditioned, as in nurses, by the early phantasy-situations. Unconsciously, the nurse associates the patients' and relatives' distress with that experienced by the people in her phantasy-world, which increases her own anxiety and difficulty in handling it.

Patients and relatives have very complicated feelings towards the hospital, which are expressed particularly and most directly to nurses, and often puzzle and distress them. Patients and relatives show appreciation, gratitude, affection, respect; a touching relief that the hospital copes; helpfulness and concern for nurses in their difficult task. But patients often resent their dependence; accept grudgingly the discipline imposed by treatment and hospital routine; envy nurses their health and skills; are demanding, possessive, and jealous. Patients, like nurses, find strong libidinal and erotic feelings stimulated by nursing care, and sometimes behave in ways that increase the nurses' difficulties, e.g. by unnecessary physical exposure. Relatives may also be demanding and critical, the more so because they resent the feeling that hospitalisation implies inadequacies in themselves. They envy nurses their skill and jealously resent the nurse's intimate contact with 'their' patient.

In a more subtle way, both patients and relatives make psychological demands on nurses which increase their experience of stress. The hospital is expected to do more than accept the ill patient, care for his physical needs, and help realistically with his psychological stress. The hospital is implicitly expected to accept and, by so doing, free patients and relatives from certain aspects of the emotional problems aroused by the patient and his illness. The hospital, particularly the nurses, must allow the projection into them of such feelings as depression and anxiety, fear of the patient and his illness, disgust at the illness and necessary nursing tasks. Patients and relatives treat the staff in such a way as to ensure that the nurses experience these feelings instead of, or partly instead of, they themselves, e.g. by refusing or trying to refuse to participate in important decisions about the patient and so forcing responsibility and anxiety back on the hospital. Thus, to the nurses' own deep and intense anxieties are psychically added those of the other people concerned. As we became familiar with the work of the hospital, we were struck by the number of patients whose physical condition alone did not warrant hospitalisation. In some cases, it was clear that they had been hospitalised because they and their relatives could not tolerate the stress of their being ill at home.

The nurse projects infantile phantasy-situations into current work-situations and experiences the objective situations as a mixture of objective reality and phantasy. She then re-experiences painfully and vividly in relation to current objective reality many of the feelings appropriate to the phantasies. In thus projecting her phantasy-situations into objective reality, the nurse is using an important and universal technique for mastering anxiety and modifying the phantasy-situations. Through the projection, the individual sees elements of the phantasy-situations in the objective situations that come to symbolise the phantasy-situations.[11] Successful mastery of the objective situations gives reassurances about the mastery of the phantasy-situations. To be effective, such symbolisation requires that the symbol *represents* the phantasy object, but *is not equated* with it. Its own distinctive, objective characteristics must also be recognised and used. If, for any reason, the symbol and the phantasy object become almost or completely equated, the anxieties aroused by the phantasy object are aroused in full intensity by the symbolic object. The symbol then ceases to perform its function in containing and modifying anxiety.[12] The close resemblance of the phantasy and objective situations in nursing constitutes a threat that symbolic representation will degenerate into symbolic equation and that nurses will consequently experience the full force of their primitive infantile anxieties in consciousness. Modified examples of this phenomenon were not uncommon in this hospital. For example, a nurse whose mother had had several gynaecological operations broke down and had to give up nursing shortly after beginning her tour of duty on the gynaecological ward.

By the nature of her profession the nurse is at considerable risk of being flooded by intense and unmanageable anxiety. That factor alone, however, cannot account for the high level of anxiety so apparent in nurses. It becomes necessary to direct attention to the other facet of the problem, that is to the techniques used in the nursing services to contain and modify anxiety.

DEFENSIVE TECHNIQUES IN THE NURSING SERVICE

In developing a structure, culture, and mode of functioning, a social organisation is influenced by a number of interacting factors, crucial among which are its primary task, including such environmental relationships and pressures as that involves; the technologies available for performing the task; and the needs of the members of the organisation for social and psychological satisfaction, and, above all, for support in the task of dealing with anxiety.[13, 14, 15] In my opinion, the influence of the primary task and technology can easily be exaggerated. Indeed, I would prefer to regard them as limiting factors, i.e. the need to ensure viability through the efficient performance of the primary task and the types of technology available to do this set limits to possible organisation. Within these limits, the culture, structure, and mode of functioning are determined by the psychological needs of the members.[16]

The needs of the members of the organisation to use it in the struggle against anxiety lead to the development of socially structured defence mechanisms, which appear as elements in the structure, culture, and mode of functioning of the organisation.[17] An important aspect of such socially structured defence mechanisms is an attempt by individuals to externalise and give substance in objective reality to their characteristic psychic defence mechanisms. A social defence system develops over time as the result of collusive interaction and agreement, often unconscious, between members of the organisation as to what form it shall take. The socially structured defence mechanisms then tend to become an aspect of external reality with which old and new members of the institution must come to terms.

In what follows I shall discuss some of the social defences that the nursing service has developed in the long course of the hospital's history and currently operates. It is impossible here to describe the social system fully, so I shall illustrate only a few of the more striking and typical examples of the operation of the service as a social defence. I shall confine myself mainly to techniques used within the nursing service and refer minimally to ways in which the nursing service makes use of other people, notably patients and doctors, in operating socially structured mechanisms of defence. For convenience of exposition, I shall list the defences as if they are separate, although, in operation, they function simultaneously and interact with and support each other.

Splitting up the nurse–patient relationship

The core of the anxiety situation for the nurse lies in her relation with the patient. The closer and more concentrated this relationship, the more the nurse is likely to experience the impact of anxiety. The nursing service attempts to protect her from the anxiety by splitting up her contact with patients. It is hardly too much to say that the nurse does not nurse patients. The total work-load of a ward or department is broken down into lists of tasks, each of which is allocated to a particular nurse. She performs her patient-centred tasks for a large number of patients, perhaps as many as all the patients in the ward, often 30 or more in number. As a corollary, she performs only a few tasks for, and has restricted contact with, any one patient. This prevents her from coming effectively into contact with the totality of any one patient and his illness and offers some protection from the anxiety this arouses.

Depersonalisation, categorisation, and denial of the significance of the individual

The protection afforded by the task-list system is reinforced by a number of other devices that inhibit the development of a full person-to-person relationship between nurse and patient, with its consequent anxiety. The implicit aim of such devices, which operate both structurally and culturally, may be described as a kind of depersonalisation or elimination of individual distinctiveness in both nurse and patient. For example, nurses often talk about patients, not by name, but by bed numbers or by their diseases or a diseased organ, 'the liver in bed 10' or 'the pneumonia in bed 15'. Nurses themselves deprecate this practice, but it persists. Nor should one underestimate the difficulties of remembering the names of say 30 patients on a ward, especially the high-turnover wards. There is an almost explicit 'ethic' that any patient must be the same as any other patient. It must not matter to the nurse whom she nurses or what illness. Nurses find it extraordinarily difficult to express preferences even for types of patients or for men or women patients. If pressed to do so, they tend to add rather guiltily some remark like 'You can't help it'. Conversely, it should not matter to the patient which nurse attends him or, indeed, how many different nurses do. By implication it is the duty as well as the need and privilege of the patient to be nursed and of the nurse to nurse, regardless of the fact that a patient may greatly need to 'nurse' a distressed nurse and nurses may sometimes need to be 'nursed'. Outside the specific requirements of his physical illness and treatment, the way a patient is nursed is determined largely by his membership of the category patient and minimally by his idiosyncratic wants and needs. For example, there is one way only of bed-making, except when the physical illness requires another; only one time to wash all patients in the morning.

The nurses' uniforms are a symbol of an expected inner and behavioural uniformity;

a nurse becomes a kind of agglomeration of nursing skills, without individuality; each is thus perfectly interchangeable with another of the same skill-level. Socially permitted differences between nurses tend to be restricted to a few major categories, outwardly differentiated by minor differences in insignia on the same basic uniform, an arm stripe for a second-year nurse, a slightly different cap for a third-year nurse. This attempts to create an operational identity between all nurses in the same category.[18] To an extent indicating clearly the need for 'blanket' decisions, duties and privileges are accorded to categories of people and not to individuals according to their personal capacities and needs. This also helps to eliminate painful and difficult decisions, e.g. about which duties and privileges should fall to each individual. Something of the same reduction of individual distinctiveness exists between operational sub-units. Attempts are made to standardise all equipment and layout to the limits allowed by their different nursing tasks, but disregarding the idiosyncratic social and psychological resources and needs of each unit.

Detachment and denial of feelings

A necessary psychological task for the entrant into any profession that works with people is the development of adequate professional detachment. He must learn, for example, to control his feelings, refrain from excessive involvement, avoid disturbing identifications, maintain his professional independence against manipulation and demands for unprofessional behaviour. To some extent the reduction of individual distinctiveness aids detachment by minimising the mutual interaction of personalities, which might lead to 'attachment'. It is reinforced by an implicit operational policy of 'detachment'. 'A good nurse doesn't mind moving.' A 'good nurse' is willing and able without disturbance to move from ward to ward or even hospital to hospital at a moment's notice. Such moves are frequent and often sudden, particularly for student nurses. The implicit rationale appears to be that a student nurse will learn to be detached psychologically if she has sufficient experience of being detached literally and physically. Most senior nurses do not subscribe personally to this implicit rationale. They are aware of the personal distress as well as the operational disturbance caused by over-frequent moves. Indeed this was a major factor in the decision to initiate our study. However, in their formal roles in the hierarchy they continue to initiate frequent moves and make little other training provision for developing genuine professional detachment. The pain and distress of breaking relationships and the importance of stable and continuing relationships are implicitly denied by the system, although they are often stressed personally, i.e. non-professionally, by people in the system.

This implicit denial is reinforced by the denial of the disturbing feelings that arise within relationships. Interpersonal repressive techniques are culturally required and typically used to deal with emotional stress. Both student nurses and staff show panic about emotional outbursts. Brisk, reassuring behaviour and advice of the 'stiff upper lip', 'pull yourself together' variety are characteristic. Student nurses suffer most severely from emotional strain and habitually complain that the senior staff do not understand and make no effort to help them. Indeed, when the emotional stress arises from the nurse's having made a mistake, she is usually reprimanded instead of being helped. A student nurse told me that she had made a mistake that hastened the death of a dying patient. She was reprimanded separately by four senior nurses. Only the headmistress of her former school tried to help her as a person who was severely distressed, guilty, and frightened. However, students are wrong when they say that senior nurses do not understand or feel for their distress. In personal conversation with us, seniors showed considerable understanding and sympathy and often remembered surprisingly vividly some of the agonies of their own training. But they lacked confidence in their ability to handle emotional stress in any way other than by repressive techniques, and often said, 'In any case, the students won't come and talk to us.' Kindly, sympathetic handling of emotional stress between staff and student nurses is, in any case, inconsistent with traditional nursing roles and relationships, which require repression, discipline, and reprimand from senior to junior.[19]

The attempt to eliminate decisions by ritual task-performance

Making a decision implies making a choice between different possible courses of action and committing oneself to one of them; the choice being made in the absence of full factual information about the effects of the choice. If the facts were fully known, no decision need be made; the proper course of action would be self-evident. All decisions are thus necessarily attended by some uncertainty about their outcome and consequently by some conflict and anxiety, which will last until the outcome is known. The anxiety consequent on decision-making is likely to be acute if a decision affects the treatment and welfare of patients. To spare staff this anxiety, the nursing service attempts to minimise the number and variety of decisions that must be made. For example, the student nurse is instructed to perform her task-list in a way reminiscent of performing a ritual. Precise instructions are given about the way each task must be performed, the order of the tasks, and the time for their performance, although such precise instructions are not objectively necessary, or even wholly desirable.[20]

If several efficient methods of performing a task exist, e.g. for bed-making or lifting a patient, one is selected and exclusively used. Much time and effort are expended in standardising nursing procedures in cases where there are a number of effective alternatives. Both teachers and practical-work supervisors impress on the student nurse from the beginning of her training the importance of carrying out the 'ritual'. They reinforce this by fostering an attitude to work that regards every task as almost a matter of life and death, to be treated with appropriate seriousness. This applies even to those tasks that could be effectively performed by an unskilled lay person. As a corollary, the student nurse is actively discouraged from using her own discretion and initiative to plan her work realistically in relation to the objective situation, e.g. at times of crisis to discriminate between tasks on the grounds of urgency or relative importance and to act accordingly. Student nurses are the 'staff' most affected by 'rituals', since ritualisation is easy to apply to their roles and tasks, but attempts are also made to ritualise the task-structure of the more complex senior staff roles and to standardise the task-performance.

Reducing the weight of responsibility in decision-making by checks and counter-checks

The psychological burden of anxiety arising from a final, committing decision by a single person is dissipated in a number of ways, so that its impact is reduced. The final act of commitment is postponed by a common practice of checking and rechecking decisions for validity and postponing action as long as possible. Executive action following decisions is also checked and re-checked habitually at intervening stages. Individuals spend much time in private rumination over decisions and actions. Whenever possible, they involve other nurses in decision-making and in reviewing actions. The nursing procedures prescribe considerable checking between individuals, but it is also a strongly developed habit among nurses outside areas of prescribed behaviour. The practice of checking and counter-checking is applied not only to situations where mistakes may have serious consequences, such as in giving dangerous drugs, but to many situations where the implications of a decision are of only the slightest consequence, e.g. on one occasion a decision about which of several rooms, all equally available, should be used for a research interview. Nurses consult not only their immediate seniors but also their juniors and nurses or other staff with whom they have no functional relationship but who just happen to be available.

Collusive social redistribution of responsibility and irresponsibility

Each nurse must face and, in some way, resolve a painful conflict over accepting the responsibilities of her role. The nursing task tends to evoke a strong sense of responsibility in nurses, and nurses often discharge their duties at considerable personal cost. On the other hand, the heavy burden of responsibility is difficult to bear consistently, and nurses are tempted to give it up. In addition, each nurse has wishes and impulses that would lead to irresponsible actions, e.g. to scamp boring, repetitive tasks or to become libidinally or emotionally attached to patients. The balance of opposing forces in the conflict varies between individuals, i.e. some are naturally 'more responsible' than others, but the conflict is always present. To experience this conflict fully and intrapsychically would be extremely stressful. The intrapsychic conflict is alleviated, at least as far as the conscious experience of nurses are concerned, by a technique that partly converts it into an interpersonal conflict. People in certain roles tend to be described as 'responsible' by themselves and to some extent by others, and in other roles people are described as 'irresponsible'. Nurses habitually complain that other nurses are irresponsible, behave carelessly and impulsively, and in consequence must be ceaselessly supervised and disciplined. The complaints commonly refer not to individuals or to specific incidents but to whole categories of nurses, usually a category junior to the speaker. The implication is that the juniors are not only less responsible now than the speaker, but also less responsible than she was when she was in the same junior position. Few nurses recognise or admit such tendencies. Only the most junior nurses are likely to admit these tendencies in themselves and then justify them on the grounds that everybody treats them as though they were irresponsible. On the other hand, many people complain that their seniors as a category impose unnecessarily strict and repressive discipline, and treat them as though they have no sense of responsibility.[21] Few senior staff seem able to recognise such features in their own behaviour to subordinates. Those 'juniors' and 'seniors' are, with few exceptions, the same people viewed from above or below, as the case may be.

We came to realise that the complaints stem from a collusive system of denial, splitting, and projection that is culturally acceptable to, indeed culturally required of, nurses. Each nurse tends to split off aspects of herself from her conscious personality and to project them into other nurses. Her irresponsible impulses, which she fears she cannot control, are attributed to her juniors. Her painfully severe attitude to these impulses and burdensome sense of responsibility are attributed to her seniors. Consequently, she identifies juniors with her irresponsible self and treats them with her own harsh disciplinary attitude to her irresponsible self and expects harsh discipline. There is psychic truth in the assertion that juniors are irresponsible and seniors harsh disciplinarians. These are the roles assigned to them. There is also objective truth, since people act objectively on the psychic roles assigned to them. Discipline is often harsh and sometimes unfair, since the multiple projection also leads the senior to identify all juniors with her irresponsible self and so with each other. Thus, she fails to discriminate between them sufficiently. Nurses complain about being reprimanded for other people's mistakes while no serious effort is made to find the real culprit. A staff nurse[22] said, 'If a mistake has been made, you must reprimand someone, even if you don't know who really did it.' Irresponsible behaviour was also quite common, mainly in tasks remote from direct patient-care. The interpersonal conflict is painful, as the complaints show, but is less so than experiencing the conflict fully intrapsychically, and it can more easily be evaded. The disciplining eye of seniors cannot follow juniors all the time, nor does the junior confront her senior with irresponsibility all the time.

Purposeful obscurity in the formal distribution of responsibility

Additional protection from the impact of specific responsibility for specific tasks is given by the fact that the formal structure and role system fail to define fully enough who is responsible for what and to whom. This matches and objectifies the obscurity about the location of psychic responsibility that inevitably arises from the massive system of projection described above. The content of roles and the boundaries of roles are very obscure, especially at senior levels. The responsibilities are more onerous at this level so that protection is felt as very necessary. As described above, the content of the role of the student nurse is rigidly prescribed by her task-list. However, in practice, she is unlikely to have the same task-list for any length of time. She may, and frequently does, have two completely different task-lists in a single day.[23] There is therefore a lack of stable person-role constellations, and it becomes very difficult to assign responsibility finally to a person, a role, or a person-role constellation. We experienced this obscurity frequently in our work in the hospital, finding great difficulty, for example, in learning who should make arrangements or give permission for nurses to participate in various research activities.

Responsibility and authority on wards are generalised in a way that makes them non-specific and prevents them from falling firmly on one person, even the sister. Each nurse is held to be responsible for the work of every nurse junior to her. Junior, in this context, implies no hierarchical relationship, and is determined only by the length of time a student nurse has been in training, and all students are 'junior' to trained staff. A student nurse in the fourth quarter of her fourth year is by implication responsible for all other student nurses on the ward; a student nurse in the third quarter of her fourth year for all student nurses except the previous one, and so on. Every nurse is expected to initiate disciplinary action in relation to any failure by any junior nurse. Such diffused responsibility means, of course, that responsibility is not generally experienced specifically or seriously.

The reduction of the impact of responsibility by delegation to superiors

The ordinary usage of the word 'delegation' in relation to tasks implies that a superior hands over a task and the direct responsibility for its detailed performance to subordinates, while he retains a general, supervisory responsibility. In the hospital, almost the opposite seems to happen frequently, i.e. tasks are frequently forced upwards in the hierarchy, so that all responsibility for their performance can be disclaimed. In so far as this happens, the heavy burden of responsibility on the individual is reduced.

The result of many years of this practice are visible in the nursing service. We were struck repeatedly by the low level of tasks carried out by nursing staff and students in relation to their personal ability, skill, and position in the hierarchy. Formally and informally, tasks are assigned to staff at a level well above that at which one finds comparable tasks in other institutions, while the tasks are organised so as effectively to prevent their delegation to an appropriate lower level, e.g. by clarifying policy. The task of allocating student nurses to practical duties was a case in point. The detailed work of allocating student nurses was carried out by the first and second assistant matrons[24] and took up a considerable proportion of their working-time. In our opinion, the task is, in fact, such that, if policy were clearly defined and the task appropriately organised, it could be efficiently performed by a competent clerk part-time under the supervision of a senior nurse, who need spend little time on it.[25] We were able to watch this 'delegation upwards' in operation a number of times as new tasks developed for nurses out of changes resulting from our study. For example, the senior staff decided to change the practical training for fourth-year nurses so that they might have better training than formerly in administration and supervision. This implied, among other things, that they should spend six months continuously in one operational unit during which time they would act as understudy-cum-shadow to their sister or the staff nurse. In the circumstances, personal compatibility was felt to be very important, and it was suggested that the sisters should take part in the selection of the fourth-year students for their own wards. At first, there was enthusiasm for the proposal, but as definite plans were made and the intermediate staff began to feel that they had no developed skill for selection, they requested that, after all, senior staff should continue to select for them as they had always done. The senior staff, although already overburdened, willingly accepted the task.

The repeated occurrence of such incidents by mutual collusive agreement between superiors and subordinates is hardly surprising considering the mutual projection system described above. Nurses as subordinates tend to feel very dependent on their superiors in whom they psychically vest by projection some of the best and most competent parts of themselves. They feel that their projections give them the right to expect their superiors to undertake their tasks and make decisions for them. On the other hand, nurses, as superiors, do not feel they can fully trust their subordinates in whom they psychically vest the irresponsible and incompetent parts of themselves. Their acceptance of their subordinates' projections also conveys a sense of duty to accept their subordinates' responsibilities.

Idealisation and underestimation of personal developmental possibilities

In order to reduce anxiety about the continuous efficient performance of nursing tasks, nurses seek assurance that the nursing service is staffed with responsible, competent people. To a considerable extent, the hospital deals with this problem by an attempt to recruit and select 'staff', i.e. student nurses, who are already highly mature and responsible people. This is reflected in phrases like 'nurses are born not made' or 'nursing is a vocation'. This amounts to a kind of idealisation of the potential nursing recruit, and implies a belief that responsibility and personal maturity cannot be 'taught' or even greatly developed. As a corollary, the training system is mainly orientated to the communication of essential facts and techniques, and pays minimal attention to teaching events oriented to personal maturation within the professional setting.[26] There is no individual supervision of student nurses, and no small group teaching event concerned specifically to help student nurses work over the impact of their first essays in nursing practice and handle more effectively their relations with patients and their own emotional reactions. The nursing service must face the dilemma that, while a strong sense of responsibility and discipline are felt to be necessary for the welfare of patients, a considerable proportion of actual nursing tasks are extremely simple. This hospital, in common with most similar British hospitals, has attempted to solve this dilemma by the recruitment of large numbers of high-level student nurses who, it is hoped, are prepared to accept the temporary lowering of their operational level because they are in training.

This throws new light on the problem of the 30 per cent to 50 per cent wastage of student nurses in this and other British hospitals. It has long been treated as a serious problem and much effort has been expended in trying to solve it. In fact, it can be seen as an *essential* element in the social defence system. The need for responsible semi-skilled staff greatly exceeds the need for fully trained staff, e.g. by almost four to one in this hospital. If large numbers of student nurses do *not* fail to finish their training, the nursing profession risks being flooded with trained staff for whom there are no jobs. The wastage is, therefore, an unconscious device to maintain the balance between staff of different levels of skill while all are at a high personal level. It is understandable that apparently determined efforts to reduce wastage have so far failed, except in one or two hospitals.

Avoidance of change

Change is inevitably to some extent an excursion into the unknown. It implies a commitment to future events that are not entirely predictable and to their consequences, and inevitably provokes doubt and anxiety. Any significant change within a social system implies changes in existing social relationship and in social structure. It follows that any significant social change implies a change in the operation of the social system as a defence system. While this change is proceeding, i.e. while social defences are being re-structured, anxiety is likely to be more open and intense.[27] Jaques (1955) has stressed that resistance to social change can be better understood if it is seen as the resistance of groups of people unconsciously clinging to existing institutions because changes threaten existing social defences against deep and intense anxieties.

It is understandable that the nursing service, whose tasks stimulate such primitive and intense anxieties, should anticipate change with unusually severe anxiety. In order to avoid this anxiety, the service tries to avoid change wherever possible almost, one might say, at all costs, and tends to cling to the familiar even when the familiar has obviously ceased to be appropriate or relevant. Changes tend to be initiated only at the point of crisis. The presenting problem was a good example of this difficulty in initiating and carrying through change. Staff and student nurses had for long felt that the methods in operation were unsatisfactory and had wanted to change them. They had, however, been unable to do so. The anxieties and uncertainties about possible changes and their consequences inhibited constructive and realistic planning and decision. At least, the present difficulties were familiar and they had some ability to handle them. The problem was approaching the point of breakdown and the limits of the capacities of the people concerned when we were called in. Many other examples of this clinging to the inappropriate familiar could be observed. For example, changes in medical practice and the initiation of the National Health Service have led to more rapid patient turnover, an increase in the proportion of acutely ill patients, a wider range of illness to be nursed in each ward, and greater variation in the work-load of a ward from day to day. These changes all point to the need for increasing flexibility in the work organisation of nurses in wards. In fact, no such increase in flexibility has taken place in this hospital. Indeed, the difficulty inherent in trying to deal with a fluctuating work-load by the rather rigid system described above has tended to be handled by increased prescription and rigidity and by reiteration of the familiar. As far as one could gather, the greater the anxiety the greater the need for such reassurance in rather compulsive repetition.

The changing demands on nurses described above necessitate a growing amount of increasingly technically skilled nursing care. This has not, however, led to any examination of the implicit policy that nursing can be carried out largely by semi-qualified student nurses.

COMMENTARY ON THE SOCIAL DEFENCE SYSTEM

The characteristic feature of the social defence system, as we have described it, is its orientation to helping the individual avoid the experience of anxiety, guilt, doubt, and uncertainty. As far as possible, this is done by eliminating situations, events, tasks, activities, and relationships that cause anxiety or, more correctly, evoke anxieties connected with primitive psychological remnants in the personality. Little attempt is made positively to help the individual confront the anxiety-evoking experiences and, by so doing, to develop her capacity to tolerate and deal more effectively with the anxiety. Basically, the potential anxieties in the nursing situation are felt to be too deep and dangerous for full confrontation, and to threaten personal disruption and social chaos. In fact, of course, the attempt to avoid such confrontation can never be completely successful. A compromise is inevitable between the implicit aims of the social defence system and the demands of reality as expressed in the need to pursue the primary task.

It follows that the psychic defence mechanisms that have, over time, been built into the socially structured defence system of the nursing service are, in the main, those which by evasion give protection from the full experience of anxiety. These are derived from the most primitive psychic defence mechanisms. Those mechanisms are typical of the young infant's attempts to deal, mainly by evasion, with the severe anxieties aroused by the interplay of his own instincts that are intolerable at his immature age.[28]

Individuals vary in their extent to which they are able, as they grow older, to modify or abandon their early defence mechanisms and develop other methods of dealing with their anxieties. Notably, these other methods include the ability to confront the anxiety-situations in their original or symbolic forms and to work them over, to approach and tolerate psychic and objective reality, to differentiate between them and to perform constructive and objectively successful activities in relation to them.[29] Every individual is at risk that objective or psychic events stimulating acute anxiety will lead to partial or complete abandonment of the more mature methods of dealing with anxiety and to regression to the more primitive methods of defence. In our opinion, the intense anxiety evoked by the nursing task has precipitated just such individual regression to primitive types of defence. These have been projected and given objective existence in the social structure and culture of the nursing service, with the result that anxiety is to some extent contained, but that true mastery of anxiety by deep working-through and modification is seriously inhibited. Thus, it is to be expected that nurses will persistently experience a higher degree of anxiety than is justified by the objective situation alone. Consideration in more detail of how the socially structured defence system fails to support the individual in the struggle towards more effective mastery of anxiety may be approached from two different but related points of view.

I will first consider how far the present functioning of the nursing service gives rise to experiences that in themselves reassure nurses or arouse anxiety. In fact, as a direct consequence of the social organisation, many situations and incidents arise that clearly arouse anxiety. On the other hand, the social system frequently functions in such a way as to deprive nurses of necessary reassurance and satisfactions. In other words, the social defence system itself arouses a good deal of secondary anxiety as well as failing to alleviate primary anxiety. I shall illustrate these points with some typical examples.

Threat of crisis and operational breakdown

From the operational point of view, the nursing service is cumbersome and inflexible. It cannot easily adapt to short- or long-term changes in conditions. For example, the task-list system and minutely prescribed task-performance make it difficult to adjust work-loads when necessary by postponing or omitting less urgent or important tasks. The total demands on a ward vary considerably and at short notice according to factors like types and numbers of patients and operating days. The numbers and categories of student nurses also vary considerably and at short notice. Recurrent shortages of second-year or third-year nurses occur while they spend six weeks in the school; sickness or leave frequently reduce numbers. The work/staff ratio, therefore, varies considerably and often suddenly. Since work cannot easily be reduced, this generates considerable pressure, tension, and uncertainty among staff and students. Even when the work/staff ratio is satisfactory, the threat of a sudden increase is always present. The nurses seem to have a constant sense of impending crisis. They are haunted by fear of failing to carry out their duties adequately as pressure of work increases. Conversely, they rarely experience the satisfaction and lessening of anxiety that come from knowing they have the ability to carry out their work realistically and efficiently.

   The nursing service is organised in a way that makes it difficult for one person, or even a close group of people, to make a rapid and effective decision. Diffusion of responsibility prevents adequate and specific concentration of authority for making and implementing decisions. The organisation of working groups makes it difficult to achieve adequate concentration of necessary knowledge. For example, the task-list system prevents the breakdown of a ward into units of a size that allows one person to be fully acquainted with what is going on in them and of a number that allows adequate communication between them and to the person responsible for co-ordinating them. In a ward, only the sister and the staff nurse are in a position to collect and co-ordinate knowledge. However, they must do this for a unit of such size and complexity that it is impossible to do it effectively. They are, inevitably, badly briefed. For example, we came across many cases where the sister did not remember how many nurses were on duty or what each was supposed to do, and had to have recourse to a written list. Such instances cannot be attributed primarily to individual inadequacy. Decisions tend to be made, therefore, by people who feel that they lack adequate knowledge of relevant and ascertainable facts. This leads to both anxiety and anger. To this anxiety is added the anxiety that decisions will not be taken in time, since decision-making is made so slow and cumbersome by the system of checking and counter-checking and by the obscurity surrounding the localisation of responsibility.

Excessive movement of student nurses

The fact that a rise in work/staff ratios can be met only within very narrow limits by a reduction in the work-load means that it is often necessary to have staff reinforcements, usually, to move student nurses. The defence of rigid work organisation thus appears as a contributory factor to the presenting problem of student-allocation. The unduly frequent moves cause considerable distress and anxiety. Denial of the importance of relationships and feelings does not adequately protect the nurses, especially since the moves most directly affect student nurses, who have not yet fully developed these defences. Nurses grieve and mourn over broken relationships with patients and other nurses; they feel they are failing their patients. One nurse felt compelled to return to her previous ward to visit a patient who, she felt, had depended a great deal on her. The nurse feels strange in her new surroundings. She has to learn some new duties and make relationships with new patients and staff. She probably has to nurse types of illness she has never nursed before. Until she gets to know more about the new situation she suffers anxiety, uncertainties, and doubts. Senior staff estimate that it takes a student two weeks to settle down in a new ward. We regard this as an underestimate. The suddenness of many moves increases the difficulty. It does not allow adequate time for preparing for parting and makes the parting more traumatic. Patients cannot be handed over properly to other nurses. Sudden transfers to a different ward allow little opportunity for psychological preparation for what is to come. Nurses tend to feel acutely deprived by this lack of preparation. As one girl said, 'If only I had known a bit sooner that I was going to the diabetic ward, I would have read up about diabetics and that would have helped a lot.' Janis (1958) has described how the effects of anticipated traumatic events can be alleviated if an advance opportunity is provided to work over the anxieties. He has described this as the 'work of worrying', a parallel concept to Freud's concept of the 'work of mourning' (Freud, 1949). The opportunity to work over the anticipated traumata of separation is, in the present circumstances, denied to nurses. This adds greatly to stress and anxiety.

This situation does indeed help to produce a defensive psychological detachment. Students protect themselves against the pain and anxiety of transfers, or the threat of transfers, by limiting their psychological involvement in any situation, with patients or other staff. This reduces their interest and sense of responsibility and fosters a 'don't care' attitude of which nurses and patients complain bitterly. Nurses feel anxious and guilty when they detect such feelings in themselves, and angry, hurt, and disappointed when they find them in others. 'Nobody cares how we are getting on, there is no team spirit, no one helps us.' The resulting detachment also reduces the possibility of satisfaction from work well done in a job one deeply cares about.

Under-employment of student nurses

Understandably, since work-loads are so variable and it is difficult to adjust tasks, the nursing service tries to plan its establishments to meet peak rather than average loads. As a result, student nurses quite often have too little work. They hardly ever complain of overwork and a number complained of not having enough work, although they still complained of stress. We observed obvious under-employment as we moved about the wards, in spite of the fact that student nurses are apt to make themselves look busy doing something and talk of having to look busy to avoid censure from the sister. Senior staff often seemed to feel it necessary to explain why their students were not busier, and would say they were 'having a slack day' or they 'had an extra nurse today'.

Student nurses are also chronically under-employed in terms of level of work. A number of elements in the defence system contribute to this. Consider, for example, the assignment of duties to whole categories of student nurses. Since nurses find it so difficult to tolerate inefficiency and mistakes, the level of duties for each category is pitched low, i.e. near to the expected level of the least competent nurse in the category. In addition, the policy that makes student nurses the effective nursing staff of the hospital condemns them to the repetitive performance of simple tasks to an extent far beyond that necessary for their training. The performance of simple tasks need not of itself imply that the student nurse's role is at a low level. The level depends also on how much opportunity is given for the use of discretion and judgement in the organisation of the tasks – which, when, and how. It is theoretically possible to have a role in which a high level of discretion is required to organise tasks that are in themselves quite simple. In fact, the social defence system specifically minimises the exercise of discretion and judgement in the student nurse's organisation of her tasks, e.g. through the task-list system. This ultimately determines the under-employment of many student nurses who are capable of exercising a good deal of judgement and could quickly be trained to use it effectively in their work. Similar under-employment is obvious in senior staff connected, for example, with the practice of delegating upwards.

Under-employment of this kind stimulates anxiety and guilt, which are particularly acute when under-employment implies failing to use one's capacities fully in the service of other people in need. Nurses find the limitations on their performance very frustrating. They often experience a painful sense of failure when they have faithfully performed their prescribed tasks, and express guilt and concern about incidents in which they have carried out instructions to the letter, but, in so doing, have practised what they consider to be bad nursing. For example, a nurse had been told to give a patient who had been sleeping badly a sleeping-draught at a certain time. In the interval he had fallen into a deep natural sleep. Obeying her orders, she woke him up to give him the medicine. Her common sense and judgement told her to leave him asleep and she felt very guilty that she had disturbed him. One frequently hears nurses complain that they 'have' to waken patients early in the morning to have their faces washed when they feel that the patients would benefit more by being left asleep. Patients also make strong complaints. But 'all faces must be washed' before the consultant medical staff arrive in the wards in the morning. The nurses feel they are being forced to abandon common-sense principles of good nursing, and they resent it.

Jaques (1956) has discussed the use of discretion and has come to the conclusion that the level of responsibility experienced in a job is related solely to the exercise of discretion and not to carrying out the prescribed elements. Following that statement, we may say that the level of responsibility in the nurse's job is minimised by the attempt to eliminate the use of discretion. Many student nurses complain bitterly that, while ostensibly in a very responsible job, they have less responsibility than they had as senior schoolgirls. They feel insulted, indeed almost assaulted, by being deprived of the opportunity to be more responsible. They feel, and are, devalued by the social system. They are intuitively aware that the further development of their capacity for responsibility is being inhibited by the work and training situation and they greatly resent this. The bitterness of the experience is intensified because they are constantly being exhorted to behave responsibly, which, in the ordinary usage of the word in a work-situation, they can hardly do. In fact, we came to the conclusion that senior staff tend to use the word 'responsibility' differently from ordinary usage. There is an essential conflict between staff and students that greatly adds to stress and bitterness on both sides. Jaques (1956) has stated that workers in industry cannot rest content until they have reached a level of work that deploys to the full their capacity for discretionary responsibility. Student nurses, who are, in effect, 'workers' in the hospital for most of their time, are certainly not content.

Deprivation of personal satisfaction

The nursing service seems to provide unusually little in the way of direct satisfaction for staff and students. Although the dictum 'nursing should be a vocation' implies that nurses should not expect ordinary job satisfaction, its absence adds to stress. Mention has already been made of a number of ways in which nurses are deprived of positive satisfactions potentially existent in the profession, e.g. the satisfaction and reassurance that comes from confidence in nursing skill. Satisfaction is also reduced by the attempt to evade anxiety by splitting up the nurse–patient relationship and converting patients who need nursing into tasks that must be performed. Although the nursing *service* has considerable success in nursing patients, the individual nurse has little direct experience of success. Success and satisfaction are dissipated in much the same way as the anxiety. The nurse misses the reassurance of seeing a patient get better in a way she can easily connect with her own efforts. The nurse's longing for this kind of experience is shown in the excitement and pleasure felt by a nurse who is chosen to 'special' a patient, i.e. to give special, individual care to a very ill patient in a crisis situation. The gratitude of patients, an important reward for nurses, is also dissipated. Patients are grateful to the hospital or to 'the nurses' for their treatment and recovery, but they cannot easily express gratitude in any direct way to individual nurses. There are too many and they are too mobile. The poignancy of the situation is increased by the expressed aims of nursing at the present time, i.e. to nurse the whole patient as a person. The nurse is instructed to do that, it is usually what she wants to do, but the functioning of the nursing service makes it impossible.

Sisters, too, are deprived of potential satisfactions in their roles. Many of them would like closer contact with patients and more opportunity to use their nursing skills directly. Much of their time is spent in initiating and training student nurses who come to their wards. The excessive movement of students means that sisters are frequently deprived of the return on that training time and the reward of seeing the nurse develop under their supervision. The reward of their work, like the nurse's, is dissipated and impersonal.

The nursing service inhibits in a number of ways the realisation of satisfactions in relationships with colleagues. For example, the traditional relationship between staff and students is such that students are singled out by staff almost solely for reprimand or criticism. Good work is taken for granted and little praise given. Students complain that no one notices when they work well, when they stay late on duty, or when they do some extra task for a patient's comfort. Work-teams are notably impermanent. Even three-monthly moves of student nurses would make it difficult to weld together a strong, cohesive work-team. The more frequent moves, and the threats of moves, make it almost impossible. In such circumstances, it is difficult to build a team that functions effectively on the basis of real knowledge of the strengths and weaknesses of each member, her needs as well as her contribution, and adapts to the way of working and type of relationship each person prefers. Nurses feel hurt and resentful about the lack of importance attached to their personal contribution to the work, and the work itself is less satisfying when it must be done not only in accordance with the task-list system but also with an informal, but rigid, organisation. A nurse misses the satisfaction of investing her own personality thoroughly in her work and making a highly personal contribution. The 'depersonalisation' used as a defence makes matters worse. The implied disregard of her own needs and capacities is distressing to the nurse, she feels she does not matter and no one cares what happens to her. This is particularly distressing when she is in a situation fraught with risks and difficulty and knows that sooner or later she will have great need of help and support.

Such support for the individual is notably lacking throughout the whole nursing service within working relationships. Compensation is sought in intense relationships with other nurses off-duty. [30] Working-groups are characterised by great isolation of their members. Nurses frequently do not know what other members of their team are doing or even what their formal duties are; indeed, they often do not know whether other members of their team are on duty or not. They pursue their own tasks with minimal regard to colleagues. This leads to frequent difficulties between nurses. For example, one nurse, in carrying out her own tasks correctly by the prescription, may undo work done by another nurse also carrying out her tasks correctly by the prescription, because they do not plan their work together and co-ordinate it. Bad feeling usually follows. One nurse may be extremely busy while another has not enough to do. Sharing out of work is rare. Nurses complain bitterly about this situation. They say 'there is no team spirit, no one helps you, no one cares'. They feel guilty about not helping and angry about not being helped. They feel deprived by the lack of close, responsible friendly relations with colleagues. The training-system, orientated as it is to information-giving, also deprives the student nurse of support and help. She feels driven to acquire knowledge and pass examinations, to become 'a good nurse', while at the same time she feels few people show real concern for her personal development and her future.

The lack of personal support and help is particularly painful for the student nurse as she watches the care and attention given to patients. It is our impression that a significant number of nurses enter the profession under a certain confusion about their future roles and functions. They perceive the hospital as an organisation particularly well-equipped to deal with dependency needs, kind and supportive, and they expect to have the privilege of being very dependent themselves. However, because of the categorisation, they find that they are denied the privilege except on very rare occasions, notably when they go sick themselves and are nursed in the hospital.

I go on now to consider the second general approach to the failure of the social defences to alleviate anxiety. This arises from the direct impact of the social defence system on the individual, regardless of specific experiences, i.e. from the more directly psychological interaction between the social defence system and the individual nurse.

Although, following Jaques, I have used the term 'social defence system' as a construct to describe certain features of the nursing service as a continuing social institution, I wish to make it clear that I do not imply that the nursing service *as an institution* operates the defences. Defences are, and can be, operated only by individuals. Their behaviour is the link between their psychic defences and the institution. Membership necessitates an adequate degree of matching between individual and social defence systems. I will not attempt to define the degree but state simply that if the discrepancy between social and individual defence systems is too great, some breakdown in the individual's relation with the institution is inevitable. The form of breakdown varies, but, in our society, it commonly takes the form of a temporary or permanent break in the individual's membership. For example, if the individual continues to use his own defences and follows his own idiosyncratic behaviour patterns, he may become intolerable to other members of the institution who are more adapted to the social defence system. They may then reject him. If he tries to behave in a way consistent with the social defence system rather than his individual defences, his anxiety will increase and he may find it impossible to continue his membership. Theoretically, matching between social and individual defences can be achieved by a re-structuring of the social defence system to match the individual, by a re-structuring of the individual defence system to match the social, or by a combination of the two. The processes by which an adequate degree of matching is achieved are too complicated to describe here in detail. It must suffice to say that they depend heavily on repeated projection of the psychic defence system into the social defence system and repeated introjection of the social defence system into the psychic defence system. This allows continuous testing of match and fit as the individual experiences his own and other people's reactions.[31]

The social defence system of the nursing service has been described as an historical development through collusive interaction between individuals to project and reify relevant elements of their psychic defence systems. However, from the point of view of the new entrant to the nursing service, the social defence system at the time of entry is a datum, an aspect of external reality to which she must react and adapt. Fenichel makes a similar point (1946). He states that social institutions arise through the efforts of human beings to satisfy their needs, but that social institutions then become external realities comparatively independent of individuals which affect the structure of the individual. The student nurse is faced with a particularly difficult task in adapting to the nursing service and developing an adequate match between the social defence system and her psychic defence system. It will have been made clear that the nursing service is very resistant to change, especially change in the functioning of its defence system. For the student nurse, this means that the social defence system is to an unusual extent immutable. In the process of matching between the psychic and social defence systems, the emphasis is heavily on the modification of the individual's psychic defences. This means in practice that she must incorporate and operate the social defence system more or less as she finds it, re-structuring her psychic defences as necessary to match it.

An earlier section described how the social defence system of the hospital was built of primitive psychic defences, those characteristic of the earliest phases of infancy. It follows that student nurses, by becoming members of the nursing service, are required to incorporate and use primitive psychic defences, at least in those areas of their life-space which directly concern their work. The use of such defences has certain intrapsychic consequences. These are consistent with the social phenomena already referred to in other contexts in this paper. I will describe them briefly to complete the account. These defences are oriented to the violent, terrifying situations of infancy, and rely heavily on violent splitting which dissipates the anxiety. They avoid the experience of anxiety and effectively prevent the individual from confronting it. Thus, the individual cannot bring the content of the phantasy anxiety situations into effective contact with reality. Unrealistic or pathological anxiety cannot be differentiated from realistic anxiety arising from real dangers. Therefore, anxiety tends to remain permanently at a level determined more by the phantasies than by the reality. The forced introjection of the hospital defence system, therefore, perpetuates in the individual a considerable degree of pathological anxiety.

The enforced introjection and use of such defences also interferes with the capacity for symbol formation. The defences inhibit the capacity for creative, symbolic thought, for abstract thought, and for conceptualisation. They inhibit the full development of the individual's understanding, knowledge, and skills that enable reality to be handled effectively and pathological anxiety mastered. Thus the individual feels helpless in the face of new or strange tasks or problems. The development of such capacities presupposes considerable psychic integration, which the social defence system inhibits. It also inhibits self-knowledge and understanding and with them realistic assessment of performance. The deficient reality sense that follows from the defence system also interferes with judgement and provokes mistakes. The individual is confronted with them when it is too late and a sense of failure, increased self-distrust, and anxiety ensue. For example, mistakes, guilt, and anxiety arise from following out the prescriptions rather than applying the principles of good nursing. This situation particularly affects belief and trust in positive impulses and their effectiveness to control and modify aggression. Anxiety about positive aspects of the personality is very marked in nurses, e.g. fear of doing the wrong thing, expectation of mistakes, fear of not being truly responsible. The social defences prevent the individual from realising to the full her capacity for concern, compassion, and sympathy, and for action based on these feelings which would strengthen her belief in the good aspects of herself and her capacity to use them. The defence system strikes directly, therefore, at the roots of sublimatory activities in which infantile anxieties are re-worked in symbolic form and modified.

In general, one may say that forced introjection of the defence system prevents the personal defensive maturation that alone allows for the modification of the remnants of infantile anxiety and diminishes the extent to which early anxieties may be re-evoked and projected into current real situations. Indeed, in many cases, it forces the individual to regress to a maturation level below that which she had achieved before she entered the hospital. In this, the nursing service fails its individual members desperately. It seems clear that a major motivational factor in the choice of nursing as a career is the wish to have the opportunity to develop the capacity for sublimatory activities in the nursing of the sick, and through that to achieve better mastery of infantile anxiety situations, modification of pathological anxiety, and personal maturation.

It may be interesting, in view of this, to add one further comment on wastage. It seems more serious than number alone suggests. It appears to be the more mature students who find the conflict between their own and the hospital defence system most acute and are most likely to give up training. Although the research objectives did not permit us to collect statistics, it is our distinct impression that among the students who do not complete training are a significant number of the better students, i.e. those who are personally most mature and most capable of intellectual, professional, and personal development with appropriate training. Nurses often talked of students who had left as 'very good nurses'. No one could understand why they had not wanted to finish their training. We had the opportunity to discuss the matter with some students who were seriously considering leaving. Many said they still wanted to nurse and found it difficult to formulate why they wanted to leave. They suffered from a vague sense of dissatisfaction with their training and the work they were doing and a sense of hopelessness about the future. The general content of the interviews left little doubt that they were distressed about the inhibition of their personal development. There is also a striking difference in the personalities of groups of students at different stages of training. We do not attribute all of this difference to the effects of training. Some of the differences appear to arise from self-selection of students to give up training. If we are correct in this impression, the social defence system impoverishes the nursing service for the future, since it tends to drive away those potential senior staff whose contribution to the development of nursing theory and practice would be greatest. Thus the wheel turns full circle and the difficulty in changing the system is reinforced. It is the tragedy of the system that its inadequacies drive away the very people who might remedy them.

SUMMARY AND CONCLUDING COMMENTS

This paper has presented some data from a study of the nursing service of a general teaching hospital. Its specific purpose was to consider and, if possible account for the high level of stress and anxiety chronic among nurses. In following through the data, it was suggested that the nature of the nurse's task, in spite of its obvious difficulties, was not enough to account for the level of anxiety and stress. Consequently, an attempt was made to understand and illustrate the nature of the methods the nursing service provide for the alleviation of anxiety, i.e. its social defence system, and to consider in what respects it failed to function adequately. The conclusion reached was that the social defence system represented the institutionalisation of very primitive defence mechanisms, a main characteristic of which is that they facilitate the evasion of anxiety, but contribute little to its true modification and reduction.

In concluding, I wish to touch briefly on a few points that space does not permit me to elaborate. I have considered only incidentally the effect of the defence system on the efficiency of task performance, apart from stating that it does permit the continuing performance of the primary task of the service. It will have been apparent, however, that the nursing service carries out its task inefficiently in many respects, e.g. it keeps the staff/patient ratio unduly high, it leads to a significant amount of bad nursing practice, it leads to excessive staff turnover, and it fails to train students adequately for their real future roles. There are many other examples. Further, the high level of anxiety in nurses adds to the stress of illness and hospitalisation for patients and has adverse effects on such factors as recovery rates. A recent investigation (Revans, 1959) has connected recovery rates of patients quite directly with the morale of nursing staff. Thus the social structure of the nursing service is defective not only as a means of handling anxiety, but also as a method of organising its tasks. These two aspects cannot be regarded as separate. The inefficiency is an inevitable consequence of the chosen defence system.

This leads me to put forward the proposition that the success and viability of a social institution are intimately connected with the techniques it uses to contain anxiety. Analogous hypotheses about the individual have long been widely accepted. Freud put forward such ideas increasingly as his work developed (1948). The work of Melanie Klein and her colleagues has given a central position to anxiety and the defences in personality development and ego-functioning (1948b). I put forward a second proposition, which is linked with the first, namely, that an understanding of this aspect of the functioning of a social institution is an important diagnostic and therapeutic tool in facilitating social change. Bion (1955) and Jaques (1955) stress the importance of understanding these phenomena and relate difficulties in achieving social change to difficulty in tolerating the anxieties that are released as social defences are re-structured. This appears closely connected with the experiences of people, including many social scientists, who have tried to initiate or facilitate social change. Recommendations or plans for change that seem highly appropriate from a rational point of view are ignored, or do not work in practice. One difficulty seems to be that they do not sufficiently take into account the common anxieties and the social defences in the institution concerned, nor provide for the therapeutic handling of the situation as change takes place. Jaques (1955) states that 'effective social change is likely to require analysis of the common anxieties and unconscious collusions underlying the social defences determining phantasy social relationships'.

The nursing service presents these difficulties to a high degree, since the anxieties are already very acute and the defence system both primitive and ineffectual. Efforts to initiate serious change were often met with acute anxiety and hostility, which conveyed the idea that the people concerned felt very threatened, the threat being of nothing less than social chaos and individual breakdown. To give up known ways of behaviour and embark on the unknown were felt to be intolerable. In general, it may be postulated that resistance to social change is likely to be greatest in institutions whose social defence systems are dominated by primitive psychic defence mechanisms, those which have been collectively described by Melanie Klein as the paranoid-schizoid defences (Klein, 1952a, 1959). One may compare this socio-therapeutic experience with the common experience in psycho-analytic therapy, that the most difficult work is with patients whose defences are mainly of this kind, or in phases of the analysis when such defences predominate.

Some therapeutic results were achieved in the hospital, notably in relation to the presenting symptom. A planned set of courses has been prepared for student nurses, which jointly ensures that the student nurses have adequate training and that the hospital is adequately staffed. Interestingly, it was in preparing these courses that objective data were calculated for the first time about discrepancies between training and staffing needs. For example, to give adequate gynaecological training the gynaecological wards would have to carry four times too many staff; to keep the operating theatres staffed, the nurses would have to have one and a half times too much theatre experience for training. Before this time, the existence of such discrepancies was known, but no one had collected reliable statistical data, a simple matter, and no realistic plans had been made to deal with them. To prevent emergencies from interfering with the implementation of the planned courses, a reserve pool of nurses was created whose special duty was to be mobile and deal with them. A number of other similar changes were instituted dealing with other problems that emerged in the course of the investigation.[32] The common features of these changes, however, were that they involved minimal disturbance of the existing defence system. Indeed, it would be more correct to say that they involved reinforcing and strengthening the existing type of defence. Proposals were made for more far-reaching change, involving a re-structuring of the social defence system. For example, one suggestion was that a limited experiment be done in ward organisation, eliminating the task-list system and substituting some form of patient assignment. However, although the senior staff discussed such proposals with courage and seriousness, they did not feel able to proceed with the plans. This happened in spite of our clearly expressed views that, unless there were some fairly radical changes in the system, the problems of the nursing service might well become extremely serious. The decision seemed to us quite comprehensible, however, in view of the anxiety and the defence system. These would have made the therapeutic task of accomplishing change very difficult for both the nursing service and the therapist.

The full seriousness of the situation is not perhaps clear without considering this hospital in the context of the general nursing services in the country as a whole. The description of the hospital makes it seem a somewhat serious example of social pathology, but within the context of other general hospital nurse-training schools it is fairly typical. Nothing in our general experience of hospitals and nursing leads us to believe otherwise (Skellern, 1953; Sofer, 1955; Wilson, 1950). There are differences in detail, but the main features of the structure and culture are common to British hospitals of this type and are carried in the general culture and ethic of the nursing profession. The hospital studied has, in fact, high status. It is accepted as being one of the better hospitals of its type.

The nursing services in general have shown a similar resistance to change in the face of great changes in the demands made on them. There can be few professions that have been more studied than nursing, or institutions more studied than hospitals. Nurses have played an active part in initiating and carrying out these studies. Many nurses have an acute and painful awareness that their profession is in a serious state. They eagerly seek solutions, and there have been many changes in the expressed aims and policy of the profession. There have also been many changes in the peripheral areas of nursing, i.e. those which do not impinge very directly or seriously on the essential features of the social defence system. Against that background, one is astonished to find how little basic and dynamic change has taken place. Nurses have tended to receive reports and recommendations with a sense of outrage and to react to them by intensifying current attitudes and reinforcing existing practice.

An example of a general nursing problem that threatens crisis is the recruitment of nurses. Changes in medical practice have increased the number of highly technical tasks for nurses. Consequently, the level of intelligence and competence necessary for a fully trained and efficient nurse is rising. The National Health Service has improved the hospital service and made it necessary to have more nurses. On the other hand, professional opportunities for women are expanding rapidly and the other professions are generally more rewarding than nursing in terms of the opportunity to develop and exercise personal and professional capacities as well as in financial terms. The increasing demand for high-level student nurses is therefore meeting increasing competition from other sources. In fact, recruiting standards are being forced down in order to keep up numbers. This is no real solution, for too many of the recruits will have difficulty in passing the examinations and be unable to deal with the level of work. Many of them, on the other hand, would make excellent practical nurses on simpler nursing duties. So far, no successful attempt has been made in the general hospitals to deal with this problem, e.g. by splitting the role of nurse into different levels with different training and different professional destinations.

It is unfortunately true of the paranoid-schizoid defence systems that they prevent true insight into the nature of problems and realistic appreciation of their seriousness. Thus, only too often, no action can be taken until a crisis is very near or has actually occurred. This is the eventuality we fear in the British general hospital nursing services. Even if there is no acute crisis, there is undoubtedly a chronic state of reduced effectiveness, which in itself is serious enough.

NOTES

* *Human Relations*, 13 (2): 95–121. Reprinted with permission of The Tavistock Institute.
  1 I wish to express my appreciation of the research opportunities provided by the hospital. I am grateful to many members of the medical and lay staff who gave us freely of their time and ideas. I am especially grateful to the nursing staff and students. They admitted us generously into close contact with their work, their satisfactions, and their difficulties, although this sometimes involved disclosing painful professional and personal matters. Senior nursing staff spent many hours with me studying data and their interpretation, so that together we might formulate conclusions and plans for action. For them, this was a difficult and distressing process which required considerable courage. It challenged their personal and professional ethics, often led to their feeling personally and professionally criticised, and seemed to point to directions of development that they found impossible to follow. I appreciate greatly their co-operation in this difficult task and am grateful for the insights they help to develop. Finally, I am indebted to the hospital for permission to publish the research material in this paper.
  2 The nursing body that controls nurse-training.
  3 A sample check of actual duration showed that 30 per cent of student moves took place less than 3 weeks after the previous move and 44 per cent less than 7 weeks.
  4 It is a feature of a therapeutic study of this kind that much of the most significant research

material emerges in its later stages when the emphasis of the work shifts from diagnosis to therapy. Presentation and interpretation of data, and work done on resistances to their acceptance, facilitate the growth of insight into the nature of the problem. This extends the range of information seen to be relevant to its solution, and helps overcome personal resistances to the disclosure of information. An impressing feature of the study here reported was the way in which, after a spell of working on the data, the senior nursing staff themselves were able to produce and execute plans directed towards dealing with their problems.

5 There is much evidence from other fields that such phenomena express a disturbed relation with the work situation and are connected with a high level of tension. See, for example, Hill & Trist (1953).

6 My colleague, G. F. Hutton, in analysing the data from another hospital study, as yet unpublished, drew attention to the descent of modern hospitals from orders of nursing sisters. These early hospitals were entirely administered by nurses. Doctors and priests were necessary and important visitors, but visitors only. They met special needs of patients but had no administrative responsibility. The tradition of what Hutton called 'nurse-directed communities' remains strong, in spite of the complexity of organisation of modern hospitals and the number and diversity of patient-centred staff.

7 Throughout this paper I follow the convention of using fantasy to mean conscious fantasy, and phantasy to mean unconscious phantasy.

8 In my description of infantile psychic life, I follow the work of Freud, particularly as developed and elaborated by Melanie Klein. A brief but comprehensive summary of her views may be found in her papers 'Some Theoretical Conclusions Regarding the Emotional Life of the Infant', Klein (1952b) and 'Our Adult World and its Roots in Infancy', Klein (1959).

9 For a further description of the process of building the inner world see Klein (1952b and 1959).

10 For a description of some patients' concepts of illness see Janis (1958) where there is also an account of how working through the fantasy may relieve the anxiety.

11 Klein (1948b) stresses the importance of anxiety in leading to the development of symbol-formation and sublimation.

12 Segal (1957) uses the terms symbolic representation and symbolic equation. In developing this distinction, she stresses the acute anxieties experienced by patients in whom the symbol does not merely represent the phantasy object but is equated with it. She illustrates from the material of two patients for both of whom a violin was a phallic symbol. For one patient the violin *represented* the phallus and violin-playing was an important sublimation through which he could master anxiety. For the other more deeply disturbed patient, the violin was *felt to be* the phallus and he had had to stop playing because he could not touch a violin in public.

13 Bion (1955) has put forward a similar concept in distinguishing between the sophisticated or work group concerned with a realistic task and the basic-assumption group dominated by primitive psychological phenomena; the two 'groups' being simultaneously operative aspects of the same aggregation of people.

14 The importance of anxiety and defences against it have been much stressed in psychoanalytical theories of personality development. Freud's earliest works show his interest and he develops his theory in later work (Freud, 1955, 1948). The central developmental role of anxiety and defences has, more recently, been much stressed by Melanie Klein and her colleagues (Klein, 1952b, 1948b).

15 For a fuller discussion of the primary task and related factors see Rice (1958).

16 The different social systems that have developed under long-wall coal-mining conditions, using the same basic technology, are a good example of how the same primary task may be performed differently using the same technology when social and psychological conditions are different. They have been discussed by Trist & Bamforth (1951).

17 Jaques (1955) has described and illustrated the operation of such socially structured defence mechanisms in an industrial organisation. The term is his.

18 In practice it is not possible to carry out these prescriptions literally, since a whole category of nurses may temporarily be absent from practical duties on formal instruction in the nursing school or on leave.

19 See *Human Relations*, pp. 104–5, for an account of how these roles and relationships arise.

20 Bion (1955), in describing the behaviour of groups where the need to be dependent is dominant, has commented on the group's need for what he calls a 'bible'. It is not perhaps surprising to find that, in the hospital, whose primary task is to meet the dependency needs of patients, there should be a marked need for just such definitive prescription of behaviour.

21 This has long been a familiar complaint in British hospitals and emerged as a central finding in a number of nursing studies.

22 A staff nurse is a fully qualified nurse who is the sister's deputy.

23 There are usually 3 different lists of tasks in a ward, numbered 1, 2 and 3, and a student nurse may well be Number 1 in the morning and Number 2 in the afternoon, e.g. if the Number 2 of the morning goes off duty in the afternoon.

24 The nurses third and fourth in seniority in administration.

25 Arrangements are almost complete for the re-structuring of the task along such lines.

26 This is connected also with the attempt to eliminate decision-making as far as possible. If there are no decisions to be made, the worker simply needs to *know* what to do and how to do it.

27 This is a familiar experience while the individual's defences are being re-structured in the course of psycho-analytic therapy.

28 I will enumerate briefly here some of the most important of these defences. In doing so, I follow the work of Freud as developed by Melanie Klein (1952b, 1959). The infant makes much use of splitting and projection, denial, idealisation, and rigid, omnipotent control of himself and others. These defences are, at first, massive and violent. Later, as the infant becomes more able to tolerate his anxiety, the same defences continue to be used but are less violent. They begin to appear also in what are perhaps more familiar forms, e.g. as repression , obsessional rituals, and repetition of the familiar.

29 Or, expressed otherwise, the capacity to undertake sublimatory activities.

30 By tradition a nurse finds her closest nurse friends in her 'set', i.e. the group with which she started training. Friendship between nurses in different sets is culturally unacceptable. But nurses in the same set spend little working-time together except in their short spells in formal instruction.

31 Paula Heimann (1952) gives a description of these important processes, through which both psychic and external reality are modified.

32 For example, the revised training programme for fourth-year students.

REFERENCES

Bion, W. R. (1955). Group dynamics: a review. In Melanie Klein, Paula Heimann, R. E. Money-Kyrle (eds.), *New directions in psycho-analysis*. London: Tavistock Publications; New York: Basic Books.

Fenichel, O. (1946). *The psychoanalytic theory of the neuroses*. New York: Norton.

Freud, S. (1948). *Inhibitions, symptoms and anxiety*. London: Hogarth Press & Institute of Psycho-analysis.

Freud, S. (1949) Mourning and melancholia. *Collected papers*, Vol. IV, pp. 152–70. London: Hogarth Press & Institute of Psycho-analysis.

Freud, S. (1955). Studies on hysteria. Standard Edition, Vol. II, pp. 1–251. London: Hogarth Press & Institute of Psycho-analysis.

Heimann, P. (1952). Certain functions of introjection and projection in earliest infancy. In *Development in psycho-analysis*. London: Hogarth Press & Institute of Psycho-analysis.

Hill, J. M. M., & Trist, E. L. (1953). A consideration of industrial accidents as a means of with-drawal from the work situation. *Hum. Relat.* 6, 357–80.

Janis, I. L. (1958) *Psychological stress: psycho-analytic and behavioural studies of surgical patients.* London: Chapman & Hall.

Jaques, E. (1955). Social systems as a defence against persecutory and depressive anxiety. In *New directions in psycho-analysis.* London: Tavistock Publications; New York: Basic Books.

Jaques, E. (1956). *Measurement of responsibility: a study of work, payment, and individual capacity.* London: Tavistock Publications; Cambridge, Mass.: Harvard Univ. Press.

Klein, M. (1948a). The psychogenesis of manic-depressive states. In *Contributions to psycho-analysis (1921–1945).* London: Hogarth Press & Institute of Psycho-analysis.

Klein, M. (1948b). The importance of symbol formation in the development of the ego. *Contributions to psycho-analysis (1921–1945).* London: Hogarth Press & Institute of Psycho-analysis.

Klein, M. (1952a). Notes on some schizoid mechanisms. in *Developments in psycho-analysis.* London: Hogarth Press & Institute of Psycho-analysis.

Klein, M. (1952b). Some theoretical conclusions regarding the emotional life of the infant. In *Developments in psycho-analysis.* London: Hogarth Press & Institute of Psycho-analysis.

Klein, M. (1959). Our adult world and its roots in infancy. *Hum. Relat.* 12, 291–303. Also reprinted as Tavistock Pamphlet No. 2, London: Tavistock Publications, 1960.

Menzies, I. E. P. (1951). *Technical report on a working conference for public health nurses, Noordwijk, the Netherlands,* 1950. World Health Organisation.

Revans, R. W. (1959). *The hospital as an organism: a study in communications and morale.* Preprint No. 7 of a paper presented at the 6th annual International Meeting of the Institute of Management Sciences, September 1959, Paris. London, New York, Paris, Los Angeles: Pergamon Press.

Rice, A. K. (1958). *Productivity and social organization: the Ahmedabad experiment.* London: Tavistock Publications.

Segal, H. (1957). Notes on symbol formation. *Int. J. psycho-anal* 38. 391–7.

Skellern, E. (1953). *Report on the practical application to ward administration of modern methods in the instruction and handling of staff and student nurses.* London: Royal College of Nursing.

Sofer, C. (1955). Reactions to administrative change: a study of staff relations in three British hospitals. *Hum. Relat.* 8, 291–316.

Trist, E. L., & Bamforth, K. W. (1951). Some social and psychological consequences of the long-wall method of coal-getting. *Hum. Relat.* 4, 338.

Wilson, A. T. M. (1950). Hospital nursing auxiliaries. *Hum. Relat.* 3, 1–32.

PART TWO

Conceptualising practice

Chapter 7

Uncovering the knowledge embedded in clinical nursing practice

PATRICIA BENNER

Introduction

In contemporary nursing, Patricia Benner's exposition of the hidden skills which experienced nurses bring to their practice has taken a unique place. Her book *From Novice to Expert: excellence and power in clinical nursing practice,* first published in America in 1984, continues to be cited, stocked and borrowed from nursing libraries in great numbers. In this book, and other work, Benner argues that nurses and others have failed to take sufficient notice of the valuable knowledge that gradually accumulates over time with the practice of any applied discipline. Her evidence for such an argument is drawn from a huge amount of documentary data from nurses talking in depth about their practice and in particular about their experiences in assessment and decision making. From such a range of accounts, she devises not only a typology of different aspects of what she terms practical knowledge, but takes on the now familiar classification of novice, advanced beginner, competent, proficient and expert nurse. The problem solving of a proficient or expert nurse, she argues, differs from that of a beginning or competent nurse: the expert grasps each situation as a whole, can draw on past concrete situations, and can quickly identify the core characteristics of a problem without 'wasteful consideration of a large number of irrelevant options'. The less-expert nurse relies on conscious, methodical analysis of each problem. Expertise greatly enhances the effectiveness of practitioners because they can, for example, recognise and act on a subtle deterioration in a patient before documentable changes in vital signs are noted. Often such perceptions are highly contextual, and Benner borrows the term 'connoisseurship' to describe this skill born of experience. From her understanding of 'experience' she explicitly excludes the reinforcement of prejudice in its negative sense, and argues that 'only when an event refines, elaborates, or disconfirms . . . foreknowledge does the event deserve the term 'experience'.

Her work parallels other contemporary reflections on the nature of professional expertise and the (apparently) different forms that knowledge can take. These would include Donald Schön's well-known investigations into 'reflective practice' and other discussions of 'tacit knowledge' or 'craft knowledge'. Benner herself draws on a model of skills acquisition (Dreyfus, H. and S. Dreyfus 1980 *A Five-Stage Model of the Mental Activities Involved in Directed Skill Acquisition*. Berkeley, CA., Operations Research Center Report). Such investigations perhaps have their roots in the post-Second World War questioning of the procedures and status of science by historians and philosophers of science, such as Thomas Kuhn and Michael Polanyi, and philosopher Martin Heidegger. The confidence in its own rationality that Europe might have felt, as the seat of the Enlightenment, was clearly shaken by the advent of the war and all its accompanying horror. During the period, many articulated an unease that the status of formalised, propositional knowledge, epitomised, perhaps, by scientific knowledge, had gained such social ascendancy. Groups that had associated their activities with such realms of knowledge could, it was argued, gain esteem, influence and reward as a result. These challenges to established views were naturally attractive to groups who had been excluded from the privilege that such claims to knowledge afforded. Among them were feminists and occupational groups, including teachers and nurses, who felt that predominant hierarchies of knowledge had rendered their own highly contextual, even intuitive, modes of making judgements dubious. To enhance the status of their own cognitive activities was an essential part of raising not only their own social position, but the self-esteem and self-awareness of their members.

The popularity of Benner's work can be understood in this context. It offered an authoritative blend of empirical evidence and philosophical grounding, and all this was lent a moral urgency by the understanding of nursing as a significant, humanistic practice. Not that Benner's desire for professional advancement is covert; she argues that part of the need for nurses to make explicit the implicit and articulate the details of their expert 'know-how' is that 'clinical expertise has not been adequately described or compensated (financially rewarded) in nursing, and the lag in description contributes to the lag in recognition and reward'. But in the process of articulating this embedded knowledge, many nurses have come to better value their own skills and activity.

Benner's work stands out in a period characterised by a drive toward high-level theory in nursing — at least in the American nursing literature. Although she sees no necessary conflict in knowledge development in nursing being both a theoretical advance and a charting of practical expertise, it is interesting to note that it is her work rather than the various models and theories that emerged during the 1970s and 1980s that has continued to have such widespread appeal.

BENNER, P. (1984)

Uncovering the knowledge embedded in clinical nursing practice*

Nursing practice has been studied primarily from a sociological perspective. Thus, we have learned much about role relationships, socialisation, and acculturation in nursing practice. But, we have learned less about the knowledge embedded in actual nursing practice – i.e., that knowledge that accrues over time in the practice of an applied discipline. Such knowledge has gone uncharted and unstudied because the differences between practical and theoretical knowledge have been misunderstood (Carper, 1978; Collins & Fielder, 1981). What's missing are systematic observations of what nurse clinicians learn from their clinical practice.

Nurses have not been careful record keepers of their own clinical learning. Although many single case studies have been published, few clinical comparisons of multiple case studies or clinical observations across patient populations exist. This failure to chart our practices and clinical observations has deprived nursing theory of the uniqueness and richness of the knowledge embedded in expert clinical practice. Well-charted practices and observations are essential for theory development.

This book will examine the differences between practical and theoretical knowledge; provide examples of competencies identified from the study of nursing practice; describe aspects of practical knowledge; and outline strategies for preserving and extending that knowledge. First, however, let us take an overall look at the nature of that knowledge and how it is acquired.

Differences between practical and theoretical knowledge

Theory is a powerful tool for explaining and predicting. It shapes questions and allows the systematic examination of a series of events. Theorists try to identify the necessary and sufficient conditions for the occurrence of real situations. By establishing interactional causal relationships between events, scientists come to 'know that.' Philosophers of science such as Kuhn (1970) and Polanyi (1958), however, observe that 'knowing *that*' and 'knowing *how*' are two different kinds of knowledge. They point out that we have many skills (know how) that are acquired without 'knowing *that*' and, further, that we cannot always theoretically account for our know-how for many common activities such as riding a bicycle or swimming. To state it differently, some practical knowledge may elude scientific formulations of 'knowing that.' And 'know-how' that may challenge or extend current theory can be developed ahead of such scientific formulations. Therefore, knowledge development in an applied discipline consists of extending practical knowledge (know-how) through theory-based scientific investigations and through the charting of the existent 'know-how' developed through clinical experience in the practice of that discipline.

KNOWLEDGE EMBEDDED IN EXPERTISE

Expertise develops when the clinician tests and refines propositions, hypotheses, and principle-based expectations in actual practice situations. Experience, as it is used here (Heidegger, 1962; Gadamer, 1970), results when preconceived notions and expectations are challenged, refined, or disconfirmed by the actual situation. Experience is therefore a requisite for expertise. For example, the problem solving of a proficient or expert nurse differs from that of the beginner or competent nurse, as described in Chapter 2. This difference can be attributed to the know-how that is acquired through experience. The expert nurse perceives the situation as a whole, uses past concrete situations as paradigms, and moves to the accurate region of the problem without wasteful consideration of a large number of irrelevant options (Dreyfus, H., 1979; Dreyfus, S., 1981). In contrast, the competent or proficient nurse in a novel situation must rely on conscious, deliberate, analytic problem solving of an elemental nature.

Expertise in complex human decision making, such as nursing requires, makes the interpretation of clinical situations possible, and the knowledge embedded in this clinical expertise is central to the advancement of nursing practice and the development of nursing science. Not all of the knowledge embedded in expertise can be captured in theoretical propositions, or with analytic strategies that depend on identifying all the elements that go into the decision (Benner & Benner, 1979). However, the intentions, expectations, meanings, and outcomes of expert practice can be described, and aspects of clinical know-how can be captured by interpretive descriptions of actual practice.

EXTENDING PRACTICAL KNOWLEDGE

Clinical knowledge is gained over time, and clinicians themselves are often unaware of their gains. Strategies are needed to make clinical know-how public so it can be extended and refined. Six areas of practical knowledge were identified: (1) graded qualitative distinctions; (2) common meanings; (3) assumptions, expectations, and sets; (4) paradigm cases and personal knowledge; (5) maxims; and (6) unplanned practices. Each area can be studied using ethnographic and interpretive strategies initially to identify and extend practical knowledge.

Expert nurses, for instance, learn to recognise subtle physiological changes. They can recognise signs of impending shock before documentable changes in vital signs are apparent and can discriminate the need for imminent resuscitation efforts prior to vascular collapse or dramatic vital sign change. Many examples of early recognition and early warnings by expert nurses are documented in this book – e.g., pulmonary embolus, or early stages of septic shock. These finely tuned abilities come from many hours of direct patient observation and care.

Often the perceptual grasp of a situation is context dependent; that is, the subtle changes take on significance only in light of the patient's past history and current situation. Polanyi (1958) calls this perceptual, recognitional ability of the expert clinician, 'connoisseurship.' Descriptive and interpretive recording of this connoisseurship uncovers clinical knowledge. Nurses need to collect examples of their recognitional abilities and describe the context, meanings, characteristics, and outcomes of their connoisseurship. This will enable them to refine their skills and to demonstrate or illustrate the qualitative distinctions they have come to recognise. Much of this takes place naturally as nurses compare their judgments of qualitative distinctions such as tonicity in a premature infant or the 'feel' of a contracted uterus in contrast to one that is firm because of clots.

Graded qualitative distinctions can be elaborated and refined only as nurses compare their judgments in actual patient care situations. For example, intensive care nursery nurses compare their assessment of muscle tone so that they can come to consistent appraisals of tonicity. Nurses evaluating wound healing compare their descriptive language as patient examples present themselves. Often, special descriptive terms will develop to describe these qualitative distinctions. However, unless steps are taken to systematically compare the meaning of these terms in actual situations, communication will break down.

This aspect of clinical knowledge (connoisseurship) is often overlooked in the quest to learn the latest technological procedures. An inordinate amount of attention is given to learning the latest technology and procedures rather than to in-depth skill acquisition in clinical judgment.

COMMON MEANINGS

As illustrated in the competencies presented in Chapters 4 and 5, nurses working with common issues in health and illness, birth and death, develop common meanings about helping, recovery, and coping resources in these human situations. For example, one common meaning uncovered in this study is that nurses typically try to develop a sense of 'possibility' for their patients even in the most deprived circumstances and even when this sense of possibility may mean only a pain-free afternoon or even acceptance of pain or death.

Nurses learn from families and patients a range of responses, meanings, and coping options in the most extreme situations. These common meanings evolve over time and are shared among nurses. They form a tradition. Understanding these meanings *without* rendering them meaningless through decontextualised analysis can provide a seedbed for systematic study and for further development of practice and theory. Common meanings become apparent when narrative accounts of diverse clinical situations are given with the intentions, context, and meanings intact.

ASSUMPTIONS, EXPECTATIONS, AND SETS

Accounts of practical situations presented in narrative form with the context intact are laden with assumptions, expectations, and 'sets' that may not be a part of formally recognised knowledge. When a narrative account is examined for the assumptions and expectations underlying the assessment or interventions, new questions can be generated for further refinement, development, and testing. For example, from having observed the clinical course of many similar and dissimilar patients, nurses may learn to expect a certain course of events without ever formally stating those expectations. These expectations may show up only in clinical practice and not in known abstractions or generalisations.

Nurses also develop global sets about patients. Gestalt psychologists define 'set' as a predisposition to act in certain ways in particular situations. Sets are accrued over time and may be even more elusive than the specific expectations or assumptions that are often apparent to the outside observer. Sets constitute the orientation toward the situation and thus alter how the situation is perceived and described. Sets can sometimes be uncovered, though they can never be completely explicit because the very act of making them explicit will change their function.

One strategy for making sets more visible is borrowed from cross-cultural studies where different 'sets' for the same situation become apparent when communication breaks down or actions do not make sense to people with divergent cultural backgrounds. Deliberate cross-cultural experiments can be created through nurses' comparing critical incidents from their practice and the ways in which they approach a clinical situation.

Divergent approaches and breakdowns in communication about the same clinical situation may point to different sets. For example, different sets were apparent in two nurses' descriptions of identifying and managing a patient crisis until physician assistance was available. One nurse had worked in a setting where nurse-physician trust and communication were high, whereas the other nurse worked in a setting where distrust was the norm and physicians even refused to sign verbal orders. Consequently, the nurse working in the latter situation did not approach a medically urgent patient situation with the same set or sense of possibility as the nurse working in the highly collaborative setting. Discovering assumptions, expectations, and sets can uncover an unexamined area of practical knowledge that can then be systematically studied and extended or refuted.

PARADIGM CASES AND PERSONAL KNOWLEDGE

Heidegger (1962) and Gadamer (1975) define experience as the turning around of preconceptions that are not confirmed by the actual situation. The precondition for perceiving a situation is a foreknowledge or set, and in clinical practice this foreknowledge is often well formed by theory, principles, and prior experience. Only when the event refines, elaborates, or disconfirms this foreknowledge does the event deserve the term 'experience.' As a nurse gains 'experience,' clinical knowledge that is a hybrid between naive practical knowledge and unrefined theoretical knowledge develops. A particular experience may be powerful enough to stand out as a paradigm case (Benner & Wrubel, 1982). Many of the exemplars presented in later chapters were paradigm cases for the nurses who presented them.

Proficient and expert nurses develop clusters of paradigm cases around different patient care issues (see Chapter 2, pp. 27–36), so that they approach a patient care situation using past concrete situations much as a researcher uses a paradigm. Past situations stand out because they changed the nurse's perception. Past concrete experience therefore guides the expert's preconceptions and actions and allows for a rapid perceptual grasp of the situation. This kind of advanced clinical knowledge is more comprehensive than any theoretical sketch can be, since the proficient clinician compares past whole situations with current whole situations.

Some paradigm cases are sufficiently simple and dramatic that they can be transmitted as case studies and taken up as paradigms by the learner (Benner & Wrubel, 1982). Expert clinical teachers present paradigm cases that transmit more than can be conveyed through abstract principles or guidelines. But in order for students to learn from another person's paradigm case, they must actively rehearse or imagine the situation. Simulations can be even more effective because they require action and decisions from the learner. In addition, simulations provide the learner with opportunities to gain paradigm cases in a guided way.

However, many paradigm cases are too complex to be transmitted through case examples or simulations, because it is the particular interaction with the individual learner's prior knowledge that creates the 'experience' – that is, the particular refinement or turning around of preconceptions and prior understanding. Polanyi (1958) calls this a transaction with personal knowledge. Each person brings his own particular history, intellectual commitments, and readiness to learn to a particular clinical situation. The transactions created by this personal knowledge and the clinical situation then determine the actions and decisions that are made. This is why a clinical discipline needs expert clinicians to model this dynamic transaction between personal knowledge and the clinical situation.

Experienced nurses can readily bring to mind clinical situations that altered their approach to patient care. Through a systematic record and study of these paradigm cases, it is possible to extend the knowledge that is embedded there.

MAXIMS

Experts pass on cryptic instructions that make sense only if the person already has a deep understanding of the situation. Polanyi (1958) calls these instructions 'maxims' (Dreyfus, 1982; Benner, 1982; Benner & Wrubel, 1982). For example, intensive care nurses point cryptically to subtle changes in premature infants' respiratory status that will make sense only to one who has had a range of experience in observing respiratory status in premature infants. Polanyi (1958) uses the example of maxims in sports. The experienced golfer or tennis player is told to 'keep your eye on the ball,' whereas it would make no sense to give the beginner the same message.

Expert nurse clinicians can learn much from the maxims they are able to pass on to one another. However, the outside observer and less expert nurse can also gain clues about areas of clinical knowledge – particularly perceptual knowledge that is cloaked in maxims. Collecting maxims can be a beginning point for identifying an area of clinical judgment.

UNPLANNED PRACTICES

The nursing role in hospitals and extended care facilities has expanded largely through unplanned practices and interventions delegated by the physician and other health care workers. This unplanned delegation might be termed delegation by default. For example, a new treatment or diagnostic regimen is introduced and because of the element of risk involved, the treatment or regimen must be administered and monitored by physicians. But frequently the nurse is given the responsibility for doing this because it is the nurse who is present at the patient's bedside.

These handed-down practices have multiple ramifications for nursing practice. For example, nurses have become experts in titrating and weaning patients from vasopressors and antiarrhythmic drugs, but this knowledge has not been systematically described or studied. Perceptions and clinical judgments are altered as a result of acquiring a new skill, yet these changes will continue to go undocumented and unrecognised unless nurses study these changes and the resultant 'know-how' that develops in their own practice.

SUMMARY AND CONCLUSIONS

A wealth of untapped knowledge is embedded in the practices and the 'know-how' of expert nurse clinicians, but this knowledge will not expand or fully develop unless nurses systematically record what they learn from their own experience. Clinical expertise has not been adequately described or compensated in nursing, and the lag in description contributes to the lag in recognition and reward. Furthermore, adequate description of practical knowledge is essential to the development and extension of nursing theory. Nursing science has much to gain from nurses who compare their graded qualitative judgments and who describe and document their observations, sets, paradigm cases, maxims, and their changing practices. There is much to learn and appreciate as practicing nurses uncover common meanings acquired as a result of helping, coaching, and intervening in the significantly human events that comprise the art and science of nursing.

NOTES

*From Novice to Expert: Excellence and Power in Clinical Nursing Practice. Upper Saddle River, NJ, Prentice-Hall, pp. 1–12. Reprinted with permission of Prentice-Hall.

Chapter 8

(Re)writing ethnography

The unsettling questions for nursing research raised by post-structural approaches to 'the field'

TRUDY RUDGE

Introduction

Nursing's historical research tradition has been embedded within social science. Every country has its distinctive research tradition and culture. But Australia has embraced critical theory and postmodernism with unparalleled enthusiasm. Geographical distance, perhaps combined with a profound scepticism of convention, help to explain the extraordinary excellence of social science theorising in this field. This paper exemplifies the post-structuralist project in nursing. It delineates the researcher/researched positioning within one observational record in research into nurse–patient interactions focusing on one particular nursing procedure. The title is playfully laden with ambiguity. It is both about writing as well as the problematic nature of 'writing up' ethnographic research. It poses uncomfortable questions about researchers as settlers, colonising 'the field', claiming its contents as their own. The complexities introduced by professionals and the different identities that they bring to the research are also opened up to interrogation. Disrupting such notions and finding an ethical path through by 'unsettling' the field is considered both in a literal and metaphorical way. Finally, the field is shown to have an extra layer of ambiguity, exemplified in a surgical site for dressing wounds.

Rudge rejects the notion of positivist ethnographic research which locates the participant observer as an objective commentator. But she does not advocate post-structuralism in its stead as an unproblematic solution. Instead she reformulates the concept of 'the field' by drawing attention to the dual role of the nurse as researcher and practitioner in observing and recording data as a participant observer of practice. It is here therefore that the role of nurse and researcher coalesce into nurse–researcher from which nursing research arguably receives its richest meaning.

The paper opens with Edward Said's eulogy on the virtues of the intellectual as nomad, forever on the move, never settling to colonise or claim in an endless quest for wonder. Rudge draws an analogy with her experience as a nurse researcher, in which her identity both as nurse and researcher shifted shape in the process of writing the research itself. But nothing, it seems either in her education as a nurse or research training as an anthropologist, had prepared her for the different shifts of identity that would follow. To understand this we need to take account of the history of ethnography itself. Ethnography as a method has come under fire for its espousal of so-called master narratives. According to this view the heroic ethnographer strives to achieve mastery over knowledge, motivated often by an unconscious desire for access to and power over that culture. Such an approach relies upon the researcher entering the field as an outsider, creating a record unavailable for negotiation. Within this formulation the power relations between researcher and researched are fixed rather than fluid. Like the conductor or choirmaster, the researcher modulates the voices, regulates the rhythm and interpretive possibilities within the score.

Rudge rejects both the ethics and aesthetics of this 'classic' model as much too neat and tidy. Hers is a more dynamic, open-ended model, involving interplay, even improvisation, between researchers and participants. In musical terms it is one that fits jazz rather than classical forms. No longer the (mere) faithful recorder of data in the field, the researcher has access to the different perspectives and positions that reframing the recording of field notes brings to the research. Rudge therefore renders the position of the researcher in ethnography problematic. She argues that observational records are texts, created as much by the researcher as the participants in research. The notes in this instance are derived from observation of a dressing procedure for a patient in a burns ward. What Rudge draws out clearly and cleverly are the different voices evident in the notes and the different positions afforded by them in the research. At first the researcher is positioned as a scientifically informed onlooker as well as a researcher requiring contextual details on the history of the patient and the nurse's clinical judgement and decision-making process about the dressing itself. The nurse self-locates both as a resource to the patient and researcher, while recognising the researcher as a nurse who understands 'clinical trade' talk and the significance of the use of such jargon terms as 'practised eye'. Rudge asks, through her notes, who is talking here? Is it nurse, researcher or nurse–researcher? Throughout her field notes, she finds that boundaries become blurred and are constantly in play. Yet at other times she seems to write herself out of the script. But never does she disappear. The notes are designed to record the different dynamics between nurse and patient. In doing so they also reveal the differential positioning of the researcher by the nurse either with, away from or in what Rudge refers to as a 'privileged blurred' position. Informants were important actors in influencing the research process through such positioning. The patient–researcher relationship threw up further questions too. Here the researcher was often caught between the patient and other nurses, sometimes as confidant, confessor or conduit to care. The latter in particular raised ethical issues about confidentiality and the dilemma of disclosure that privileged proximity to the patient's own position brings with it. Rudge seemed to side with sociologist Geertz's own scepticism of the truth claims of the 'ethnographic gaze' by acknowledging that ethnography is as much about writing as it is about participation in the field.

It is rare to find accounts of research as revelation, but Rudge's is a good example.

What she trains our attention on as 'readers' of research is a force, sometimes sinister, which we would rather ignore than acknowledge – the power relations within the text and their inescapababality. In doing so Rudge plays out post-structuralist theorising within nursing, but plays that back into ethnography with elegance and relevance. In this way she provides a point of contact, a conversational conduit into and contribution to post-structuralist debates in this area. Her solution or at least parting shot is uplifting, even romantic: 'I would rather position myself as one who wonders, not colonizes; travels with 'the researched' rather than conquering the field; and recognizes how we all have come to live with not excavate, the field of nursing' (p. 152).

RUDGE, T. (1996)

(Re)writing ethnography: the unsettling questions for nursing research raised by post-structural approaches to 'the field'*

INTRODUCTION

> A [researching nurse] is like a shipwrecked person who learns how to live in a certain sense *with* the land, not *on* it, not like Robinson Crusoe whose goal is to colonise his little island, but more like Marco Polo, whose sense of the marvellous never fails him, and who is always a traveller, a provisional guest, not a freeloader, conqueror, or raider (p. 43–44).[1]

This is a story from the field that explores dynamics that are inherent in the research process and embedded in the 'texts' of ethnography. It outlines how, as a researcher, I came to recognise that I was not like Robinson Crusoe, rather I positioned myself, and was positioned by others, more like the guest and traveller suggested by Said.[1] As a nurse, researching nursing, it became only too apparent that 'the nurse' within me, a nursing subjectivity, was a crucial aspect of my participation in 'the field'. Such positioning frequently blurred and unsettled my, in hindsight, rather naive conceptualisation of ethnographic research. How I wrote the observational record, how the nurses and patients used these notes, and how the notes recorded my positioning became a source of unsettling and challenging thoughts about the research process.

All of my studies, reading and preparation for this research did not prepare me for how these records told me as much about 'the researcher' as they did 'the researched'. Exploring my field notes for authorial positioning led to a fuller understanding of the ethics of research, the perspective and rhetoric embedded in the notion of participant observation, as well as a way in which to incorporate post-structural perspectives into the research process itself. What follows in this paper is some discussion of current understandings about participant observation and ethnographic research. I will then explore, through the examination of one field observation, the different positionings evidenced within the field notes. The observation that formed the basis of this paper was two and half hours in duration, due to part of the observation being some discussion with the patient and the nurse after the dressing procedure had been completed.

THE DISAPPEARING FIELD

As an undergraduate student of anthropology during the late 70s and early 80s, I witnessed what appeared to be the expansion of ethnography into the analysis of deviant, but colourful sub-cultures, or rural backwaters, of 'late monopoly capitalist' society. There was much soul searching on the ethics of applied anthropology (given its work with mining companies; more recently with various Land Councils), on the ethics of 'doing the natives', and on the ethics of covert research or the exploitation of the host culture as part of an academic career. Ethnography, as a research process and outcome, continued to cross disciplinary boundaries, forming alliances with psychology, medicine and law, as well as spawning enclaves of cultural analysis in geography, history, education, and even stronger links with its epistemological roots in philosophy.

Indeed, women anthropologists using feminist perspectives re-analysed exotic cultures from women's point of view, reconceptualised the concepts of the economic exchange of women, sexuality and social taboos, and kinship practices, and highlighted the importance of race and class as confounding and compounding factors on women's position. It was always obvious to me that the debates about knowledge construction and underpinning epistemological positions were central to anthropology's understanding of its 'field'. Was it appropriate to analyse primitive culture from the perspective of structural marxism? Were Western feminist perspectives, predicated as they were on different structural realities, the appropriate approach for 'island' cultures? How could ethnographers consistently deny the cultural imperialism of white ethnographies of African cultures, which disavowed the effect of tribal affiliations in Africa's political context or the central role of apartheid in the political economy of South Africa? Indeed, all of these questions challenged anthropology's assumptions.

(RE)WRITING THE FIELD

Writing in 1992, Hammersley questioned where ethnography was going and the problematic nature of its assuming a critical inflection.[2] Hammersley doubted whether such moves would overcome the problems of validity and relevance, which he considered accompanied the ethnographic method. He suggested, similar to Simon and Dippo[3] and Carr and Kemmis,[4] that participant or practitioner research may overcome ideological distortions and power imbalances currently embedded in this research process. In summing up ethnography's future, Hammersley suggested that both participant observeration and ethnographies might need to be re-thought, or even renamed, to more accurately represent the form of research entailed. Furthermore, Hammersley suspected that the deconstruction of the dichotomy of quantitative/qualitative research methods would further destabilise its position within the domain of qualitative research.

Even such 'classical' ethnographers as Geertz[5] are currently challenging how interpretation of discourses of informants occurs and how the field notes are considered, as well as the ethnography itself. In opening up 'the field' for consideration as a text, Clifford welcomed this critique of empiricism and its attendant privileging of the 'ethnographic gaze' (see also Clough,[7] Van Maanen,[8] Clifford[9]).[6] Further, Clifford asserted, the time that it has taken for this critique to surface is indicative of how strong the belief is, within the social sciences, in ethnography's purported transparency and congruence with reality and experience. The role language played in the method was masked by a position that asserted that ethnography was simply 'writing reduced to method: keeping good field notes, making accurate maps, "writing up" results' (p. 2).[6] As Geertz,[10] Clifford[6] and Pratt[11] all suggested, ethnography is as much about writing as it is participation in the 'field'. Such writing contains the personal narrative of the participants, both direct and interpreted by the researcher, the narrative of the researcher's journey and the narrative of the research outcomes themselves.[11] As such, Clifford contended that ethnography, as text, invents culture rather than fully representing cultural reality described within its texts.[6] He further argued, along with Tyler,[12] that ethnographies are constructed according to particular textual rules set by the academy, and represent 'ethnographic fictions' (see Geertz[10]), which cannot claim to be 'truth' or to accurately correspond with the culture written about in the text. Consequently, ethnographic writings can, at best, claim to be partial in that they are 'something made or fashioned',[6] but also in the sense put forward by Gore[13] and Ellsworth[14] that they are representations both partial and partisan.

As Clough asserted with regard to the current textual practices and narratives in sociology, not only does the narrative construction of ethnography construct an empirical reality, it 'enacts for sociological discourse the authority of the storyteller, in the figure of *the heroic ethnographer* . . . Ethnography is the productive icon of empirical scientific authority' (p. 2, emphasis added).[7] With the dissolution of its colonial 'field' as I outlined earlier,[6] ethnography, both as process and outcome, has been problematised for its ethnocentric focus; for its unquestioning belief in the unitary nature of the ethnographer 'subject'; and for the primacy afforded the knowledge produced by such a unitary 'subject' ethnographer.[7]

Clough considered that while acknowledging the dissolution of the field of ethnography, Clifford did not sufficiently extend his analysis to explain the interrelationship between narrative and empirical reality. She claimed that the desire for unity of the subject remains unacknowledged within ethnographic works. Clough highlighted how post-modern reflections on desire, which has embedded within it an awareness of how such desire is unconsciously motivated, suggests that both ethnographer and informant are motivated by unconscious desire in the 'picture' they present (see Bourdieu[15]). To conceive of these texts as unaffected by such desire, Clough argued, is to deny how we construct such narratives. Further, Pratt suggested that the dominant metaphors of ethnography, that is participant observation, data collection and cultural description, are imbued with unconscious desires of mastery over knowledge and appropriation of the cultures described within them.[11] More problematically for nurses researching nursing, these metaphorical positions assume continuation of 'the outsider' standpoint.

But can we, as Clough suggested, open ethnography and its textual records if we view them as but textual mediations of reality? Does this open paths to new forms of text, new forms of resistance to the hegemonic discourses that seek closure and empirical certainty? Would such contestation and constitution of the various subject positions open to the 'ethnographic hero' prevent premature closure of the textual record of such inquiry? The result she suggested would be 'textual fields' of resistant knowledges, openly partial and partisan. What follows is an attempt to open up one such record, to explore the positionings evident within it and to detect the influences upon that record. Voices within a particular text are evidence of positions afforded within them.[16] Similarly, they are evidence of the power relations underpinning language use in the formation of knowledge or truth claims as they relate these to espoused positions. In exploring my field notes for positionings within them, I will raise more questions than answers. Marcus suggested that application of post-modernism and poststructuralism result in 'messy texts'. These texts resist totalising effects of traditional ethnography, and in opening field notes to this critique I suggest that this record, even before analysis, conveys much about the messiness of research.

RESEARCHER PRESENCE: POSITIONED BY THE RESEARCHED AND THE RESEARCH

The notes are from an observation of a dressing procedure for a patient in a burns unit. The patient had been in the unit for two months, and six days prior to my observation he had undergone his third debridement and skin grafting. He had been showered, clean dressings had been applied to his still burnt skin, and he was back in bed to have his recent skin grafts receive their second radical trimming and clean up. In the case notes, it was noted that the patient's newer areas of grafting needed trimming, and some assessment was made of the areas that required further grafting. The nurse doing this had worked in the unit for six years. I had been present in the unit for three months and focusing on this patient since the first week of his admission to the ward. At this stage, I had had several informal discussions with the nurse, and had been present at most of the dressings this patient had undergone since his first week in hospital. What follows is an excerpt from my records for this patient.

> Today Gary's dressing is to be done by Susan. The first parts of the dressing were done in the bathroom, that is Gary washed under the shower and parts of the dressing were then done in his room. The areas that had recently been operated on now these new grafts could be more extensively trimmed and cleaned up as they were more stable and therefore need to be attended to by a more senior nurse. The parts which needed to be attended were his flanks and the areas on his arms. Susan waited until Gary was back in bed to do them as they were quite extensive. She explained to me that what she is doing is an extended clean up of the areas of graft which were over some areas which

were granulating, areas of graft which were in fact doubled up and radical trimming and cleaning up of serious ooze which had built up around some grafts. She explained to Gary that these areas needed to be cleaned up as they could become infected or would not heal properly. I asked her why she was doing it because a GNP had helped Gary with his shower. She said that it needed a practised eye, one that could see the difference between the various types of skin that were now evident on Gary's grafted areas. Some of the areas might need new skin grafts or would need some attention which unless you knew what you were looking at you would not see that it actually needed cleaning up. Also some of the grafts were quite fragile and easily damaged and this took some practice to work out whether they should stay or be cleaned up.

Nursing researcher or nurse–researcher

This extract from my field notes shows some of the voices evident in the notes, and the positioning afforded within them. This was the first time that I had worked with this nurse, but certainly not the first time that we had talked. I have largely written the observation in narrative form: a story of a particular nurse doing a particular patient's dressing. Within the talk at the beginning of the dressing, the nurse positioned herself as someone who needs to provide information to both the patient and to me. She has provided different types of information though. For me, she has provided information that suggests that I understand the language of wound care, speaking to me about serous ooze, granulating tissue and trimming grafts. Her assumption is that I understand the scientific framing of the dressing and the actual timing of this extensive 'trimming'. Such talk positions me as informed with the basic understanding of the process, and with an understanding of wound healing and graft care requirements. At the same time, she is also aware of my 'information' needs as a researcher, explaining why she had come to do this dressing even though that day the patient was cared for by a first-year registered nurse.

It is this desire for information that of course drives most research that we undertake. To be aware of how we use this information is perhaps the key issue here. The notes contain a signal to me of an aspect of the care which I need to take note of; its primacy indicated by its situation at the beginning of the observation notes. The idea of experience and knowledge alluded to in the nurse's use of the term 'the practised eye' came to be one of the key aspects of care that differentiated nurses from each other. However, my noting of difference and positioning, as well as experience, does not surface unintentionally – it is loaded with desire. I am searching for such occurrences because of the post-structural theoretical perspectives and literature about nursing practice informing my research. But as is also evident, this was solicited by my inquiry as to why this nurse was doing this dressing. As Clough suggested it is difficult to explicate whose desire is surfacing here.[7] Why did I ask the question? Was I seeking to confirm something I had noted before? Why did the nurse answer in the way that she did?

There are other influences evident in this section of the record. Indeed, in the record it is apparent that I am observing the wound as well as the dressing process itself. I explain in the field notes about grafts and how the wound looks in that 'areas which were granulating, areas of graft which were in fact doubled up and needed radical trimming and cleaning up of serous ooze which had built up around some grafts'. But the question I ask of this record is, 'who is talking here'. Is it nurse, researcher or nurse–researcher? All through the field notes, I find instances of this blurring of boundaries in my positioning within the textual record. It seems that at times, I am positioning myself within the knowledge system of wound care 'science' and that my notes speak with this voice. At other times, the nurses position me as co-worker with 'special' information needs about the processes within the unit. In this observation record, the nurse assumes some form of knowledge, but when I ask her why she is actually doing the dressing she provides me with vital confirmation, not only about what the dressing entails but about an element of the nurses' work which would come to be pivotal in differentiating what was happening on the unit.

Moreover, in 'traditional' ethnography, there is a position for this nurse. She is a 'key' informant, someone who assists the ethnographer to mark out the significant parts of the research observations, as well as assist in discussion about these observations. These moments of insight are evident in the observational record by the way in which I privilege them at the beginning of the record, or highlight them by turning my record from a description of the observation into an interpretation of what I see and hear.

RESEARCHER ABSENCE: SILENCING BY THE RESEARCH

It is also evident from this observational record and the discussion afterwards that I actively change my own positioning. At times, my presence in the notes disappears. When and how this happens is the key to understanding the position of researcher.

> While she was cleaning the area with saline, forceps and fine scissors, the nurse took the opportunity to point out to the patient the sort of things that he needed to do to get going again. Susan: For example, because your hands have been grafted, you need to use your hands. One of the ways you can do this is to put the cream on yourself (this was the Nutra-D cream that is used to keep the grafted skin supple and moisturised). When you do this you will have to get used to opening the jar, and used to the feel of putting on the cream and having to reach behind to stretch your arms and shoulders. This will help to get your body used to moving again. You'll get used to how your new skin feels and to learn how much pressure it can take as well as what feels right and what doesn't. It's all part of getting used to the way things would feel like now . . . This will double up as good exercise for your hands and help to get the fine movement back in your fingers. Having to stretch to get to awkward areas will help in getting the movement back into your arms and shoulders. Gary: Yes I have started to do that a bit more. But it still hurts and

I don't really know what I can do. Susan: I know. But the longer you leave it, the longer it will take to get moving again. You might have to work against some of the pain. We can give you some lighter pain relief to help and each day will get easier because you will be able to move easier than the day before.

THE PARADOX OF RESEARCHER SILENCE

The notes relate the conversation in detail (only an excerpt is shown here), with the voices of the nurse and patient taking the main part of the notes. My presence is recorded only in my observation of what they were doing at the time they were having this conversation. Such absences can be identified throughout my observational field notes. This raises the question of how and why I disappear. My main aim in this research was to observe and analyse nurse–patient interactions during the processes of wound care, thus to intervene with my own observations or talk would be to prejudice this aspect of the research process. My silence is essential so that I can analyse, as an outsider, an interaction between nurse and patient. Evidenced within the observation is a nurse at work with a patient, seeking to have him understand his role in his recovery, but at the same time providing him with information about the recovery process and how the nursing staff can assist with this. I noted the talk in order to provide evidence of the textually mediated practice of nurses and patients; to explore the discursive framing of their talk as social practice to uncover the assumptions and taken-for-granted background to their work,[18] just as I am observing to see how this impacts on nursing practice.

But what of the post-structural researcher who would insist that the researcher, and their paradigmatic influence, is never absent? Well, it is evident I am not. Paradoxically, I am present in my absence, because this is a central focus of my research. I am present by the special position accorded to such interactions within my research notes; in the record of nurses discussing a particular patient's wound care, psychosocial needs, pain relief measures; in the detail of conversations between nurses and patients; in the detail of conversations I had with patients about the care provided for them. I am present in how I talk about the climate of the interaction, how I observe the reaction of the patient or nurses within the conversations, and in the questions I ask about the observation or in more formal interviews. The questions come from my research perspective and the focus that my observations came to take. I am apparent also in the focus on not so much what explicitly happened in each dressing but the noted differences, how each nurse approached the dressing, and what they and the patients said to each other and to me.

In informal discussion with this nurse, she picked up on the idea of experience and how this allowed her to provide the patient with examples of what could happen and how he could help himself. This nurse was able to identify, when we talked later, how she has changed her practices to take opportunities to talk with patients about their treatment, their progress and what they can do to help themselves – in effect, how she negotiates interaction with patients. Discussion based around the observational record also allowed the nurse to identify how her way of doing 'procedures' had changed over time and now took place in a way very different from when she had first worked in the unit.

Such discussion highlighted for me how, in working with each nurse, I needed to keep alert on how each nurse positioned me during the observation. Not all nurses were able to position me 'with' them. Some wanted me to be the distant observer, working hard to ignore my presence, others thought I needed information about the science of wound care, and others talked to me and to the patient, and positioned me in what I came to interpret as a privileged 'blurred' position. I came to view what happened to me during each dressing as an indicator of 'comfort' level with my presence, which some nurses came to terms with and others did not. Sometimes, the nurse putting me into the position of 'fly on the wall' became a part of the discussion of the observational record, and came to be a way of identifying their own comfort with their position of nurse practitioner. The effect of my presence showed, as Street has suggested, the problematic nature of visibility in nursing practice.[19]

Many of these nurses were still coming to terms with work on the unit, and when we talked about the dressing afterwards, they would often point out why they had not answered patient questions or had not taken this time to interact with the patient in other ways. Others, more comfortable with their work and with my presence, incorporated me into discussions, at different levels and in differing ways, viewing my needs as different from theirs and different from the patients. Such positioning is evident in the different way that the nurse talked to me and to the patient. In this way, it became apparent to me that nurses and patients who were being observed were actively positioning me, taking account of me. Such effects would imply that Hammersley's critique of ethnographic method has some substance. It would also suggest that desire 'to inform' is continuously problematic (see Bourdieu[15]), and to consider that informants are not 'present', or neutral, in the information they give is to deny the effects of research on 'the researched' and their lives.

PATIENT AND RESEARCHER PRESENCE: RESEARCHER AS IN BETWEEN

Indeed, these interpretations of the observed practices acted, for most nurses, as ways of focusing discussion we had that led to very fruitful insights for us. As I highlighted, the nurse was able to say how, when she read the observation, she wondered if she had not been too hard on the patient at that time. We talked about how difficult it is to choose the 'right' moment to provide some forms of information, and how difficult it was to motivate these patients. This next excerpt highlights what I specifically identify as 'different' in this observation.

> This was the first time that anyone had suggested this to the patient and in some ways he told me that he was taken aback by it. He said that part of not doing anything had come from not being sure as to what he could do and that no-one else had told him this.

On looking back through my field notes I confirmed that no other nurse had informed him of his part in his recovery, or had chosen the dressing time as an opportunity to do this. Many had asked him to wash himself; very few ever said why. But in talking with the patient about what was said, it was also a time for him to share some of the ways he was feeling at this particular time. Because each of the patients who agreed to participate in this study became the focus of my study at that time, each of them 'became' very used to my presence. They also often positioned me as confidante, always it seemed to me as 'nurse' someone they could talk to about what was happening and how they felt, and in some respects as someone outside of the care situation. I do not, however, wish to gloss this situation. Not all patients were as open, or told me everything, but they did position me as an outsider who had a different perspective from the nurses providing them with care.

This was a very difficult position for me to take, one circumscribed and inscribed with ethical dilemmas, which abound in such research. On the one hand, I was positioned as confidante (which may at times place me outside of the nursing position and with the patient), and conversely it was also apparent that patients were always aware that I was a nurse as well. Using my notes in this way opened up very different forms of discussion with patients and nurses, and made evident the different positions open to them in the situation. In talking about this observation, the patient told me of the context of his feelings at the time. He was lonely, homesick and depressed. He was worried about his wife and children and told me that he felt guilty about the way in which the accident had interfered with and endangered his life – a deeply 'personal' response. What became apparent to me from these talks with patients was that their talk signalled a 'resistant' positioning and discourse.[16, 20] Such talk gave me their positioning, and indeed how complex this was. The patient described a positioning of a 'life on hold', away from his familiar environment, at a moment when he was feeling 'down' and coming to terms with his part in his recovery. It is also obvious that his positioning is fragmented by the incident, by his responsibilities at home, by the uncertainties that surround the entire healing process.

In some ways I was privileged with both sides of the story. However, alerted to the idea of desire, I sometimes wondered whether patients confided in me so that I could act as a bridge. It was always possible that discussions about how they felt at that time were therapeutic in their outcomes. At other times, I believed that the patient used these discussions as interpretive bridges, in the belief that such information would inevitably get back to the nurses. But should I pass such information on? How would this position me, and was what we were talking about to remain in confidence between me and the patient?

CONCLUSION

This paper has outlined researcher/researched positioning evidenced within one observational record in research into nursing–patient interactions focused on one nursing procedure. What it exposes is how researcher positionings are not static, neither is the position of informant or participant. It also suggests that researching in the clinical context as a nurse means it is difficult to remove oneself from the research, even when nurses locate you as outside of the event. As author of such notes, it is important to recognise 'author' positions, as well as 'researched' positions, in the discursive framings of such notes. They not only indicate power relations within the text, but also the dynamics in the positionings by all participants in the research.[21] To deny effects of any one of these positions is to disavow the desire for mastery of the field evident when maintaining the 'outsider' researcher positioning of traditional ethnography.

While I recognise that this is but one record in a long study, I believe it does provide evidence of how a 'post' positioning challenges the myth of objectivity. Such analysis also renders problematic research that seeks to remove 'the nurse' from research within nursing. As this research focused on a single nursing procedure, much of the day-to-day work within the unit escaped analysis. As Marcus would suggest, in seeking a research focus and by (re)analysis of field notes it becomes evident how much of this record 'remains the surplus of difference beyond, and perhaps because of our circumscription' (p. 567).[17] Marcus warned that research will only provide a partial and partisan 'reality'. In troubling the transparency and congruence of these notes, I would position myself as one who wonders, not colonises; travels with 'the researched' rather than conquering the field; and recognises how we all have come to live with, not excavate, the field of nursing.

ACKNOWLEDGEMENTS

My thanks to the nurses who welcomed me into their working lives and allowed me to observe and talk with them about their practice, even during frantic moments. My thanks also to the patients who allowed me to observe and question them about their experiences during their time in the unit.

NOTES

* *Nursing Inquiry* 3 (3): 146–52. Reprinted with permission of Blackwell Science.

1 Said E. *Representations of the Intellectual*, London: Vintage, 1994.

2 Hammersley M. *What's Wrong with Ethnography: Methodological Explorations*. London: Routledge, 1992.

3 Simon R & Dippo D. On critical ethnographic work. *Anthropology and Educational Quarterly* 1986; 17: 195–202.

4 Carr W & Kemmis S. *Becoming Critical: Knowing through Action Research*. Victoria: Deakin University Press, 1986.

5 Geertz C. Making experience, authoring selves. In: Turner VW & Bruner EM (eds). *The Anthropology of Experience*. Urbana: University of Illinois, 1986.

6 Clifford J. *The Predicament of Culture*. Cambridge: Harvard University Press, 1988.

7 Clough PT. *The End(s) of Ethnography: From Realism to Social Criticism*. Newbury Park: Sage, 1992.

8 Van Maanen J. *Tales of the Field: On Writing Ethnography*. Chicago: University of Chicago Press, 1988.

9 Clifford J & Marcus GE (eds). *Writing Culture: The Poetics and Politics of Ethnography*. Berkeley: University of California Press, 1986.

10 Geertz C. *Local Knowledge: Further Essays in Interpretive Anthropology*. New York: Basic Books, 1983.

11 Pratt ML. Fieldwork in common places. In: Clifford J & Marcus GE (eds). *Writing Culture: The Poetics and Politics of Ethnography*. Berkeley: University of California Press, 1986.

12 Tyler S. Post-modern ethnography: From document of the occult to occult document. In: Clifford J & Marcus GE (eds). *Writing Culture: The Poetics and Politics of Ethnography*. Berkeley: University of California Press, 1986.

13 Gore J. What can we do for you? What *can* 'we' do for 'you'? Struggling over empowerment in critical feminist pedagogy. In: Luke C & Gore J (eds). *Feminism and Critical Pedagogy*. New York: Routledge, 1992.

14 Ellsworth E. Why doesn't this feel empowering? Working through the repressive myths of critical pedagogy. In: Luke C & Gore J (eds). *Feminism and Critical Pedagogy*. New York: Routledge, 1992.

15 Bourdieu P. *Outline of a Theory of Practice*. Cambridge: Cambridge University Press, 1977.

16 Cheek J & Rudge T. Webs of documentation: the discourse of case notes. *Australian Journal of Communication*, 1994; 21(2): 41–52.

17 Marcus GE. What comes (just) after 'Post'? The case of ethnography. In: Denzin NK & Lincoln YS (eds). *Qualitative Methods*. New York: Sage, 1994; 563–574.

18 Fairclough N. *Language and Power*. London: Longman, 1989.

19 Street AF. *Inside Nursing: A Critical Ethnography of Clinical Nursing Practice*. New York: State University of New York Press, 1992.

20 Buchbinder D. *Masculinities and Identities*. Melbourne: Melbourne University Press, 1994.

21 Bruni N. Reshaping ethnography: contemporary post-positivist possibilities. *Nursing Inquiry* 1995; 2: 44–52.

Chapter 9

Knowing the body and embodiment

Methodologies, discourses and nursing

JOCALYN LAWLER

Introduction

Jocalyn Lawler has become well known in nursing circles for her writing about the body. In her first book, *Behind the Screens, Somology and the Problem of the Body*, published in 1991, she made two key arguments. The first was that formal knowledge in our culture has not developed simply as a passive response to what there is to be known, but can be understood as being influenced by the social and psychological characteristics of the individuals in those sections of society that are mostly concerned with, and in control of, society's institutions of investigation and knowledge. In Europe and the West, certainly since the classical Greek era, which established many of our foundations of thought and culture, it has been men who have tended to occupy these positions, and of course most other positions of power and influence. A great many writers, Lawler among them, have argued that the Greeks, most notably the philosopher Plato, have presented the physical body (and the whole physical realm to some extent) as a, if not *the*, source of weakness and problems for humanity. This would be quite different from the more integrated way that the body is figured in, for example, the ancient Jewish texts of what has become the Old Testament. (Interestingly, Lawler does not mention the Hebrew sense of knowing as having sexual relations with someone in her review of definitions of the verb to know.)

Affluent Greek society, at least so we understand, was one in which slaves, many of whom were captives of war, and to some extent women, were expected to look after the practicalities of physical life, leaving men to rule and philosophise undistracted. The reason for this apparent refusal of men to identify with their embodied existence has never been established, and there are exceptions to it, but it can be seen as a strong force in much of subsequent Western philosophical and cultural development. It finds famous expression in seventeenth-century French philosopher Descartes' analytical distinction between mind and body, and his view of the mind and consciousness as centre and essence of personhood. This sharp, hierarchical distinction has come to be known as Cartesian dualism. Such dualism has been a powerful influence on the development of anatomical study of the body and medical knowledge which, to some extent, grew from such study.

Emotions, again possibly since Plato's influence, have become identified with the body, and understood as a source of problems, and consigned a subservient place to the mind.

Lawler's second argument in *Behind the Screens* was to do with the nature of nurses' involvement with the bodies and bodily products of their patients. Drawing on the insights of anthropologist Mary Douglas, she argued that the taboo nature of, for example, excrement and blood, has come to define the social standing and (in)visibility of nursing.

All of this is a long preamble to Lawler's present chapter, which is a more theoretical critique of contemporary discourses on, or ways of 'knowing' and talking about, the body and how some of these discourses operate and have been taken on by nurses, in ways that do not do justice to the complexity of nursing, its focus on personal relationships, or, ultimately, serve its best interests.

She argues first that, instead of a well-developed and integrated understanding of the lived experience of embodiment, we have inherited from male-shaped institutions of learning fragmented and detached collections of altogether unhelpful partial accounts of the body. This is particularly unhelpful for nurses, whose work, of course, is immersed in bodily awareness and concerns. What is even more regrettable, according to Lawler, is that nurses, out of a need for the social power and capital that goes with establishment and respect within intellectual institutions, have adopted generally conventional approaches when developing their own bodies of knowledge. In this chapter, she looks at two such systems of knowledge, first economic analyses of health care and second the 'objective' style of writing about disease and those people receiving medical or nursing care.

She argues that economic discourses have seduced nurses into attempts to formalise nursing care in a way which may be useful to finance managers and government economists, but which is inadequate, inappropriate and alienating for nurses themselves. Economic discourses, she argues, lie behind many quality assurance initiatives and drives to develop nursing diagnoses. Because these systems of knowledge have taken on ascendancy, nurses have become drawn to them in order to represent and argue for the importance of their own work. About the second, the valuing of scientific detachment in writing about health and illness, she suggests that because nursing is a practice in which relationships with the bodies of patients are always (hopefully) undertaken in the strong context of awareness of and feeling for the experiences of that body, any approach to knowledge in this context which ignores such an important awareness cannot but be anathema to good nursing. She gives examples of the way that the extreme distress associated with, for example, unwanted drug effects and medical mistakes, can never be anything but erased within these detached styles of writing.

Although some may disagree with her views, Lawler has opened up awareness and debate about the body in nursing, and articulated important issues with relevance for all nurses.

LAWLER, J. (1997)

Knowing the body and embodiment – methodologies, discourses and nursing*

INTRODUCTION

In this chapter I would like to consider the issue of how we, as relative newcomers to the formal academy, are being invited to formalise our knowing and researching of the body and embodiment within dominant discourses. It is my argument that our know-ing and our discourse(s) should both reflect and affect the manner of our practice as nurses. However, our recorded discourses and formalised knowing are more reflective of influences external to nursing than the practice of nursing as it might emerge from clinical practice settings.

The central question I want to explore here is this: how are we, as nurses, to know and understand the body and embodiment as researchable topics of fundamental importance to the discipline? I am taking it as self-evident that the body and embod-iment *are* central concerns of nursing.

The physical body is studied, in pieces, in a number of different disciplines, but embodiment has attracted much less attention. Where embodiment (the experience of the lived body) has been studied, it has been predominantly a topic for philosophy inquiry in which matters of the intellect and consciousness have been central. Embodiment in its more encompassing sense (beyond the intellect) has a history as a relatively silent and ignored matter, unlike the object body. There are two main reasons why this has been the case: first, dominant discourses of the modern period have sub-merged the subjective in the quest for objective and 'value free' (pure) knowledge; and second, the academy, which is powerfully masculinised, has found topics such as emo-tions and feelings to be troublesome (Lawler 1991a).

As we have moved more into the realm of the postmodern, which focuses (in part) on the human subject(ive), scholars in feminism, sociology, and nursing are looking more comprehensively at the embodied realm of human existence. They are looking beyond consciousness, thinking and rational thought, to explore hitherto margin-alised and moralised domains (see for example *Sexy Bodies*, Grosz & Probyn 1996, which emphasises the carnal experiences of feminism).

Nursing knowledge and much of its practice have been silenced and rendered rel-atively invisible because of 'the problem of the body' and this is a function of two things: first, knowledges of the body have been theoretically and epistemologically fragmented; and second, our cultures and way of life have rendered the body private and unspeakable (Lawler 1990, 1991b: 1–3). I want to re-visit and extend my earlier discussion of the problem of the body by focusing on the discourses and disciplinary practices that help sustain epistemological fragmentation, in particular the positivist discourses of science and economics. It will be my argument that, as discourses which take the stance of objectivity, they necessarily submerge the personal and subject(ive); and that, as disciplines which hinge on what is quantifiable, they make it difficult for us to formalise our knowing about embodiment and nursing. That aspect of the problem of the body, which relates to the private and taboo nature of nursing work, will not be discussed in any detail here.

My discussion draws on Foucault's notions of power/knowledge and 'games of truth' as they are embedded in, and mediated by, typifying practices within and among the formal disciplines in the academy. Games of truth were described by Foucault as 'an ensemble of rules for the production of the truth'; the resultant 'truth' itself is, therefore, a function of the rules and principles of its production and inseparable from the discourses employed to communicate it (see Foucault's interview with Fornet-Betancourt et al in *The Final Foucault* 1988).

The tensions which surround the question of how to articulate nursing's knowledges[1] of the body and embodiment (and other aspects of our discipline) centre on which games of truth will best render nursing known, knowable, and researchable. We have three identifiable means from which to choose and through which we have operated with varying degrees of success: (i) the biomedical sciences and scientific discourses generally, including the social sciences, which are all predominantly derived from the academy and sustained by it; (ii) economically driven discourses that pervade the market place and the state; and (iii) practising nursing and reflecting on it. The first two of these are positivistic, reductive, predictive and probabilistic; in that they are alike and indistinguishable. However, knowing derived from practising nursing and reflecting on it and from studies of the experience of illness and embodiment are emerging as narrative in form, irreducible, personalised, contextual, and meaningful only as a gestalt; these ways of knowing are not necessarily predictive or probabilistic.

While the discourses and disciplinary practices of the biomedical and social sciences offer nursing ways to articulate its knowledges, which are relatively useful and helpful, they are not entirely adequate. What economics offers nursing as a practice based discipline is less appealing and potentially damaging. What I want to focus on here is the tension between, and choices inherent in, articulating (or performing) our knowing in these different and differing ways.

SCIENTIFIC DISCOURSES, THE PROBLEM OF THE BODY, AND KNOWING IN NURSING

The 'traditional' sciences, which have their origins in the academy, pursue knowledge, often for its own sake; in this sense, the sciences and nursing are in sympathy with each other in so far as nursing seeks to validate itself by articulating a discrete body of knowledge. On other matters, predominantly methodologies and models of knowing, nursing and the sciences have less in common. Nursing knowledges, like many other knowledges, can be made to look familiar to those who are accustomed to positivist/scientific discourses. And we might also, perhaps, use their terminology and conceptual basis; in many respects, we already do, particularly in areas where we share common concerns, for example in areas such as anatomy, physiology, biochemistry and the workings of the material world. But turning nursing into look-alike scientific knowledge can be misleading and it can construct epistemic faslehoods that are to nursing's disadvantage.

Most particularly, we want to know about what takes place between the nurse and the patient as people who are often situated as captives together. The patient is captive in the dysfunctional and/or sick(ly) body or with an embodied problem[2] and the nurse is captive with the patient, often for hours or days on end, or until death occurs. As captives, their worlds are necessarily brought together and focused on more immediate concerns and on ways in which experiences can be endured and transcended. It is possible to understand some of these experiences, both for the patient and the nurse, within the conceptual and discursive space of captivity about which we know little except in so far as it relates to matters over which the state presides.

The practice of nursing relies on many different ways of knowing and many kinds of knowledge nursing knowledges. Consequently, the nature of nursing knowledges and emerging disciplinary practices mean that borrowings, while necessary, will not suffice for nursing because so much of what we know comes from both being a nurse and doing nursing; that is, nursing's knowledges are ontological (and felt), intellectual, performed and expressed. Therefore, we want and need to talk differently about some of the same things that concern disciplines with which we share those common concerns and whose methodologies and discourses we have borrowed and, at times, appropriated.

Knowing, scientific discourses, the body and embodiment

I would like to make some observations about the multiple meanings of the verb, to know, and its adjectival form, knowing, that we might consider in the light of how we want to know the body and embodiment in nursing. The verb, *to know*, is said to mean:

> 1 to perceive or understand as fact or truth, or apprehend with clearness and certainty . . . [or] 2. to have fixed in the mind or memory; *to know a poem by heart* . . . [or] 3. to be cognisant or aware of; to be acquainted with (a thing, place, person, etc.), as by sight, experience, or report . . . [or] 4. to understand from experience or attainment [e.g.] . . . how to make something . . . [or] 5. to be able to distinguish, as one from another . . . [or] 6. **not to know from Adam**, not to recognise (someone) . . . [or] 7. **know chalk from cheese**, to be able to note differences . . . [or] 8. **know the ropes** . . . to know the details or methods of any business or the like etc. (*The Macquarie Dictionary* 1991).

There are several observations that can be highlighted in these forms of knowing. First, the research community does not equally value these different forms; second, some ways to know are sensitive to context, experience(s) and the passage of time; third, some are inherently unstable and changeable[3] while others are more enduring and robust;[4] and fourth, some forms can be expressed in language and others cannot. However, those forms which can be encased in language are the most pervasive and, according to Foucault, the most powerful. Also, some forms of knowledge are affected by our memories, cognitive/intellectual activities (or decline), readings and research, and others change only in relation to life circumstances, periods of emotional turbulence, profound shocks, and examination of self and the meaning of life. Yet we live in a world that places relatively more value on forms of knowledge which can be externalised, verbalised, and often in nursing – proselytised, if not evangelised! As economic rationalism and late-stage capitalism manifest themselves in the so-called 'information' age, knowledge has also become a commodity to be commercialised and traded.

The adjectival form *knowing* takes on more subtle and socially constructed qualities than the verb *to know*, but again with a relatively dominant emphasis on the intellect. For example, *knowing* is said to mean:

> 1. shrewd, sharp, or astute; often affecting or suggesting shrewd or secret understanding of matters: *a knowing glance*. 2. having knowledge or information; intelligent; wise. 3. conscious; intentional; deliberate (*The Macquarie Dictionary* 1991).

We cannot talk of knowing and knowledge in isolation from *what* we know; nor can we ignore the social significance and political consequences of that knowing. I want to turn now to that issue and focus on the several questions: (i) what do we know about the body and embodiment?; (ii) how have we come to know them and render them knowable matters; (iii) how do we talk about them ?; (iv) what do we know that we do not or cannot admit to our formal discourses; and (v) what have we silenced?

If knowledge is both the source of power and inseparable from it and the discourses which mediate it (Foucault 1980), our knowledges of the body and embodiment are indeed powerful. However, our knowing has been, and continues to be, affected by regulation and control often through its transformation into dominant discourses which are recognised and respected in the academy but which are not necessarily inherently suited to nursing. In another context, I have argued that

> Academic traditions of western patriarchy create illusions about knowledge and ways to know which make nursing seem inherently untidy. Nursing is concerned with things, like feelings and emotions and the body, which the academy has difficulty in accommodating . . . [A]spects of the human condition which make people uncomfortable, but which are central concerns of nursing, are in danger of being marginalised and disenfranchised because the traditions of the academy operate to transform them into something less threatening to the established order.
>
> As a consequence of the dominant ideas of that established order in the academy, nursing has been presented with a kind of 'Sophie's choice' about the location of its knowledge and the methods which may be used to articulate and research that knowledge. Nurses have been asked to choose between the seeable and the feelable . . . [but we] must address both lived and material reality (Lawler 1991a: 13).

We have many more opportunities to formalise our knowing and teaching (see Brown & Seddon 1996) of the physical body as a biological and medical entity than we do as embodiment or the-person-in-the-body because the latter are inherently sub-jective. Typically, scientific discourse relies heavily on a form of objectivity which invites distance and detachment rather than engagement with the subjective – in effect excluding or minimising the potential effect(s) of the subjective. In this kind of knowing space, the body is the object of examination, inspection, and investigation as a physical thing like any other mechanical and biophysical machine whose malfunctions are identified and corrected. Running repairs and replacements are the order of things – much like a motor vehicle – as long as you can get the replacement parts or fix the original ones, you can keep the machine going. If we, as nurses, want and need to know the human body in this way, and we do in some respects, how are we to relate our knowledge of it to others and what will be the manner of our discourse?

If nursing evolves its disciplinary practices and discourses for knowing of the body in terms which typify the natural and biomedical sciences, the body will be anony-mous, de-personalised, passive, and, inevitably, reduced to the sum of its malfunctioning parts and related remedies. Furthermore, embodiment will not feature at all. Those are the inescapable consequences because the methodologies and dis-courses of these sciences would invite us and, seemingly, demand of us that we research and record our knowledge of the physical body in this way (see Parker & Gardner 1992).

To illustrate my point, I will turn to a report on events which are, in some respects, medical mistakes but which are reported, in Australia, as adverse drug reactions (Adverse Drug Reactions Advisory Committee 1994:2–3). I am referring to the gel, Dinoprostone (Prostin E2 Vaginal Gel) which was recently approved ' . . . for induc-tion of labour in pregnant women at or near term who have favourable induction features and who have a singleton pregnancy with a vertex presentation' (p. 2). The report continues:

> 10 October 1993 . . . [the Committee] had received 5 reports of suspected uterine reactions associated with dinoprostone. Four of these reports described uterine perforation, which in 2 women, led to hysterectomy. In at least 2 of these cases, dinoprostone was not used in accordance with the approved indications.
>
> In one case uterine rupture occurred about 2 hours after application of the gel whereas in other case it occurred more than 24 hours later. In a third case, although no uterine hypertonia was detected clinically, fetal bradycardia and persistent transverse lie (contraindicated) necessitated laparotomy. It was then found that uterine rupture had occurred intrapartum and the baby was lying within the mother's abdomen. In the fourth case, dinoprostone was administered twice to a woman who had a previous delivery by Caesarean section (contraindicated). Abdominal pain and fetal bradycardia led to an emergency Caesarean section with delivery of a stillborn baby and the obser-vation that the uterine scar had ruptured. In a further report, although there was no uterine rupture, the patient experienced 4 hours of myometrial

hypercontractility and hypertonus after the application of the gel (Adverse Drug Reactions Advisory Committee 1994:2).

There are many aspects of this report which invite critique and comment. However, I want to highlight the way in which these events are related to us – the readers and potential knowers about 'adverse drug reactions'. First, and most obviously, this is a relatively typical report of the scientific/medical findings, albeit in the context of 'adverse drug reactions'. Second, the discourse is typically scientific, it is objective, precise, descriptive, and informative. Third, the narrative appears in third person passive prose – we know only that this is a story of 'adverse' events involving women in an advance state of pregnancy. We do not know anything else about them; they have no personas and no distinguishing features except for the particular bodily arrangements of two of the women which constitute contraindications. These are not women in the more complete sense of the word; rather, they are cases of women's pregnant bodies and the bodies of babies, one of which is dead.

The manner of the reporting speaks to the scientific community and in that sense, it is unremarkable. Another reading of this report of 'adverse drug reactions' raises the question: in what way does the discourse of this report differentiate these women from cases involving any other large mammal – a sheep, a cow, a horse? If we want to know the body as a physical and physiological entity, are we, as nurses, also obliged to articulate our knowledge impersonally, objectively, dispassionately, and with detachment? What are the consequences if we do, and what are the consequences if we do not? Is there a space between these two epistemological and discursive worlds?

It is reasonable to assume that the experience of myometrial hypercontractility and hypertonus is both painful and distressing, but the manner of the reporting does not allow for the ontological features of these conditions to be discussed because the subjective is silenced. We read nothing of the pain, distress and suffering of these women because the reported events are contextualised not around the women, but the drug. If there is such little space for the subject(ive) in the scientised knowledge/discourse of biomedicine, what, if any space does it allow for the subject(ive) in practice?

The most remarkable aspect of this report, however, is that the gel is constituted as the causal agent, and not the person or persons who prescribed it. And it is safe to assume, in these cases, that self-medication is not an issue. If we read this report with a view to the properties of narrative (see Polkinghorne 1988) we are invited by the manner of the discourse in the report to ascribe agentivity to the gel, leaving silent the matter of who prescribed and/or administered it.

However, if we take Kenneth Burke's view, we would read this story differently; he argued that 'well-formed stories . . . are composed of a pentad of an actor [or actors], an action, a goal, a scene, and an instrument – plus trouble' (Kenneth Burke 1945 cited in Bruner 1990:50). So, if we read about these 'adverse drug reactions' from the perspective of Burke's description of a good story, we would re-cast the gel not as the agent, but as the instrument. Who then, we might ask, is the actor? If we view the discourse of this report from a narrative frame of reference, we render the objectivity of scientific discourse problematic for disciplines such as nursing, which are concerned with human experience, embodiment and intersubjective interaction.

It is not my argument that biomedicine is inherently unconcerned with the human condition; rather, it is to propose that the manner of a typifying and dominant discourse is reflective of typifying and dominant practice. In the case of medical practice, allegiance to the rational-scientific model, with its emphasis on practising on the physical, object(ive) world, has led to dehumanising trends when applied to the object(ive) body of the patient – a pattern of medical care that some of their own profession have criticised (see, for example, Kleinman 1988, Moore 1991, Little 1995). Kleinman has argued, for example, that ' . . . a medical or scientific perspective . . . doesn't help us to deal with the problem of suffering' (1988:28). It would be possible to re-read Kleinman's statement to mean that these perspectives do not deal with embodiment; nor does the discourse of biomedicine allow for it as a mainstream concern. The same can be said of the discourse of economics in so far as it is being used to structure misleading language and thinking about nursing practice(s), which I will address later in this chapter.

Scientific reporting, the person(al), and third person passive prose

Scientific discourse does not allow the person to enter the story, except in the passive voice and, consequently, it does not allow for embodiment or the non-material world. In that sense, therefore, scientific methodologies, in so far as they are inseparable from the discourses which typify them, are inadequate for nursing; they may allow us to know the body, but not in a way which provides space for an understanding of embodiment – and I argue that we cannot have one without the other (Lawler 1991b). Scientific discourse is inadequate for nursing's understanding of the body as a physical thing because we do not have the ideological, practical, philosophical or epistemological liberty to stand apart and distant from it; nursing is also concerned with the embodied other as a human being and that concern is interactive, contextual and intersubjective.

Put another way, if nursing is a form of practice in which the object and experienced body are integrated in the context of particular patients and their nursing care (Lawler 1991b), such matters cannot adequately be conveyed in the discourse typical of scientific reporting. Not only does a scientific perspective, unlike nursing, place primary emphasis on the physical body and the physical (non-experiential) world generally, it is conducted in third person passive prose; and this form of prose reflects the assumption that, in science, objectivity is a necessary condition for good research.

Another example from the literature highlights the same problem of scientific/medical methodologies and discourses as they apply in psychiatry, which is, presumably, a little closer to the person and a little more resistant to distancing discourse. The case report, which I use to illustrate this point concerns a young Ethiopian woman who became anorexic following a period of imprisonment and torture (Fahy et al 1988). The report tells us that she is 22 years old, 157 centimetres tall and that, at the time of admission, she weighed 39 kilograms. Her history included vomiting, which began at the age of 16 when she was imprisoned, interrogated and tortured about the involvement of her father and brother in political activities. She was imprisoned for six months, during which time her father was executed and she was subjected to beatings and 'on one occasion, a blood-stained rag was stuffed into her mouth to prevent her screaming' (p. 385). After this event, she had 'vomited blood-streaked material and when she attempted to eat, vomited repeatedly. She said that at the time, eating had reminded her of the rag in her mouth' (p. 385).

The report continues to detail her medical, psychiatric and life histories which included: weight loss, 'abnormal eating and vomiting'; work with refugees; qualifying as a pharmacist; and her migration to the UK where she came to the attention of the group who eventually reported her case in the literature. The report contains a brief section called 'investigations' in which we are told that 'on physical examination, extensive scarring was found across both her breasts. There were scars on her elbows and dorsal surfaces of the feet from previous lash-injuries'. She had a number of other investigations of her gastrointestinal system, a CAT scan of her head, and a psychometric assessment including an assessment of her attitudes to eating.[5] All were within normal limits. We are then told relatively more about her mental state and progress, that she was placed on an antidepressant medication, and that there was 'a nursing regime of a kind formulated for patients with anorexia nervosa, but in this case beginning with a liquid diet' (pp. 385–6).

While not wanting to take this report out of context – because it is principally concerned with reporting an unusual and atypical aetiology for anorexia nervosa – the manner of the reporting is such that perforce, the woman's story is objectified and so is she. Allowing for the complexities of body/self interplays in anorexia nervosa and the authors' attention to details relevant to her social being, the reading which these authors – all men (in so far as one can tell from given names) – make of her condition and progress is taken predominantly from the physical body. We learn little about what meanings the woman makes of her experiences, diagnosis, situation or embodied being. The report reads as if the discourse of scientific/psychiatric reporting takes priority over the embodied experiences and subjective meanings which the woman herself might relate.

This is not a situation isolated to the scientific and medical communities, but one which is also apparent in the discourses which appear in some nursing literature. Such literature demonstrates the tensions between the customs of scientific and 'academic' reporting, which have been adopted to a greater or lesser extent in nursing, and in matters in which the subject(ive) is central. This tension is most apparent in situations where third person passive prose is used to relate knowing in which the subjective experience of the other is the central theme. The mismatch between the chosen discourse for reporting and the subject matter it concerns often sounds quaint, if not superficial or artificial and possibly patronising. The central problem is quite simple: the phenomenon under investigation is subjective experience relating to us in objective prose.

I have taken an example from *Nursing Science Quarterly* (Coward 1990) to demonstrate my point. This example illustrates the limitations of third person passive prose and the problems of 'objective' reporting for some ways of knowing in nursing. The report is titled, 'The lived experience of the self-transcendence in women with advanced breast cancer'. It was an exploratory study, the purpose of which was to describe women's experiences of self-transcendence, that is, reaching out beyond oneself. We are told in the article that:

> The research was planned and conducted using the phenomenological research method as described by Colaizzi (1978). The first step was for *the researcher* to examine *her* presuppositions about the topic to be investigated. In *her* experience with seriously ill patients, *she* had been puzzled by the considerable variation in the manner people faced illness [emphasis added] (Coward 1990:163).

We can ask: who is this anonymous person called 'the researcher'?; what is her intention – as a phenomenological researcher – in entering into the meaning world of the other?; is this how she wanted to tell this story or did she feel obliged, compelled or required to tell her story of this research from the detached viewpoint of the third person?' is this what she has been taught about the 'proper' way to represent herself as a researcher?; or was this the only way she could tell the story and get her work published?[6] These are not trivial questions; rather, they are fundamental issues about how we want to articulate and represent our practice and how we want to build our discourse and disciplinary practices in nursing.

When we, as nurses, use ourselves as the therapeutic agent in an interactive and person-to-person sense, scientific discourse is unavailable to us to articulate such matters publicly and formally; we – the practitioners – are relatively silent, silenced, and invisible. Third person passive prose creates distance, removes reference to the personal and subjective, and disallows the articulation of matters at the core of nursing practice. And that does not begin to address those aspects of nursing practice that cannot be framed in words, formalised, or encapsulated in *any* form of discourse because they are felt, perceived, experienced and known in an embodied and shared way.[7] However, while the discourses of biomedical and social sciences do not accommodate embodied and felt knowledge formally, they are recognised and acknowledged, albeit informally, peripherally, and inadequately. In economic discourse such recognition is usually absent.

Economic discourse, nursing, and the embodied other

I want to focus here on the impact on nursing of economically derived and economically driven discourses and disciplinary practices. Economic discourses, because they do not account for embodiment and personal meaning making, with which the experience of health and illness are centrally concerned, are inadequate[8] for, and detrimental to, the evolution of discourses for nursing practice. Also, as positivist approaches,[9] they are methodologically inadequate for studying embodiment and nursing. Economic discourses and methodologies have distracted and misled us, and worse – have seduced us into formalising our knowing of the physical body and nursing care in a form which is more meaningful and useful to economists and managers than it is to practising nurses, scholars and researchers. Our knowledge of embodiment and our dealings with the person-in-the-body, however, cannot find an authentic and authenticable space in economic discourse and games of truth; that is another compelling reason to reject them as inadequate and inappropriate for nursing.

In the last three decades, the discourses, concerns and disciplinary practices of economics – especially economic rationalism – have gradually but progressively invaded our everyday social and working lives, language, daily news reports, media commentary and politicians' addresses on 'the state of the nation'. Some have argued that economic rationalism, in the western world in particular, has taken priority over political and social order – a trend unaccompanied by serious debate about its consequences (see Cordery 1995). Nursing and health care, like other public sector institutions, have been affected and, in some respects, transformed by economic rationalist philosophies, policies and practice(s) – also without much debate or sustained criticism.

In the contexts of the practice setting where the financial and resource management of clinical services is a major issue, nursing has virtually no viable alternative, in the current climate, than to adopt paradigms and discourses of market economics as the dominant means with which to articulate nursing matters when there is a need to communicate to non-nurses about resource issues. This is an economic imperative; without the means to speak about nursing in the language of economics, nursing is vulnerable to erosion and to relative impoverishment in the provision of nursing services.

Being able to communicate about nursing in economic discourse, however, does not guarantee protection from the erosion of nursing services both in numerical and other ways. In some respects it may contribute to erosion, especially if there is no acceptance of the extent to which aspects of nursing cannot be reduced to, or rendered meaningful as, entities that can be measured for productivity, cost effectiveness and efficiency. The question of value (and cost) in this context is operationalised in its monetary sense; the more generic and socially constructed notion of value is irrelevant in economic discourses, though it has a token presence in the rhetoric of 'quality care', 'best practice' and the like.

Problems of economic discourse and games of truth for nursing

At their most fundamental level, the purposes and intentions of economic games of truth and economically derived discourses are not the articulation of clinical matters so that we might better understand the practice of nursing. Rather, they are designed for cost control, the allocation of resources and the relatively arbitrary, but allegedly objective, business of assigning monetary values to factors which are constitutive of economic understandings of health care systems and their resource utilisation. Economically derived discourses, which pervade public discussion at the political level, also have been adopted and inculcated into the language and texts of nursing, most particularly those which originate in the USA. Such texts, however, are typically devoid of critiques which would problematise these trends and issues, and they show little sensitivity to the relevance of these writings in other countries or cultures (see Lawler 1991c). Rather, they tend to promote, 'sell', or more seriously, evangelise a particular viewpoint or way of thinking – and they are well placed to do that, given the extent to which works published in the USA saturate the international nursing literature.

It is one thing for us to borrow concepts, discourses and research methodologies to try out in nursing, or to respond pragmatically to a prevailing economic climate; it is another thing entirely to be subjected to the imposition of the discourses and methodologies of market economics on nursing which is, in many respects, concerned with matters that are embodied, interpersonal, socially constructed, human, and shared. Economically derived discourses, which underlie nursing process, nursing diagnoses, casemix, DRGs and much of the current thinking on quality in health care and outcome standards, are much more troublesome for nursing than are the biomedical and social sciences, for a number of reasons.

First, economic discourse invites us to adopt the language, concepts and methodologies of the market place to reflect matters which are clinical and practical; as a result, the practice of nursing is articulated within an imposed discourse which is not derived from the doing of nursing but from the perspective of measurement-for-the-sake-of-costing or outcome assessment. Nursing per se is not, therefore, articulated in a form inherently suited to it as a practice discipline, but in a discourse that reflects economic constructs and games of truth.

Second, within economic discourse and methodologies, nursing is at a particularly high risk because economics, like other disciplines which rely on positivist methodologies, leaves no space for many of the subtleties of nursing. Rather, important aspects of nursing practice, like aspects of the body and embodiment (see Lawler 1991b), are constituted by their absence and silence, or by a form of words that diminishes them. A good example of how nursing is diminished in this way can be found in Reeve's (1993) report, *Coherent & Consistent Quality Assurance & Utilisation Review Activities in Public and Private Hospitals in Australia*, in which he claims that:

> Casemix and Quality in nursing care will require careful overview of the costing process. Casemix will impact on the cost of nursing services. Sensitivity must be exercised as to the level at which this occurs. **It would not be difficult to eliminate the vital, personal elements of the art of nursing care. If costed too tightly, such a move could reduce the amount of time the nurse would have to just pass the time with a patient, a component of nursing that has been traditional and special to the profession. This would be a serious negative result for the Casemix programme which is designed to be a positive initiative. The matters need close attention. To overlook it would have serious consequences for the Quality of Care** (original emphasis) (Reeve 1993:46).

Reeve's report illustrates how we may not be able to speak of nursing in the language which is understood, or about things which are valued, by those who currently set the economic and political agenda (see Lawler 1993). What Reeve calls ' . . . just pass[ing] time with a patient' is understood and articulated differently by nurses. Taylor's 1990, 1994) work on ordinariness and the interpersonal qualities in nursing and Marck's (1990) work on therapeutic reciprocity are two particularly relevant examples of how we, as nurses, understand 'pass[ing] the time' as interactive, contextual, richly grounded in knowing the other and intended for therapeutic effect. Nurses make known their knowledge of these subtle and sophisticated matters using words and language which do not diminish either the acts or actors themselves as they are related to us.

The third reason why economic discourse is troublesome for nursing is that the main agenda for economics is the aggregation of data which leaves little space for the individual and individual experience. This is a sad irony for nursing, given the extent of our investment in promoting individualised care as a central tenet of nursing and about which so much has been written and spoken. Much of the discourse about 'individualised' care, however, has been filtered through nursing process rhetoric which is, in itself, an inherently positivistic and economically driven construct and which does not allow for embodiment or lived experience more generally (Lawler 1991b, 1991c).

Fourth, economic discourses and practices do not benefit from the humbling and sobering realities that people in clinical practice understand. Economists' knowing, like that of the general scientific community, is a rather more impersonal affair, at least in so far as it is committed to the published record.

Effects of economic discourse on nursing practice

The methodologies which stem from economics, and economic rationalist philosophies in particular, emphasise efficiency and cost effectiveness in so far as they can be made meaningful as functions of positivist, cause-and-effect, outcome oriented models. Consequently, what counts as data are decontextualised indicators by which efficiency and effectiveness can be assessed within the games of truth that typify economics. Cordery (1995) has been very critical of this approach, arguing that within economic rationalist methodologies

> [t]he rich and non reducible aspects of organised socioeconomic life – the things from which one develops a sense of identity and meaningful existence – are marginalised. This is a great irony for economic philosophy and theory, particularly when one considers the extent to which the social sciences generally – economics excepted – have moved into the postmodernist era and recognised the limitations of positivist understandings of social order (p. 357)

In Foucault's terms (1988), the games of truth within economic rationalist methodology are self-contained, circular, and apparently self-serving – and they are distinctly and powerfully modern at a time when other disciplines move to postmodern ways of knowing. In the language and methodologies of the economists and accountants, the non-quantifiable aspects of nursing, or those qualities of practice which cannot readily be measured and factored into output-oriented formulae, are particularly vulnerable. In part, this is due to what van Manen (1990:113) called *epistemological silence*, that is, 'the kind of silence we are confronted with when we face the unspeakable'.

Epistemological silence has several forms, but the form of interest to nursing, in relation to the games of truth within economics, concerns the manner in which some things are sensitive to the discourse in which they are related. This sensitivity can be illustrated by using the concept of love, which is problematic for behavioural science methodologies and discourse, but not for the discursive forms used in poetry, music and the fine arts (van Manen 1990:114–115). The same could be said of the different discursive forms employed to describe what nurses do when they talk with patients. In the economic discourse which Reeve (1993) uses, nurses' talk with patients is constituted as 'just pass[ing] the time with the patient'; but grounded in a nursing discourse, such talk becomes the rich and valuable concepts of therapeutic reciprocity (Marck 1990), ordinariness (Taylor 1990, 1994), making ordinary (Parker & Gardner 1992) and creating an environment of permission (Lawler 1991b), among other things which are yet to be articulated. Not surprisingly, these works by nurses were all conducted within interpretive paradigms and discourses and their data are in narrative form.

What nurses talk with patients about includes a wide range of apparently normal, and highly 'abnormal' subject matter which, in its own right, is worthy of serious investigation (see, for example, Bottorff & Varcoe 1995). However, the interactive and interpersonal qualities of talk(ing) itself help to transform extraordinary situations in which patients are vulnerable, uncertain, and fearful, into states which can be endured, transcended, survived, or from which it is possible to recover; such states usually centre around the dysfunctions and disfigurements of the physical body and distresses of human embodiment, fear of death, disease or the person's ability to endure suffering. These are not topics about which one 'just pass[es] the time of day' as though it is small talk of no great consequence beyond sociability.

The discourse and methodologies of economics have had a dramatic, but underrecognised, impact on nursing. Coming as they did after a period of sustained pressure to scientise nursing knowledge, economically driven constructs of nursing which are themselves based on the fundamentals of scientific methodology are just another indication of attempts to authenticate nursing within a basically patriarchal world. I have crtiticised this trend previously, arguing that

> [t]he academic discourse on the discipline [of nursing], which is dominated by the USA, has reflected a growing emphasis on the perceived 'need' to develop and scientise nursing knowledge. We have been encouraged – extolled even – by most of the North Americans and their Australian followers to embrace positivist scientific models, and with them reduction, objectification, quantification and taxonomic and linear thinking. We have been encouraged to see scientific knowledge and scientific nursing practices as universal and highly desirable features of the discipline – indeed some have gone so far as to argue that it is only through traditionally scientific methods that we can develop the knowledge base and standing (that is, the status) of the discipline. While much of nursing practice can be studied by quantification, measurement and positivist inquiry, individual patient perspectives and perceptions are also important, especially if we are committed to patient-centred care.

> But within positivist approaches patients' experiences of illness can become peripheral or unresearchable. Although nursing has, of necessity, accommodated more technologically and scientifically oriented health care, it has also retained a concern for the care and comfort of patients but, in the academic literature, this commitment has taken on some ideological, rhetorical and philosophical qualities as notions of 'scientific' nursing have tended to override non-quantifiable elements in nursing (Lawler 1991c: 214)

Dunlop's (1986) critique of how the quest to scientise the concept of caring is a classic example of how science – for the sake of science itself – has contributed to thinking and lines of argument that cannot be sustained in nursing; they are nonsensical and philosophically and epistemologically incoherent. Furthermore, attempting to scientise nursing, ipso facto, risks a potentially damaging transformation of concerns central to nursing. In the short term, and perhaps more importantly, scientising nursing can create the impression – however erroneously and unintended – either that there is little of substance in nursing practice or that nursing is another scientific approach to health care. Not all of nursing or human responses to, or experiences of, illness and health care can be explained with reference to positivist models of knowing nor within scientific or economic discourse; rather, we also look to storytelling, narrative knowing, aesthetics and personal meaning making as ways in which our worlds and practice can speak to us and for us.

The 'new' nursing language, embodiment and the body

Economically motivated demands to demonstrate nursing's effect on patient care are apparent not only in more global constructs such as the nursing process and nursing diagnosis but also in the language that accompanies them. This language is not an authentic nursing discourse but an economically derived dialect that reflects the influence of economic games of truth on nursing.

The term, 'highly dependency nursing', for example, is one of the earliest terms which is inherently economic; it derives originally from measurement of the level of nursing time required for particular categories of patients whose physical body – and what needs to be done to it by nurses – are the sources from which temporally defined demands originate. The term does not speak to particular nursing practices nor a substantive area of our knowledge base, necessarily, but to the notion of quantifiable time as it can be measured in minutes. In practice, however, high dependency nursing has come to mean a number of things to nurses and we have developed some shared sense of what a high dependency unit or patient is; the problem is that we have not yet found a more epistemologically or ontologically authentic term to replace it and, in doing so, liberate us from the language of time-and-money.

However, nursing diagnoses provide the best example not only of the imposition of economic discourse and language on nursing but also the false assumptions about the utility, for nursing, of inclusive, logico-linear and output-oriented models. Without entering into the debates about their questionable ethicality (Mitchell 1991), cultural insensitivity and North American bias (Lawler 1991c), lack of clinical support

(Dennison & Keeling 1989), and restrictive, narrow focus (Mitchell & Santopinto 1988), there are questions about their validity and conceptual clarity (Jenny 1987). More importantly, there are questions about what they exclude and silence, and whom they oppress. One particularly curious example of this pressure to 'diagnose' patients' nursing needs is the (unofficial) nursing diagnosis of 'acopia'[10] that has evolved in at least one Australian hospital. This 'condition' is manifested in a variety of ways, all of which are indicative of normal human responses to suffering and distress but which cannot be addressed within the (economically determined) resources of the nursing staff. In the context of nursing diagnoses, normality is pathologised and rendered 'a problem', in a way reminiscent of psychology's attempts to deal with coping behaviour (see Wortmann & Silver 1989). An 'acopic' patient (or relative) is often one who requires emotional support or whose lived body experience is the source of most angst.

Advocates of nursing diagnosis themselves admit that 'the implementation of nursing diagnosis in the clinical area continues to produce resistance, duplication and frustration . . . [but that] since the early 1980s, [it has] been used with increasing frequency and consistency in periodicals, textbooks, and nursing care plans' (Vincent & Coler 1990). There is, as yet, no evidence that the advent of nursing diagnosis is improving care, facilitating the work of clinicians or in any way enhancing the articulation of nursing knowledge. Rather, we are witnessing a re-run of the pattern that typified the introduction of the nursing process, which has itself been a spectacular failure when assessed against its own alleged benefits. Not only are these economically generated notions alien to practitioners, but they are also imposed, usually by the same people who write the texts and promote the use of clear plans to which Vincent and Coler (1990) refer. In terms of the more global picture, the imposition of nursing diagnosis configures the research-practice nexus 'arsy-versy' (Lawler 1991c). As a consequence, nursing, as it might emerge from clinical practice, is silenced and marginalised, and issues of central importance to patients, such as how they might interpret what is happening to them, are not afforded a space.

One of the major areas of silence is embodiment – and there are some clear and quite straightforward explanations for that. The most obvious reason is that the concept of nursing diagnosis is derived from within a biomedical and traditional scientific-reductive paradigm where the focus is the physical world, including the physical body, and on what can be observed and measured; it is also a model of rational knowledge, which necessarily excludes non-cognitive-intellectual ways of knowing. There is no real problem here, for nursing, in so far as the physical body and its biophysical malfunctions and remedies are concerned, because nursing is inescapably concerned, among other things, with the physical body and its malfunctions.

However, the biophysical model does not and cannot claim to account for aspects of practice which are contextually dependent or which have their origins within the person-in-the-body and his or her embodied experiences of illness, disease and health care. These are limitations that are not acknowledged by advocates of nursing diagnostics or health economists as important indicators of care of quality of nursing.

The real danger of nursing diagnosis lies in the false premise that it is an inclusive and comprehensive taxonomy, which potentially can account for nursing; such a proposition is untenable and excessive. For example, in their argument to introduce a unified diagnostic model for nursing, Vincent and Coler (1990) construct their case for integrating NANDA and ANA taxonomies, in part, with very selective reference to what happens in biology. What they fail to take into account is that taxonomies in biology are based on anatomy and anatomical differences, that is, physical difference. Unlike nursing, biological taxonomies do not attempt to include experiential or socially mediated phenomena. On that basis also, nursing diagnoses are manifestly inadequate as a comprehensive and inclusive taxonomic system.

Not surprisingly, the most controversial and problematic areas for developers of nursing diagnoses are those beyond biomedical parameters and the physical body, that is, the area of human responses to illness. There is a voluminous and compelling literature on the limitations of traditional scientific models for understanding humans and social life – literature that seems to have been ignored by those who continue to concoct and promote nursing diagnostics, interventions, and therapeutics.

More alarming, perhaps, is the use of the language of nursing diagnostics system as metaphors for nursing itself. The term 'nursing interventions', for example, is rapidly becoming a metaphor for nursing care, and consequently, nursing is in danger of being reduced (in terms both of its valuableness and in relation to methodology) to the sum of its repertoire of 'interventions'. There are several issues to be considered in this context: first, not all nursing can be captured in terms of interventions; and second, sometimes the best 'intervention' is not to intervene. On a more general level, speaking of nursing in the language of intervention is to suggest that nursing is inherently about intervening; whereas nursing is also about watching, waiting, and allowing nature to take its course. Nursing is about working with naturally occurring processes and is fundamentally a form of non-invasive practice. The term, 'interventions' is not a naturally derived notion in relation to nursing. Stripped of the things that nurses do at the behest of medicine or because of medical intervention, there is very little about nursing that is either invasive or interventionist.

Like other manifestations of economic rationalism in action, the games of truth of nursing diagnosis are self-contained, circular, and apparently self-serving. More importantly, they disempower and silence people on whom the games of truth are visited; this is reflected in Mitchell's (1991) argument that 'the diagnostic process encourages a professional arrogance which for some nurses is oppressive, restrictive and discomforting'. However, if one takes on nursing diagnostics, it is a 'package deal' along with managed care and other economically derived concepts about efficiency and effectiveness, which seemingly leaves nothing to chance. The package consists of the diagnosis itself to which interventions are assigned and measured as 'outcomes' – and all this is situated in the context of what is believed to be the province of care in which nursing is the accountable profession.

Nursing, however, is an inherently untidy discipline which has to straddle a very wide range of paradigms, knowledges, problems and daily contingencies and demands (Lawler 1991c); it is not, therefore, amenable to inclusive models in which everything is neat and tidy. There is another problem which is rather difficult to pin down, and that is a direct result of the games of truth which nursing diagnosis employs. The problem created by the game goes like this: if the phenomena of concern to nursing are those things which can be framed in nursing diagnoses, and if the nurse is accountable only for those things which lie within the phenomena of concern to nursing, then where does that leave those aspects of nursing practice which cannot be reflected in this non-inclusive, but allegedly inclusive, model.

How does nursing address those things which do not lend themselves to logico-linear, positivistic, rational, outcome-oriented, causal models; where does that leave meaning making, storytelling, embodiment and the embodied self – and where does that leave the patients' perspective? Taking the rhetoric and discourse of nursing diagnostics at face value, such matters must, by default, lie outside the domain of nursing as they define it. Such a proposition is a nonsense and it is dangerous.

SILENCING DISCOURSES, GAMES OF TRUTH AND THE EMERGENCE OF NURSING'S VOICE

There are aspects of the ambience and environment in which nursing takes place, which can profoundly affect patient care, but which cannot be factored into out-come-driven economic formulae; nor can they be framed in economic or scientific discourses; nor can they be disaggregated to display patient care cost at the level of the individual. There is research evidence (for example, Shields 1978, Lawler 1994) that patients take great comfort from the perceived availability of the nurse. Availability is a perceived and intangible phenomenon that relates not only to the physical availability of the nurse, but also an emotional, personal, existential availability in which patients sense that the nurse is there for them – as the embodied and vulnerable 'other' who needs protection, reassurance and support. These are things that lie outside the discourse and modalities through which economic understandings are formalised.

Likewise, availability is not a concept which can be reflected in, or talked about, as an 'intervention' in the discourse of nursing diagnostics; nor would a hypothetical nursing diagnosis 'potential to need the availability of a nurse' have much credibility because such availability is implicit in the generic provision of a nursing service. Perceiving the availability of the nurse as an embodied and interpreted sense of safety and comfort that the patient experiences; it is not necessarily a rational event but an emotional response to felt states such as fear and vulnerability. Availability, in its felt sense, does not and cannot feature in economic or scientific models of nursing.

Evidence is also emerging that the dominant discursive form about clinical nursing matters, e.g. for verbal reports, is predominantly storytelling (Parker, Gardner & Wiltshire 1992). Furthermore, there are games of truth in reporting nursing which not only silence nursing but preserve the power of medicine to pronounce various bio-physical events; that nurses also know how to pronounce is taken for granted, but silenced (Parker & Gardner 1992).

When we reflect on how we are to read and research nursing and draw some pre-liminary conclusions about how to read the physical body, lived body, the embodied self, experiences of illness and embodiment in nursing, we are left with some clear options. At the very least, we have a need to understand biophysical and biological events that affect the physical body and to do so in their discourses of origin — without that form of knowing and communication we would lose our points of anchorage with other aspects of health care. Because we also practise with living, breathing, speaking, social humans, we have a need to operate with reference to the humanities and the social sciences and to be able to speak their languages, without which we lose our points of anchorage to forms of knowing that focus on being human and embodied. Because we are schooled within western traditions, we have a need to face our ignorance of other ways of knowing and experiencing life, death, suffering and healing.

And because we are fundamentally a practice discipline and have a need to speak within, from and to the practice of nursing, we have a need to give voice to our own business. In that sense, much of nurses' business is like a women's business — it is taken for granted, it is storied, it is grounded in experiential knowing, and it has been silenced in a patriarchal world. We cannot render the body and embodiment researchable for nursing within borrowed methodologies, but we can — and have a need to — share in those knowledges in order to practise. We also have a need to see the limitations of what we borrow, or have imposed on us, and to explore ways of knowing — and ways to transmit that knowing to others — so that we reflect nursing and not nursing-through-the-words-of-others.

It is my argument that the discourses of the sciences and economics, while they have shaped and continue to shape the way we talk and think about nursing, have silenced important and central concerns for nursing. Furthermore, these influences and their games of truth cannot account for nursing. The knowledges of nursing itself are to be found in practising nursing, reflecting on it, and coming to understand ways of being which inhere in the relationships between nurse, patient and contexts in which nursing occurs. Inevitably, these knowledges will be grounded in, and will, to a large extent, need to be understood as, complex gestalts, which are temporally, environmentally and ontologically sensitive. They also will be narratives, and they will allow for expressive and meaningful engagement and contact among humans, in both physical and interpersonal senses.

NOTES

The Body in Nursing: a collection of views. Edinburgh, Churchill Livingstone. Chapter 4. Reprinted with permission of Churchill Livingstone.

1 I use the term in the plural to heighten our understandings of the multiplicities of nursing's ways of knowing. To refer to knowledge in its singular sense is to erroneously suggest that knowledge is some kind of homogenous stuff.

2 This is often the case in mental health nursing; although the problem is non-physical in the sense that we understand illnesses of the object body, many of the issues that concern people with mental illnesses are embodied, for example, feeling depressed and unable to get out of bed and face the day. Self-mutilation and self-abuse are also examples of ways in which the embodied self is caught up with states that we call mental illness.

3 A good example is knowledge about early mobility in the case of serious illness(es); within decades, nursing and medical practices have altered dramatically as concepts about the relative merits of mobility and immobility have been challenged and changed.

4 The most robust knowledge is that which is borne primarily of experience and practising, but which has, necessarily, a cognitive component. For example, one's knowledge of riding a bicycle or making a bed does not deteriorate with age; one's physical prowess, speed, and ability to perform may deteriorate, but the knowledge embedded in performed knowing may not.
5 The authors state, however, that the validity of the Eating Attitude Tests are of 'limited relevance' because their validity for Africans is uncertain.
6 Like many of my colleagues, I have been instructed by reviewers to remove the personal pronoun from research reports and I am sure I am not alone in this experience.
7 Nurses often report that there are events of experiences that they cannot describe in words; this is not to say they are inarticulate, but to indicate the limitations of language as a means of communicating about some events of experiences.
8 Not only is economic discourse inadequate for much of what nursing involves, it is also inappropriate in many circumstances.
9 I would draw a distinction here between some of the discourses of the social sciences, particularly sociology and some aspects of psychology, in which there are attempts to write in the subjective. The dominant theme within these disciplines, however, remains scientific/positivistic and reductive.
10 This term literally means not coping.

REFERENCES

Adverse Drug Reactions Advisory Committee 1994 Australian Adverse Drug Reactions Bulletin 13(1):2–3
Bottorff J L, Varcoe C 1995 Transitions to nurse-patient interactions: a qualitative ethology. Qualitative Health Research, 5(3):315–313
Brown C, Seddon J 1996 Nurses, doctors and the body of the patient: medical dominance revisited. Nursing Inquiry 3(1):30–35
Bruner J 1990 Acts of meaning. Harvard University Press, Cambridge, Mass.
Cordery C 1995 Doing more with less: nursing and the politics of economic rationalism in the 1990s. In: Gray G, Pratt R Issues in Australasian nursing 4. Churchill Livingstone, Melbourne, 355–374
Coward D D 1990 The lived experience of self-transcendence in women with advanced breast cancer. Nursing Science Quarterly 3(4): 162–69
Dennison P D, Keeling A W 1989 Clinical support for eliminating the nursing diagnosis of knowledge deficit. Image: Journal of Nursing Scholarship 21(3): 142–144
Dunlop M J 1986 Is a science of caring possible? Journal of Advanced Nursing, 11:661–670
Fahy T A, Robinson P H, Russell G F M, Sheinman B 1988 Anorexia nervosa following torture in a young African woman. British Journal of Psychiatry 153:385–387
Foucault M 1980 Michel Foucault; power/knowledge: selected interviews and other writings, 1972–1977. Harvester Press, Brighton
Foucault M 1988 The ethic of care for the self as a practice of freedom. An interview with Michel Foucault. In: Bernauer J, Rasmussen D (eds) The final Foucault. MIT Press, Cambridge, Mass
Grosz E, Probyn E 1996 Sexy bodies: the strange carnalities of feminism. Routledge, London
Jenny J L 1987 Knowledge deficit: not a nursing diagnosis. Image: Journal of Nursing Scholarship 19(4):184–185
Kleinman A 1988 The illness narratives. Suffering, healing and the human condition. Basic Books, New York
Lawler J 1990 The body, dirty work and nursing: toward understanding the invisibility of

nursing care. Proceedings of XII Annual Conference of the Royal College of Nursing, Australia, Sydney, 216–229

Lawler J 1991a What you see is not always what you get: seeing, feeling and researching nursing. Proceedings of Nursing research: pro-active vs reactive, Centre for Nursing Research & Royal College of Nursing, Australia, Adelaide, 13–21

Lawler J 1991b Behind the screens: nursing, somology, and the problem of the body, Churchill Livingstone, Melbourne

Lawler J 1991c In search of an Australian identity. In: Gray G, Pratt R (eds) Towards a discipline of nursing. Churchill Livingstone, Melbourne, 211–227

Lawler J 1993 Researching nursing: minding our language and finding our way(s). Proceedings of Research in nursing: turning points, Centre for Nursing Research, Adelaide, 1–11

Lawler J 1994 A study of adult patients' expectations of nurses and the nursing service: some surprises and issues. Proceedings of the Institute of Nurse Administrators of NSW and ACT Conference, Sydney

Little M 1995 Humane medicine, Cambridge University Press, London

Marck P 1990 Therapeutic reciprocity: a caring phenomenon. Advances in Nursing Science 131):49–59

Mitchell G J 1991 Nursing diagnosis: an ethical analysis. Image: Journal of Nursing Scholarship 23(2):99–103

Mitchell G J, Santopinto M 1988 An alternative to nursing diagnosis. The Canadian Nurse, 84(10):25–28

Moore T 1991 Cry of the damaged man. Picador, Sydney

Parker J, Gardner G 1992 The silence and the silencing of the nurse's voice: a reading of patient progress notes. Australian Journal of Advanced Nursing 9(2):39

Parker, J, Gardner, G, Wiltshire, J 1992 Handover: the collective narrative of nursing practice. Australian Journal of Advanced Nursing 9(3):31–37

Polkinghorne D E 1988 Narrative knowing and the human sciences. State University of New York Press, New York

Reeve T 1993 Coherent & consistent quality assurance & utilisation review activities in public and private hospitals in Australia. Casemix Development Programme, Canberra

Shields D 1978 Nursing care in labour and patient satisfaction: a descriptive study. Journal of Advanced Nursing 3:535–550

Taylor B J 1990 Conservation of natural resources: save ordinariness in nursing. Proceedings of XII Annual Conference of the Royal College of Nursing, Australia, Sydney, 230–249

Taylor B J 1994 Being human. Churchill Livingstone, Melbourne

The Macquarie Dictionary 1991 Macquarie University, Sydney

Van Manen 1990 Researching lived experience, State University of New York, New York

Vincent K G, Coler M S 1990 A unified nursing diagnostic model. Image: Journal of Nursing Scholarship 22(2):93–95

Wortmann C B, Silver R C 1989 The myths of coping with loss. Journal of Consulting and Clinical Psychology 57(3):349–357.

Chapter 10

Feminism, relativism and the philosophy of science

An overview

DAVID G. ALLEN

Introduction

Anyone who has ever questioned whether research involves anything more subtle than defining a problem, designing an instrument to investigate it, aiming the instrument in approximately the right direction and reading off the results will quickly realise that they face a bewildering array of unanticipated problems.

A perhaps conventional view of research is that we arrive at the most trustworthy knowledge by escaping, in our inquiry, the dangerous limitations of our individuality – our personal beliefs and 'biases', the tricks that impressions can play on us, the limitations of a partial view or too strong a commitment to a political position. The best way of avoiding this fundamental danger is to establish formalised procedures that any investigator following in our footsteps can copy and, in a sense, validate. Once these problems have been overcome, so the argument goes, we can all apprehend the world around them, or phenomena, or facts, uninfluenced by our own individuality or the social group to which we belong. This possibility means that knowledge produced in this way can claim an authority of an entirely different character from that claimed by individuals or institutions by virtue of their political power or force.

This view, as many readers will well know, has come under considerable attack in the last four decades. Many groups have asked whether the supposedly objective practices of scientific research really are politically and socially neutral, and have claimed that in effect they represent and promote, either consciously or – importantly – unconsciously, the values and views of the groups from which the practitioners of science have tended to come. Some involved in this attack differentiate *social* sciences from, for example, physical sciences, arguing that the crucial fact of investigating human affairs opens possibilities for covert political work to be done via the practices of science, and that it is simply not possible to study human activity in the same way that we might study plants or molecules. A powerful part of their argument would be that conventional science draws a boundary around knowledge, or fact, that can easily exclude the explanations or voices of those humans under study. It is interesting to note that when August Comte, founder of what he called the 'queen of the sciences', sociology, proposed an ordering of society, based on the findings of this new science, the proposed rulers were none other than sociologists, presumably because of their special access to the knowledge needed to organise members of that society.

The suggestion that class or other social characteristics can unconsciously influence the way that individuals understand the world and their place in it has been developed by Marxists, particularly French philosopher Louis Althusser whom Allen refers to in this chapter. The notion of 'ideology' or false consciousness cuts across the idea that we can simply observe the world in any neutral or entirely trustworthy way. Marx has come to be considered one of the modern 'masters of suspicion'.

As Allen notes, the key argumentative turn is that, if conventional knowledge practices can be understood as techniques of oppression, then the possibility is opened up for other practices that explicitly set out to counter such hidden oppression. These alternative approaches to the generation of knowledge go under many names, one being emancipatory research. Feminist researchers, for example, have gathered a range of compelling evidence for the implication of science in the operation of patriarchy, and have undertaken whole programmes of research aimed to counter such forces. This, if it is not already obvious, is where its relevance and appeal to nurses thinking about research lies, because the debate between these approaches to research has been played out within the area of health and illness issues. Some feel that research approximating conventional approaches to knowledge and inquiry has largely ignored or undervalued the views and experiences not only of the sick, but, many nurses argue, of nurses themselves.

The problem is that, once we abandon a belief in the possibility of objective knowledge of the world and in the reliability of procedure alone to invest our findings with authority, we enter a world where any research finding can be dismissed as simply reflecting the position of those who have carried out or commissioned the research. As Allen asks, 'how does one argue that one's own science is preferable to another form of science without lapsing back into authoritarianism?' He tackles this by looking at two issues; the problem of what counts as research *evidence*, and how we should make judgements about *explanations* for phenomena. Allen does not offer simple procedures to ensure a correct approach to either of these issues, but is more concerned that researchers are not naïve about the social conditions within which the beliefs of those we might be researching, for example, arise. He suggests, in passing, that some interpretative traditions, such as phenomenological approaches, tend to this naïvety. Some readers may well wish to take issue with this.

Allen's chapter is a good, relatively easy introduction to these debates and offers some interesting additional reading for those who wish to pursue these issues further. As he says, his suggestions are best viewed as ideas to strive for rather than prerequisites for research. Nurses who wish to turn away from conventional approaches to research knowledge will need to thoroughly understand the implications if they are to counter the challenges they are bound to receive along the way.

ALLEN, D.G. (1992)

Feminism, relativism and the philosophy of science: an overview*

INTRODUCTION

This chapter introduces some key issues in the feminist philosophy of science and attempts to increase our understanding of what a body of research based on feminist philosophy would look like.

Those of us committed to generating knowledge supportive of and consistent with emancipatory communities often find ourselves in a quandary; deeply skeptical of any claim to 'authoritative' knowledge, we often lapse into various forms of relativism. Not wanting to claim too much for our research, we claim too little. While it is important not to overgeneralise the relevance of our work for fear of its colonialist potential, we tend to implicitly accept a view that marginalises our work by leaving it either at a descriptive level or by believing its implications are limited to the context in which the study was actually conducted.

Relativism is not an option for feminists, however. Feminists and their supporters do not believe that feminism is just an *alternative* to racism, sexism, or classism (Harding, 1986; Fonow & Cook, 1991). It is *preferable*. But how does one argue that one's own science is preferable to another form of science without lapsing back into authoritarianism? Here, I will sketch out two themes that are keys to answering this question: first, what kind of scientific argument is necessary to simultaneously promote knowledge generation and protect against its oppressive potential (as well as to protect against its spread (Allen, Allman, & Powers, 1991)). A second, related theme has to do with the idea of 'explanation.' One reason so much feminist research has remained descriptive is the well-grounded fear of substituting the 'researcher's' explanation for that of the persons being researched. Women and people of color have a long, terrible history of having their explanations supplanted by those of white, male scientists. A 1990 study by Rushton that asserted African Americans are more susceptible to AIDS because of a genetic predisposition to impulsive and aggressive behavior is only the most recent in a long line of such racist scientific enterprises (Rushton, 1989; Leslie, 1989). An equally long history of medical science providing biological explanations for women's inferiority has its current permutations in left-right brain attributions (Bleier, 1986).

The various feminist critiques of science have at their core a rejection of perceived relationships between patriarchy and science (Harding, 1986; Keller, 1985). There has also been increased concern with the interaction of dominant models of science and racist and class-based oppression (Fonow & Cook, 1991). Because current critiques have demonstrated how supposedly neutral or universalising claims are shaped by the social position of scientists (among other aspects), these former 'truths' have been 'relativised.'

These critiques have raised the question of what models of science can be created or adopted to avoid oppressive relationships. But as Harding and others have noted, the critique of the theory and practices of science from feminist and critical perspectives is far more developed than any elaboration of an alternative view of science. That we are clearer about what not to do than how we should proceed shouldn't be surprising or alarming. Contemporary philosophy of science emphasises the social conditions within which scientific practices arise (Bernstein, 1983; Rorty, 1979; Benhabib, 1986). Unfortunately, few communities that have internalised the values and visions of feminism and critical theory have also generated much science. We will not know what a fully emancipatory science looks like until we have a fully emancipatory community.

This is not to suggest that we should abandon our efforts to criticise and reform science to concentrate primarily on issues of broader social justice. For one thing, the role of science in sustaining social injustices is too significant to ignore. In all likelihood, the same people who are articulating the critique of science are also addressing, in their own situations, other institutionalised practices of injustice.

What I will explore there, then, are two key issues in identifying a 'preferable' science. First, there is the question of evidence or grounds or reasons: given that we have two competing theories or truth claims, what *kind* of evidence or reasoning should we use. The supposedly neutral contents of observation are no longer unproblematic (although we certainly don't want to abandon observational data). I will argue that we cannot rely upon any single or unique set of criteria or kinds of evidence – including the beliefs of oppressed people. Instead, we can only secure our arguments by understanding the social conditions in which they are debated. In this regard, the critical and feminist perspectives on *process* and *communication* are central to the establishment of an emancipatory science (Fay, 1987; Benhabib, 1987; Fraser, 1989; Lather, 1991).

Second, there is the problem of explanation: what is involved in explaining how or why something occurred. The current emergence of interpretive traditions, especially the more phenomenological perspectives such as grounded theory, in my view, simply beg this question. On what grounds do we prefer the interpretations and explanations of one group versus those of another? Under what conditions do we trust more the *explanatory* accounts of the mentally ill individual to those of the neurobehaviorist? The shaman to the oncologist? The woman to the psychiatrist? The political commitment of feminism and the belief in its preferability as a perspective do not allow us to escape these choices. However, in addressing *explanation*, I hope merely to highlight some of the issues underlying these alternatives just mentioned and how they might influence the construction of research programs.

The importance of the issues of evidence and explanation for feminist politics can be highlighted through a brief discussion of the problem of ideology. Other terms used to refer to this same notion are: *false consciousness, internalised sexism, self-defeating discourse,* or *denial* (Althusser, 1971; Sumner, 1979; Coward, 1985; Lichtman, 1982; Benhabib & Cornell, 1987). These are all current formulations concerning why 'native' accounts are not necessarily preferable. Ideologies, we must remember, are not just sets of alternative belief systems. Some belief systems (e.g., those that value women or people of color as fully human) are, from our perspective, preferable to those that do not. The history of the term *ideology* (and its successors) embodies a notion of critique: ideologies (e.g., sociobiological notions of sexism or racism) are systematic misrepresentations or distortions (Thompson, 1984). They may be and often are fully and heartily believed and endorsed by their adherents, who need not be supposed to be acting on any conscious (or even unconscious?) bad faith. One can sincerely believe in racism even if that belief is not warranted. One can sincerely believe one is cured or is recovering, even when one is facing imminent death. One can honestly believe, as a woman, that one is genetically inferior and ought not embrace the rigors and stresses of public life.

Yet the phenomenological traditions and their adherents — as they emerge in nursing — limit us to simply describing belief systems (Lennon, 1990). The most sophisticated adherents, for example, can identify contradictions between beliefs or beliefs and actions, but, at the same time, they are relatively mute on the question of preferability or of systematic delusion. Thus, for both scientific and political reasons, we need a view of the explanation of racism and sexism that prefers Reverend Martin Luther King to Judge Clarence Thomas — Audre Lorde to Margaret Thatcher.

PROCESS CRITERIA FOR ESTABLISHING PREFERABILITY

The history of science should not be abstracted from the history of political emancipation (Harding, 1986; Forester, 1985; Foucault, 1979, 1980). The rise of modern science was part of a complex reaction to state imperialism and religious authoritarianism. The Protestant reformation that stressed individuals could read holy texts and establish their own relationships with the divine, the emergence of a merchant class as a model of social mobility, and the development of science as a form of discourse that could be used and assented to by any human being were all emancipatory projects. Like most such projects, however, they were gradually transformed into ideological straitjackets for later generations. The shattering of centralised religious authority and the social disruption of industrialisation led to a model of extreme individualism, an abstract, single person without history and community. Science developed its own priesthood to interpret the divine texts of nature to the unenlightened.

Scientific discourse and activity is a subset of broader, cultural discourse. Most philosophers since Kuhn have admitted that there is an interaction between cultural discourse and scientific discourse (Bernstein, 1983; Rorty, 1979, 1989). Harding, for instance, identifies a salient feature here which characterises much talk about science as ideological: science wants to submit every activity to causal analysis except its own! On the other hand, one can talk about the social basis for the emergence of varying forms of scientific discourse as well as the effects of these discourses on broader social practices.

The reason I introduce this perhaps obvious point is to raise the issue of rationality. Rationality, in its broadest sense, refers to arguments which are recognised as being something other than mere personal opinion or the employment of force. What characterises this difference is, of course, the heart of the matter. One factor which distorts our understanding of the preferability of feminist science is the extent to which a certain form of scientific rationality has been accepted as rationality per se. Even the term *rationality* is suspect for a feminist audience because it has been equated with specific Europatriarchal models of discourse (Bowles & Klein, 1983; Nicholson, 1989; Sayers, 1987). Feminist critiques want to acknowledge the role of emotion, for example, in rationality. One reason that scientific rationality failed to dominate European cultures to the extent that it did American discourse concerns the irrationality of fascism, which was a product of the best science of its age. The sociobiologic arguments of Darwin and his cousin Galton led directly to the ideas of racial purification. Since we manage to fight most of our wars on other people's soil, we are experientially less familiar with the horrors of these forms of scientific rationality – although during the Persian gulf war, only extreme censorship prevented it from entering the consciousness of white American. Indians who had suffered genocide in America through the virtual extermination of tribal cultures or those who suffered the perfectly rational, if nightmarish, science of the Tuskegee experiments or those who suffered imprisonment without trial and forfeiture of property for suspected Japanese ancestry during World War II find it less strange and often share feminists' suspicion of scientific rationality.

I believe that Habermas's view of democratic communicative situations and the feminist views of process can be combined to offer a model of social conditions under which truly alternative models of science can emerge and thrive – at least in Western, industrialised societies (Habermas, 1984; Fraser, 1987, 1989; Benhabib, 1986; Fay, 1987; Alford, 1985; Balbus, 1984; Love, 1991; Spivak, 1985).

In this regard, there are two sorts of communicative situations I must address. First, there is the commonplace, in which a group/community gathers to discuss issues within the contexts of relatively stable and taken-for-granted normative backgrounds. Such communicative situations might be viewed as nonrevolutionary interactions in which the social, political, and normative relationships among participants are not of primary focus. Those involved share enough common ground, perspectives, and values that the conversation can concentrate on resolving the issue and can be primarily directed away from the participants and towards the topic at hand.

Under these, most common, situations, Habermas (1984) proposes that rationality is approached through pursuit of two ideal conditions: autonomy and responsibility. Rationality refers to the confidence one can have in the outcome of the conversation. Consequently, it is not an 'all or nothing' quality. The ideal conditions of autonomy and responsibility are probably rarely if ever fully achieved. Instead, autonomy and responsibility are 'regulative ideals' towards which we constantly strive. *Autonomy*, which refers to the ability and willingness to participate openly in the conversation, requires being sufficiently self-reflective to understand one's own values, interests, needs, and inhibitions and to take them into account when interacting. *Responsibility* refers to ensuring that all participants can function autonomously by attending to group dynamics, knowledge imbalances, power differences, and so forth. Feminists have elaborated on these notions to emphasise two aspects ignored or neglected by Habermas: the *relationships*, the connectedness among participants, and the role of *emotion and intuition* understood not as threats to, but as supportive of, group rationality (Gilligan, 1889; Chinn & Wheeler, 1985; French, 1986).

Thus, when modified through the feminist insights, Habermas's notions of autonomy and responsibility are clarified and augmented to reflect the social and relational basis of communication. Autonomy is best supported in contexts within which one feels valued and loved. Responsibility requires attending to affective dimensions of interactions and to the intuitively appreciated patterns of connection and strain.

The notions of consensus and coalition are also important here; responsibility and autonomy require the balancing of separateness, difference, and connection. The more problematic this balance, the more conversations will lean toward more radical versions in which horizons are being reforged across communicatively achieved, rather than normatively secured, values. That is, the more difference there is among the values and experiences of group members, the more they will have to focus their attention on achieving a mutual understanding of individual perspectives. Value clarification must precede value negotiation. The focus will have to be first on the participants' worldviews, then on the topic at hand.

The above, then, is analogous to the distinction between Kuhn's notions of 'normal' and 'revolutionary' science (Kuhn, 1970). In normal science, conversations occur within a context of shared and taken-for-granted assumptions that allow discourse to proceed with a minimal level of self-reflection on the rules of discourse themselves. In revolutionary periods, however, the rules of logic, evidence, and normative assumptions come into dispute.[1] Feminist empiricists can often overturn sexist and racist science within the rules of normal empirical discourse; biased sampling, unclear variables, and faulty logic were among the errors in sociobiological science as critiqued by Ruth Bleier (1986).

For those who reject the empiricist paradigm, an increasingly important theme concerns the idea of 'situatedness' (Haraway, 1988; Hekman, 1990). Sometimes viewed as a form of relativism, situatedness might be better understood as one moment within the formation of discursive communities. Rather than assuming the voice of 'neutral authority' that ignores the social position of the author, 'situated discourse' locates the speaker, specifying the personal, social, and cultural perspective of the author. In the absence of interpersonal conversation, this process of situating oneself might be understood as the opening gambit in an interaction. Locating oneself permits other participants to appraise how much of a horizon of beliefs, values, and experiences they share with the author or speaker (Pratt, 1984). The more divergent the horizon of author and reader, the more 'wary' the reader is of conclusions offered; were the context interpersonal, more time and energy would be required to focus on communicatively achieved norms. It is important to emphasise that, like autonomy and responsibility, the notion of 'situating oneself' is an ideal. One can never stand apart from one's position in order to describe it: the description of one's location is itself the product of a situated consciousness. Thus, the dialogical interpretation of situatedness maintains a vital openness to challenging and revising descriptions of the social 'location' of participants.

The emphasis on situatedness reflects a historical shift away from a homogeneous set of speakers (who assumed their audience was equally homogeneous and shared their horizons). This is a product of (1) the increasing diversity of speakers (e.g., we have a more varied set of authors); (2) the awareness that the authors are not nearly diverse enough and can't be taken as unproblematically 'representative'; and (3) especially, that the results of their conversation (monologue?) are often 'applied' to individuals who were not involved in the original conversation at all.

For example, throughout the 1950s and 1960s, one could reasonably assume that the authors of scientific medical arguments were white, European males from fairly privileged social class positions. The 'results' of their science were argued and assessed within a context of similar perspectives but often 'applied' to groups (e.g., women or people of color) who were quite different and were not at all involved in the discussions of the merit of the work (Leavitt, 1984; Navarro, 1976; Waitzkin, 1983). Currently, diversification of scientific persons to include increasing numbers of women and people of color has shifted the conversation to the meta- or revolutionary level discussed above, in which the rules of discourse, of who gets to speak and under what conditions, are an important focus. Thus, academic discourse on feminist critiques of science arose. Similarly, these and others who had previously experienced the effects of having science applied to them, without full participation in its formation and review, increasingly questioned the 'universality' of its premises and conclusions.

From this perspective, situatedness is not an implicit claim to relativity (i.e., that my work would be duplicated by and could only apply to persons exactly like me and the individuals I studied). Rather, it is part of a conversation that would include an *appraisal* of both the degree to which author, readers, and consumers shared a horizon and of whether any lack of overlap would influence its acceptability.[2] In other words, situatedness is an empirical and dialogical *question*, not a conclusion. It needs to be assessed, weighed, and discussed.

The more divergent the speakers (author, reader, or consumer), the more radical the nature of the communicative situation. As Benhabib points out these radical 'discourses arise when the intersubjectivity of ethical life is *endangered*; but the very project of discursive argumentation presupposes the ongoing validity of a *reconciled* intersubjectivity' (in Rasmussen, 1990). In other words, the ideal communicative situation posited by Habermas and augmented by feminism assumes a commitment to securing intersubjective agreement through autonomy and responsibility. But in conditions of extreme difference or distrust, the premises for such discourse may not exist. This is precisely the situation in the Middle East peace conferences between Israeli and Palestinian groups; the current goal is to establish the ability and willingness to talk. This may be a precondition or a consequence of discussions of any particular topic, such as water rights or territorial control.

How do these themes address the problem of relativism? Science is inextricably linked to communities. Research must be viewed as an *argument*, as part of a dialogue within the community. Since the communities are often geographically dispersed, communication most often is through written and not interpersonal discourse. But within most Western contexts, rationality can only be assessed within the context of the communicative situation within which the dispute arose. Thus, we need to attend to the political institutions which support the community of scientists to maximise the ability for all citizens to participate therein and, by their participation, to pursue the ideals of autonomy and responsibility (Lather, 1991; Lash, 1990). One moment in this process is the requirement to 'situate' oneself, that is, to understand the position from which one speaks and to communicate that to one's audience. This permits an audience to appraise the extent to which they might expect to share a general perspective or alerts them to sources of possible divergence.

The call for critically informed action research by Thompson (1991), Lather (1991), and others is part of this same emphasis. If research, both as process and as reported, is conceived as an argument or dialogue, then it is critical that the participants include the people being researched. This involves more than simply calling them participants or coinvestigators; insofar as possible, they should be integrated into the conceptualisation, design, execution, analysis, and reporting. Nor does this imply that results need be based upon a consensus or that the subjects' accounts are uncritically privileged, but that the process and reporting of the research reflect the different voices within the project.

Consequently, faced with competing claims, the most trustworthy are those which emerge from contexts which most closely resemble those described above. Of course, such conditions are precisely those envisioned by feminists as keys to a more just Western world.

Yet, even within the communicative situation as described above, how does one decide which explanations of human activity are preferable to others?

EXPLANATION

While it is both safe and laudatory to document women's voices through various forms of phenomenological and hermeneutic inquiry (Levesque-Lopoman, 1988; Deegan & Hill, 1987), it is scientifically and politically more problematic to study *why* women say what they do. Immediately, certain specters rise from the mist: biological reductionism in which women are reduced to their reproductive organs; the nature/nurture controversy; and professional and patriarchal elitism that all too readily substitutes its understanding for women's own (Martin, 1987; Suleiman, 1986). Explanatory studies are necessary, however, to understand how to restructure social institutions so as not to reinforce or merely reframe current injustices (Thompson, 1984; Giddens, 1987; Bernstein, 1983).

Particularly apt is Anthony Giddens's theory of structuration – a theory I have used to explore the question of explanation individually and with students. Giddens (1987) offers a theory of what a comprehensive explanation would have to include. Because the theory provides a perspective on the relationship between individual action and social structures, it is especially helpful in determining the character of a comprehensive explanation. In addition, Giddens's theory permits an integration of biological information into the explanatory process, an integration which many social theories avoid or simply refuse to consider.

Further, Giddens has the advantage of familiarity with both European and British-American philosophies of science. Consequently, he endeavors to integrate disparate traditions such as Heideggerian hermeneutics, critical theory, and realist models of explanation. Since a full explanation of Giddens's model and current criticism of it are beyond the scope of this chapter, I will highlight some of its theoretical features I have found most helpful.

Three components of Giddens's model

Giddens argues that a comprehensive explanation must include three dimensions: action (what the people being studied believe they are doing and why they are doing it), unintended consequences of action (consequences that 'escaped' the knowledge of goals of the people [agents]), and unacknowledged conditions (resources that made the action possible but were not acknowledged in the actors' accounts). A terminological note is in order – I am using *people*, *agents* and *actors* as synonymous terms that presuppose linguistically competent human beings.

Action

Explanation must *begin* with an account of what the actors are doing from their own perspective (Winch, 1958; Hookway & Pettit, 1978; Little, 1991; Lennon, 1990). This involves both description and explanation. For example, describing action differentiates between walking to work, sight-seeing, or exercising to burn off calories or to reduce stress. Although the description often implies an explanation, this is not always the case. For example, the explanation of walking to work may be 'because it's Monday and I'm due there by 8:00 A.M.' or 'I'm trying to reduce pollution and save money.' Research strategies can include grounded theory or hermeneutic approaches (Roth, 1987; Madison, 1988).

Beginning with action from the actors' perspective is an asset from a critical perspective. First, it grants intelligence and agency to the people being studied; second, it makes more difficult an uncritical substitution or imposition of the researcher's explanation (Lather, 1991); third, it introduces the level of everyday activity that often provides the mediating process between 'macro' level explanations, such as gender, race, or class, and individual behavior without reducing people to passive 'effects' of social structure.

The study of action may involve several components. *Rationalisation of action* refers to the agents' abilities to provide a 'rationale' or a discursive account of what they are doing and why. *Reflexivity and monitoring of action* refers to the moment-to-moment, often subconscious, adjustment of individual behavior required to achieve a goal; for example, the motor reflexes and environmental scanning involved in walking down a sidewalk or in driving a car. Similarly, there are those adjustments that cannot be reduced to a set of discrete decisions and actions; for example, the internalised, field-dependent judgments studied by Pat Benner (Benner & Wrubel, 1989; Benner, 1985) and others. *Motivation of action* refers to the fact that action is goal directed; one is trying to keep a job and save money, lose weight, or avoid health problems. Motivation, however, need not be conscious; being socially acceptable, avoiding unpleasant feelings, and pleasing an internalised parent are all goals that may shape our behavior whether or not we recognise them consciously.

Unintentional Consequences of Action

Action, by definition, is intentional; almost all human behavior of interest (with the limited exception of purely reflexive feedback systems) is guided by goals or purposes. However, limited understanding, knowledge, and reflection result in our actions having consequences beyond our awareness or intention. I flip on a light switch intentionally to illuminate a room. My flipping on a light switch may also scare off a potential burglar or overload an electrical system and cause power outages. In another sense, I may be intending to hire only the 'best qualified' candidate for a job but unintentionally discriminate against people of color or women. In response to such situations, our legal system makes radical distinctions between intentionality and unintentionality; for example, intentionally or unintentionally causing injury or death to others. The writing of history also comes to mind here. While history used to be written as the intentional outcomes of great men or, in the case of nursing history, of great women, increasingly it is being viewed as the unintentional consequences of much smaller and less global actions.

The notion of unintentional consequences helps account for certain forms of oppression without having to postulate or rely on more problematic 'conspiracy theories.' For example, a researcher or reader needn't assume that the writers of children's books were participating in a conspiracy to limit the social potential of women by reproducing stereotypes, that is, women characters caught up in stereotypically disempowered relationships with men or other conditions. Although some writers of children's books might have been so caught up, most of those writers probably never envisioned sexism as a consequence of their art.

Unacknowledged Conditions of Action

Unacknowledged conditions are resources that make the action being studied possible, but which are not recognised within the accounts of actors. Language and the material resources of privilege are apt examples here (McIntosh, 1988).

When one asks women about their experiences of menopause and how it shapes their daily actions, the responses received depend vitally upon the women's vocabulary (Dickson, 1990). Do the women asked have access to historical 'folk wisdom' passed down by women generation after generation? How much do the women understand of the biology of menopause? How much of their view of menopause is shaped by the influence of biomedical perspectives reproduced in women's magazines? Language is a critical resource – it is central to both self-concept and the possibility of change. The U.S. government's 'termination' programs that attempted to eradicate the languages and religious practices of Native Americans, for example, were based on the realisation that control of language leads to control of populations (Swinomish Tribe, 1991). Whether meanings are expressed in verbal or nonverbal forms, they are incorporated into our understandings of ourselves and our visions of how the world might be. Consequently, regardless of whether or not the authors of children's books, the authors of college textbooks, or the writers of beer advertisements are *intentionally* sexist, their work must be challenged lest it influence the pool of meanings available for us and future generations. In this sense, much of the historical and mythological research of feminists has been directed toward recovering or creating more diverse and powerful vocabularies for women.

Tom Harkin, former 1992 presidential candidate, captured the material resources of privilege when he quipped that the problem with George Bush is that he was born on third base and thinks he hit a triple. Similarly, the racist and sexist political programs that promise, like the Colorado Ku Klux Klan leader, or Duke, Buchanan, or Bush, 'equality for everyone, special consideration for none' are racist and sexist precisely because they fail to acknowledge the resources that *already* give men and whites unearned privileges (McIntosh, 1988). Their forefathers having slaughtered American Indians to gain the very land they stand on as they speak, these politicians speak out against 'unfair' access of tribes to fishing and hunting resources. Having enslaved African Americans, passed generations of Jim Crow laws, segregated and underfunded school systems, they now decry the unfair advantages conferred by affirmative action. Having the privilege of seeing white male faces reflected at them in all media representations of success and power and, indeed, within the corridors of power themselves, they undermine the Equal Rights Amendment as unnecessary.

Another resource we rarely acknowledge due to the privilege of good health is physiological intactness. Our linguistic and physical competence is based upon adequate physical health.

As a category, the importance of unacknowledged conditions resides in its focus on the interaction between socially structured resources and individual human actions. We are not limited to just the accounts given by agents of what makes their actions possible. The symbolic and material resources of culture are critical to understanding human action and envisioning new social arrangements. Feminists have long understood this, of course, as exemplified in their efforts towards comparable worth, child care, and nonsexist media. Giddens's model simply helps us formulate and incorporate such conditions into our research programs.

CONCLUSION

As researchers, before we throw up our hands in despair, I must emphasise again that the themes discussed in this chapter should be seen as regulative ideals, as models to strive for. Giddens's model, for example, will rarely be fully incorporated into a single study; it is more helpful to think of applying it to *programs* of research. Similarly, we all conduct research under conditions usually not of our choosing, including constraints of tenure, funding sources, time, university bureaucracies, and so forth. Recall that I said we would fully understand the nature of emancipatory research only within the context of emancipatory communities. While I love my job, I am sad to report that I can't consider major research universities to be fully emancipatory either!

What the models of process and explanation provide, then, is an emerging vision of how to produce research that is resistant to the authoritarianism and imperialism of current research approaches. As we pursue these visions, we will no doubt find new ways in which our research efforts can serve oppressive purposes or discover old oppressive purposes reappearing in new forms. The only assurance available to us is commitment to participative, communicative ideals and the processes which can create and nurture them.

DISCUSSION QUESTIONS

1   Allen states that feminism cannot be relativistic because it is explicitly or implicitly presented as a *preferable* perspective. It is viewed as a 'better' perspective than, say, racist or sexist approaches to research, theory, or practice. Summarise in your own words how the concept of 'situatedness' can be used to balance the risks of relativism and authoritarianism.

2   Many feminist and phenomenological traditions emphasise the importance of women's understanding of their own lives. Research from these perspectives often elucidates women's view of, say, menopause or parenting. What are the strengths and limitations of approaches which limit themselves to explicating women's understanding of their own lives?

3   In nursing, as a health occupation, the realm of the 'biological' is often regarded as more real, less socially implicated than psycho-social or cultural realms. Apply the model of explanation based on Giddens from Allen's chapter to both Allman's chapter, 'Race, Racism, and Health,' and Henderson's chapter on sociopsychoanalytic theory and women's health to develop your own ideas about how biological ideas play a role in our research on women. You might consider developing a rationale for a research proposal on an aspect of women's health that explores the relationship between the social functions of biological discourse and a feminist perspective on social-political context.

NOTES

Critique, Resistance and Action. pp. 1–19. Reprinted with permission of Jones & Bartlett.

1   One reason the abortion debate can't proceed, for example, is that the discussion remains on the metalevel; until some common horizon is achieved, no movement is possible other than through force.

2   For example, if the author had been raised as a Methodist and the reader a Presbyterian, their horizons might diverge but not sufficiently to raise questions of mutual understanding of research on behavior interventions with Alzheimer's victims. If the research were on the role of religious beliefs in civil life, however, questions of mutual understanding might be raised.

REFERENCES

Alford, C. F. (1985). Is Jurgen Habermas's reconstructive science really science? *Theory and Society*, 14, 321–340.

Allen, D. (1986). The use of philosophical and historical methodologies to understand the concept of 'health.' In P. Chinn (Ed.), *Nursing research methodology*, (pp. 157–168). Rockville, MD: Aspen.

Allen, D. (1987). Health, objectification and alienation: Critical social theory and the process of defining and attaining health. In M. Duffy & N. Pender (Eds.), *Conceptual issues in health promotion* (pp. 128–137). A report of proceedings of a Wingspread Conference. Indianapolis: Sigma Theta Tau International.

Allen, D. (1987). Critical social theory as a model for analysing ethical issues in family and community health. *Family and Community Health* 10(1), 63–72.

Allen, D. (1989). Challenge: The influence of gender on nursing science. *Proceedings of the fifth nursing science colloquium: Strategies for theory development in nursing*, V. Boston University, 1988.

Allen, D. (1991). Applying critical social theory to nursing education. In N. Greenleaf (Ed.), *Curriculum revolution: Redefining the student-teacher relationship*. New York: National League for Nursing.

Allen, D., Allman, K. M., & Powers, P. (1991). Feminist nursing research without gender. *Advances in Nursing Science* 13(3), 49–58.

Allen, D., Diekelmann, N., & Benner, P. (1986). Three paradigms for nursing research: Methodological implications. In P. Chinn (Ed.), *Nursing research methodology* (pp. 23–38). Rockville, MD: Aspen.

Althusser, L. (1971). Ideology and ideological state apparatuses: Notes towards an investigation. In *Lenin and philosophy* (pp. 127–186). New York: Monthly Review Press.

Balbus, I. D. (1984). Habermas and feminism: (Male) communication and the evolution of (patriarchal) society. *New Political Science*, 13, 27–47.

Benner, P. (1985). Quality of life. *Advances in nursing Science*, 8(1), 1–14.

Benner, P., & Wrubel, J. (1989). *The primacy of caring*. Menlo Park: Addison-Wesley.

Benhabib, S. (1986). *Critique, norm and utopia: A study in the foundations of critical theory*. New York: Columbia University Press.

Benhabib, S. (1987). The generalised and concrete other: The Kohlberg-Gilligan controversy and moral theory. In E. F. Kittay & D. Meyers (Eds.). *Women and moral theory*, (pp. 154–177). Totowa, NJ: Rowman & Littlefield.

Benhabib, S, & Cornell, D. (Eds.). (1987). *Feminism as critique*. Minneapolis: University of Minnesota Press.

Bernstein, R. (1983). *Beyond objectivism and relativism*. Philadelphia: University of Pennsylvania Press.

Bleier, R. (1986). *Science and gender: A critique of biology and its theories about women*. New York: Pergamon Press.

Bowles, G. (1984). The uses of hermeneutics for feminist scholarship. *Women's Studies International Forum*, 7(3), 185–188.

Bowles, G., & Klein, D. (Eds.). (1983). *Theories of women's studies*. London: Routledge, Kegan & Paul.

Campbell, J., & Bunting, S. (1991). Voices and paradigms: perspectives on critical and feminist theory in nursing. *Advances in Nursing Science* 13(3), 1–15.

Card, C. (1986). Oppression and resistance: Frye's politics of reality. *Hypatia*, 1(1), 149–166.

Chinn, P. L., & Wheeler, C. E. (1985). Feminism and nursing: Can nursing afford to remain aloof from the women's movement? *Nursing Outlook*, 33(2), 74–77.

Chodorow, N. J. (1985). Beyond drive theory: Object relations and the limits of radical individualism. *Theory and Society*, 14(3), 271–319.

Collins, P. H. (1989). The social construction of black feminist thought. *Signs*, 14(4), 745–773.

Coward, R. (1985). *Female desires: How they are sought, bought and packaged*. New York: Grove Press.

Deegan, M. J., & Hill, M. (Eds.). (1987). *Women and symbolic interaction*. Boston: Allen & Unwin.

Dickson, G. L. (1990). A feminist poststructural analysis of the knowledge of menopause. *Advances in Nursing Science* 12(3), 15–31.

Fay, B. (1987). *Critical social science: Liberation and its limits*. Ithaca, NY: Cornell University Press.

Fee, E. (1986). Critiques of modern science: The relationship of feminism to other radical epistemologies. In R. Bleier (Ed.), *Feminist approaches to science* (pp. 42–56). New York: Pergamon Press.

Fonow, M. M., & Cook. J. A. (1991). *Beyond methodology: Feminist scholarship as lived research*. Bloomington: Indiana University Press.

Forester, J. (Ed.). (1985). *Critical theory and public life*. Cambridge, MA: MIT Press.

Foucault, M. (1979). *Discipline and punish: The birth of the prison*. New York: Vintage.

Foucault, M. (1980). *The history of sexuality* (Vol. I). New York: Vintage.

Fraser, N., (1987). What's critical about critical theory? The case of Habermas and gender. In S. Benhabib & D. Cornell (Eds.), *Feminism as critique* (pp. 31–56). Minneapolis: University of Minnesota Press.

Fraser, N. (1989). *Unruly practices: Power, discourse and gender in contemporary social theory*. Minneapolis: University of Minnesota Press.

French, M. (1986). Beyond power: Women, men and morals. *The Women's Review of Books*, IV(1), 20–21.

Giddens, A. (1987). *Social theory and modern sociology*. Stanford, CA: Stanford University Press.

Gilligan, C. (1989). *Making connections: The relational worlds of adolescent girls at Emma Willard school*.

Habermas, J. (1984). *The theory of communicative action* (Vols. I & II). Boston: Beacon Press.

Haraway, D. (1988). Situated knowledges: The science question in feminism and the privilege of partial perspective. *Feminist Studies*, 14(3), 575–599.

Harding, S. (1982). Is gender a variable in conception of rationality? A survey of issues. *Dialectica* 36, (2–3), 43–63.

Harding, S. (1986). *The science question in feminism*. Ithaca, NY: Cornell University Press.

Harding, S. (1987). The curious coincidence of feminine and African moralities. In E. F. Kittay & D. Meyers (Eds.), *Women and moral theory* (pp. 296–316). Totowa, NJ: Rowman & Littlefield.

Harding, S. (1989). Taking responsibility for our own gender, race, class: Transforming science and the social studies of science. *Rethinking Marxism*, 2(3), 8–19.

Hekman, S. (1990). *Gender and knowledge: Elements of a postmodern feminism*. Boston: Northeastern University Press.

Held, D., & Thompson, J. (Eds.). (1989). *Social theory of modern societies: Anthony Giddens and his critics*. New York: Cambridge University Press.

Held, V. (1985). Feminism and epistemology: Recent work on the connection between gender and knowledge. *Philosophy & Public Affairs*, 14(3), 296.

hooks, b. (1984). *Feminist theory: from margin to center*. Boston: South End Press.

Hookway, C., & Pettit, P. (Eds.). (1978). *Action and interpretation*. New York: Cambridge University Press.

Jaggar, A., & Bordo, S. (Eds.). (1989). *Gender/body/knowledge: Feminist reconstructions of being and knowing*. New Brunswick, NJ: Rutgers University Press.

Keller, E. F. (1985). *Reflections on gender and science.* New Haven, CT: Yale University Press.

Kuhn, T. (1970). *The structure of scientific revolutions* (2nd ed. enl.). Chicago: University of Chicago Press.

Lash, S. (1990). *Sociology of postmodernism.* New York: Routledge.

Lather, P. (1991). *Getting smart: Feminist research and pedagogy with/in the postmodern.* New York: Routledge.

Leavitt, J. (Ed.) (1984). *Women and health in America.* Madison: University of Wisconsin Press.

Lennon, K. (1990). *Explaining human action.* LaSalle, IL: Open Court.

Leslie, C. (1989). Scientific racism: Reflections on peer review, science and ideology. *Social science and Medicine* 31(3), 891–912.

Levesque-Lopman, L. (1988). *Claiming reality. Phenomenology and women's experience.* Totowa, NJ: Rowman & Littlefield.

Lichtman, R. (1982). *The production of desire: The integration of psychoanalysis into marxist theory.* New York: Free Press.

Little, D. (1991). *Varieties of explanation.* San Francisco: Westview Press.

Lorde, A. (1984). The uses of anger: Women responding to racism. In *Sister outsider* (pp. 124–133). Trumansburg, NY: The Crossing Press.

Love, N. S. (1991). Ideal speech and feminist discourse: Habermas revisited. *Women & Politics.* 11(3), 101–122.

Madison, G. B. (1988). *The hermeneutics of postmodernity.* Bloomington: Indiana University Press.

Manicas, P., & Secord, P. (1983). Implications for psychology of the new philosophy of science. *American Psychologist,* 399–413.

Martin, E. (1987). *The woman in the body: A cultural analysis of reproduction.* Boston: Beacon Press.

McIntosh, P. (1988). White privilege and male privilege: A personal account of coming to see correspondences through work in women's studies. Working Paper No. 189 (pp. 1–15); Wellesley College.

Navarro, V. (1976). *Medicine under capitalism.* New York: Prodist.

Nicholson, C. (1989). Postmodernism, feminism, and education: The need for solidarity. *Educational Theory,* 39(3), 197–205.

Pratt, M. B. (1984). Identity: Skin, blood, heart. In E. Bulkin, M. B. Pratt, & B. Smith (Eds.), *Yours in struggle: Three feminist perspectives on antisemitism and racism* (pp. 11–61). Brooklyn, NY: Long Haul Press.

Rasmussen, D. M. (1990). *Reading Habermas.* Cambridge, MA: Basil Blackwell.

Rorty, R. (1979). *Philosophy and the mirror of nature.* Princeton, NJ: Princeton University Press.

Rorty, R. (1989). *Contingency, irony and solidarity.* New York: Cambridge University Press.

Rose, H. (1989). Talking about science as a socialist-feminist. *Rethinking Marxism,* 2(3), 26–29.

Roth, P. (1987). *Meaning and method in the social sciences.* Ithaca, NY: Cornell University Press.

Rothenberg, P. (1990). The construction, deconstruction, and reconstruction of difference. *Hypatia,* 5(1), 42–57.

Rushton, P., & Bogaert, A. F. (1989). Population differences in susceptibility to AIDS: An evolutionary analysis. *Social Science & Medicine* 28(12), 1211–1220.

Sayers, J. (1987). Feminism and science – Reason and passion. *Women's Studies International Forum,* 10(2), 171–179.

Spivak, G. C. (1985). Feminism and Critical Theory. In P. Treichler, C. Kramarae, & B. Stafford

(Eds.), *For alma mater: Theory and practice in feminist scholarship* (pp. 119–142). Chicago; University of Illinois Press.

Street, A. F. (1989). *Thinking, acting, reflecting: A critical ethnography of clinical nursing practices.* Unpublished manuscript.

Suleiman, S. (Ed.). (1986). *The female body in western culture.* Cambridge, MA: Harvard University Press.

Sumner, C. (1979). *Reading ideologies.* New York: Academic Press.

Swinomish Tribe. (1991). *A gathering of wisdoms.* La Connor, WA: Swinomish Tribal Community.

Thompson, J. (1981). *Critical hermeneutics: A study in the thought of Paul Ricoeur and Jurgen Habermas.* New York: Cambridge University Press.

Thompson, J. (1984). *Studies in the theory of ideology.* Berkeley: University of California Press.

Thompson, J. L. (1987). Critical scholarship: The critique of domination in nursing. *Advances in Nursing Science,* 10(1), 27–38.

Thompson, J. L. (1990). Hermeneutic inquiry. In L. Moody (Ed.), *Advancing nursing research through science* (Vol. II). Newbury Park, CA: Sage.

Thompson, J. L. (1991). Exploring gender and culture with Khmer refugee women: Reflections on particpatory feminist research. *Advances in Nursing Science,* 13(3), 30–48.

Waitzkin, H. (1983). A marxist view of health and health care. In Mechanic, D., *Handbook of health, health care and the health professions* (pp. 503–528). New York: Free Press.

Wheeler, C., & Chinn, P. (1985), *Peace and power: A handbook of feminist process.* Buffalo, NY: Margaretdaughters, Inc.

Winch, P. (1958). *The idea of a social science and its relation to philosophy.* London: Routledge, Kegan Paul.

Chapter 11

Doing occupational demarcation

The boundary work of nurse managers in a district general hospital

DAVINA ALLEN

Introduction

One of the characteristics of nursing is its occupational closeness to medicine. Often this closeness is a cause of great anxiety because many nurses sense an assumption of hierarchy in the relationship between the two professions, and believe that many doctors view nurses as technicians whose role is little more than to carry out their instructions. This thorny issue stretches from the national policy level, where nursing often struggles for high-level representation in situations in which medicine appears to be admitted without question, to the relationships between individual clinicians. The effects of gender, class and education loom large, and stereotypes and propaganda abound on both sides.

One of the benefits of research, and perhaps of a 'research mentality', if such a thing exists, is its therapeutic potential. Emotive problems, such as those of professional relationships and power, can, when placed into different contexts and teased out a little, look rather different and feel less disempowering. However, the price is that sometimes – certainly not always – we emerge from the process a little less committed to any particular positions.

The paper by Davina Allen investigates the efforts of members of the nursing and medical professions to 'police the boundaries' of their occupations during the early 1990s, a crucial period of policy change in the UK. During this period, as she describes, the effects of a number of policy initiatives flowed into health care in (their usual) exquisite contradiction. Project 2000 was founded on a 'holistic' view of nursing, part of a professionalising strategy, an attempt to turn away from a preparation for practice that could centre around meeting service needs at the cost of the educational needs of the student. Partly because the new student nurses' working hours would be reduced, Project 2000 was bought at the political price of the introduction of the new Health Care Assistant (HCA), whose training was determined, not by any nursing body, but by the National Council for Vocational Qualifications. In addition, there was the impact of managerialism in the wake of the Griffiths reorganisation and the NHS and Community Care Act of 1990 which introduced the health care 'market'. Managers were eager to reduce salary costs by attention to 'skill-mix' adjustments, and many conflicting reports on this aspect of workforce composition emerged in this period. Added to this was the Junior Doctors' Hours Initiative which emerged partly as a result of much publicised cases of young doctors' exhaustion. *The New Deal* for junior doctors which was published in 1991 put limits on junior doctors' contracted working hours and recommended a reorganisation of their work. In short, pressures to cascade certain health care tasks towards a cheaper worker (from doctor to nurse; from nurse to HCA) collided with nursing's desire to establish its identity as both based on sound theoretical understanding and involved in caring for the 'whole person'.

Davina Allen's paper is important, not only because it tracks the effects of these significant policies at a local level, but also because it speaks to the debates about the 'essence' of nursing — what differentiates nursing from medicine and the contribution of other health care disciplines. In the process, she places this investigation in the context of wider research into professional demarcation, how it is achieved and how it needs to be constantly reinforced. In fact, it is this last point, the suggestion that the boundaries, and hence the character, of any occupation have to be constantly 'accomplished' rather than existing in some natural or stable way, that some readers may find a disorientating feature of her approach. Nevertheless, her evidence, drawn from hospital documentation, internal memos, interviews with staff and tape recordings of training sessions for HCAs, shows how, for example, doctors and nurses present the meaning and value of the same task in different ways in order to place that task either within or beyond the rightful boundary of their own occupation. Medical staff, she notes, typically downgraded the value of tasks such as cannulation which were devolved to nurses by emphasising their repetitive nature, while nurses drew on notions of holism to welcome them as part of appropriately holistic care. At the other boundary, between nursing and the activity of HCAs, Allen shows how senior nurses running training sessions for this new grade of worker tended to define their realm of activity in terms of whatever nursing was *not*. Its boundaries are hedged by legal threats of overstepping competence and by denial of access to the mystique of nursing 'assessment', but offering access to the technical task of collecting 'numbers' – patients' vital signs.

Allen's work shows what can be accomplished when data (and thinking about data) are placed under the organising principle of a strong theoretical context. Sociological literature on the division of labour and professional behaviour allows her to go far beyond simply summarising the words of her participants or devising more or less superficial categories to place them in. For example the so-called indermination/technicality ratio, proposed by researchers Jamous and Peloille in 1970 after work in French teaching hospitals, helps her to find significance in the way that, when task areas are being taken over by rival groups, professionals rhetorically reduce the role of these competing groups to that of 'technician' while emphasising something about their own activities as irreducible to simple technical procedures. Her research gives evidence of both doctors and nurses resorting to such a boundary-reinforcing strategy.

Allen's theoretically orientated approach allows her to understand particular activity as an example of a larger theorised phenomenon, and allows the reader to understand the events and struggles at Woodlands hospital, as well as their own experiences, in a new way.

ALLEN, D. (2000)

Doing occupational demarcation: the boundary work of nurse managers in a district general hospital*

This article analyses how nurse managers attempted to accomplish the formal boundaries of clinical nursing work in a large UK district general hospital. As a site where occupational jurisdictions are claimed and sustained, the management arena has been hitherto neglected in interactionist studies of hospital settings. The sociological eye has focused primarily on the ways in which staff in the clinical domain negotiate their occupational roles, and the formal organisational plan is typically treated as a background against which the daily constitution of work boundaries takes place. Yet, as proponents of the negotiated-order perspective have pointed out, the formal organisational structure is itself a negotiated order, even if it becomes more-or-less stable at particular points in time and/or for specific analytic purposes. In this article, I explore the ways in which nurse managers charged, inter alia, with the formalisation of nursing jurisdiction, attempted to do occupational demarcation. The strategies they employed are treated herein as examples of 'boundary-work' (Gieryn 1983, 1999). My aim is to examine the detail of these micro-political processes and to consider their contribution to the interactional accomplishment of the division of labor between nursing, medical, and support staff. I shall be using ethnographic data from a wider study (Allen 1996) into the ways in which hospital-based nurses routinely produce their work boundaries.

THE DIVISION OF LABOR – AGENCY AND STRUCTURE

Most interactionist studies of hospital workplace settings undertaken over the past thirty years owe an enormous intellectual debt to Strauss and colleagues' work on negotiated orders (Strauss 1978; Strauss et al. 1985; Strauss et al. 1964; Strauss et al. 1963). Introduced into the literature as a way of conceptualising the ordered flux found in their study of two North American psychiatric hospitals, the negotiated-order perspective attempted to address the question of how social order was maintained in the face of change. Critical of the emphasis given to formal structures and regulations which characterised the then dominant paradigm in organisational studies, Strauss et al. (1963) proposed an alternative approach in which the social order was (re)conceptualised as in-process, reconstituted continually.

In underlining the dynamic nature of social organisations, negotiated-order theorists were attempting to create an analytic space for human agency as a counterbalance to the excessive determinism of the orthodox view. Contrary to the claims of its critics (Benson 1977a, 1977b, 1978; Day and Day 1977, 1978; Dingwall and Strong 1997), however, the approach did not assume that social life was *indefinitely* negotiable. Strauss (1978) developed the concepts of 'negotiation context' and 'structural context' to sensitise researchers to those factors which shape social action. The former refers to immediate features of a social setting which enter into negotiations and directly influence their form and course; the latter relates to the circumstances which transcend the immediate negotiation context. Many of the studies undertaken within this tradition have focused on the interaction of personal processes and social structures.

> Negotiated orders refer to those arenas through which structural constraint, in the form of rules, policies, laws, normative proscription, and ideology are defined, interpreted, and incorporated into the daily activities of organisational members. (Maines and Charlton 1985: 303)

Nevertheless, negotiated-order theorists insist that while 'structures' exhibit stability at a particular point in time and/or for certain analytic purposes, ultimately they too are negotiated orders (Glaser and Strauss 1964; Maines 1977). Maines (1977, 244) cites the example of the tax structure of the United States which, on the one hand, constitutes the framework in which negotiations about tax deductions take place but which, on the other, was itself the focus of negotiation between various competing interests at the point of legislative reform. The division of labor may also be considered in an analogous way. At one level, as Freidson has pointed out,

> it seems accurate to see the division of labor as a process of social interaction in the course of which the participants are continuously engaged in attempting to define, establish, maintain and renew the tasks they perform and the relationship with others which their tasks presuppose. (Freidson 1976, 311)

At another level, however, as Freidson (1976) himself stresses, these negotiative processes are not entirely free. Social interaction may be constrained, for example, by the relative power of the participants or the material features of the negotiation context. Moreover, however central social interaction is to the division of labor, it is also the case that abstract conceptions of roles and responsibilities *are* made – in formal organisational policy and, in the case of certain occupations, in state legislature – and while they may not determine work boundaries in a straightforward way, they certainly help to fashion their contours. Although more-or-less fixed for certain purposes, these 'official' divisions of labor are themselves negotiated orders: occupational jurisdictions have to be claimed and sustained in public, legal, and workplace arenas and the particular context in which negotiations take place shapes the form that they assume (Abbott 1988).

THE SOCIAL PRODUCTION OF HOSPITAL WORK

Although its proponents emphasise that the negotiated-order perspective can be applied to all kinds of organisation, it has been most extensively employed in research on hospital settings. The interpenetration of the structural and social on the health care division of labor has been a central concern of much of this work.

A dominant theme in this literature is how formal divisions of labor are mediated in daily practice by features of the work setting. For example, a number of studies have shown how nurses are able to exert influence over doctors in relation to clinical decision making (Hughes 1988; Svensson 1996; Porter 1991). Work boundaries may also be fashioned by the hospital's temporal organisation (Zerubavel 1979). As the only occupational group in the hospital providing 24-hour care, nurses frequently find themselves crossing occupational boundaries (Evers 1982; Milman 1976; Roth and Douglas 1983; Taylor 1970; Zerubavel 1979). Work pressures are another mediator of formal jurisdictions in the hospital context (Sudnow 1967; Hughes 1980; Roth and Douglas 1983). Sudnow (1967) and Hughes (1980) describe how the development of informal practices between casualty and ambulance staff led to ambulance crews being accorded the power to declare a patient 'dead' although, legally, this should have been performed by a doctor.

Others have run the lines of emphasis in the opposite direction, highlighting the constraining effects of the hospital structure on the daily practice of health workers and the conflicts to which this gives rise (Anspach 1987, 1993; Chambliss 1997; Rosenthal et al. 1980). Anspach (1987, 1993) describes how the division of labor between nursing and medical staff in the neonatal intensive care setting leads to different perceptions of infant prognosis. Chambliss (1997) draws attention to the moral and ethical dilemmas which are created for nursing staff as a result of their position of subordination in relation to both doctors and hospital administrators. He argues that what appear as ethical arguments are, in actuality, thinly disguised turf battles.

Another theme in the ethnographic literature on hospital settings relates to the micro-political processes via which occupational boundaries are negotiated at the point of service delivery (Guillemin and Holmstrom 1986; Mesler 1989, 1991; Porter 1991; Svensson 1996). Mesler (1989, 1991) has explored the strategies clinical pharmacists employed in attempting to expand their role. He argues that by deploying 'tact and diplomacy,' 'role-taking,' and 'tactical socialisation' (1989), they were able to enlarge their jurisdiction in ways which were acceptable to nursing and medicine. Others have pointed to the importance of the workplace as the site of occupational 'identity work' (Brown 1989; Emerson and Pollner 1976). Emerson and Pollner (1976) argue that by designating certain tasks as 'shit work,' mental health workers were able to distance themselves from those activities which threatened their occupational identity, thereby marking the legitimate boundaries of their practice.

There is, then, a rich body of literature which has examined the inter-relationship of structure and agency in the social constitution of the hospital division of labor. Although we now have a much better understanding of the factors which shape work boundaries at the point of service delivery, relatively little is known about the ways in which the formal division of labor is produced by those charged with the formulation

of organisational policies and plans. Indeed, despite the claim of negotiated-order theorists that all social orders are in some sense negotiated orders, in most of the hospital
workplace studies arising from this tradition, the formal plan of work is consistently
treated as a stable 'background' feature against which shop floor negotiations take
place. Thus, while the negotiated-order perspective clearly provided an important cor-
rective to the overemphasis on formal organisational structures which characterised
traditional approaches to the field, the balance of sociological attention may now
have shifted too far the other way, thereby inverting the original error (Dingwall and
Strong 1997). The corollary is that we have only a partial understanding of the ways in
which division(s) of labor are socially constituted, and our conceptualisation of the
relationship between the formal and social organisation of hospital work remains tentative.

THE CHANGING BOUNDARY BETWEEN NURSES, DOCTORS AND SUPPORT WORKERS: POLICY CONTEXT

One possible reason for the absence of studies of formal organisational plans as negotiated orders is lack of opportunity. As negotiated-order theorists point out,
organisations are not in a permanent state of flux: they can become more or less stable
at particular points in time. It is during conditions of change, uncertainty and ambiguity, disagreement, ideological diversity, and newness and inexperience that
negotiations are most likely to arise. In the UK in the early 1990s a number of developments in medical and nursing education (General Medical Council 1993;
Department of Health and Social Security 1987; United Kingdom Central Council for
Nursing, Midwifery and Health Visiting 1987) and health policy (Department of
Health 1989) converged to provide the impetus for jurisdictional shifts at two of
nursing's key occupational boundaries: at the interface with medicine on the one
hand, and with support staff, on the other. Rekindling deep-seated historical tensions
between professional and service versions of nursing, these policy changes provided
a natural laboratory for the study of the micro-political processes via which occupational jurisdictions are socially constituted.

First there was Project 2000. This was the United Kingdom Central Council For
Nursing, Midwifery and Health's (UKCC) plan for the reform of nursing education,
structure, and practice.[1] At one level, an explicit professionalising strategy, at another,
an attempt to overcome the fragmentation and technical orientation of health provision, its proponents argued that it had the potential to overcome some of the
occupation's most persistent problems: low status, poor retention, and the lack of a
clearly defined area of expertise with a scientific basis for practice (Beardshaw and
Robinson 1990). The Project 2000 reforms were wide-ranging. Nurse education was
relocated from hospital-based schools of nursing to institutes of higher education, and
emphasis was given to education rather than training. A single portal of entry was
established by abolishing the SEN (State Enrolled) grade of nurse.[2] There was a shift
in the curriculum from an emphasis on disease to health and the introduction of a
'New Nursing' (Beardshaw and Robinson 1990) ideology which advocated a holistic,

rather than a task-oriented, approach to care.[3] Crucially, for the purposes of this article, learners' contribution to service provision was reduced from 60 to 20 percent.
Nurses in training had always been an important source of labor on hospital wards;
there was now a need to find ways of replacing their contribution.

Project 2000 was an explicitly elitist program of reform and its acceptance by the
government was initially puzzling to some observers. Similar proposals had previously
been constrained by economic realities (Dingwall et al. 1988), and the general thrust
of government policy at the time was directed at curbing professional power in the
public sector. As Rafferty (1992, 1996) has pointed out, however, historically the
success of nurse-driven policy changes can be traced to their synchronisation with
wider organisational and policy concerns and, in the case of Project 2000, there
appeared to be several possible reasons for the government's willingness to embrace
its recommendations. First, there was the specter of the 'demographic timebomb.'
During the late 1980s policy making was dominated by the prospect of having to
recruit up to half of all the suitably qualified women school leavers in order to maintain staffing and wastage levels in the National Health Service (NHS). In this context,
the creation of a small, highly skilled nursing core, supported by a pool of cheaper
workers, made for a more flexible workforce which could be deployed to meet changing demographic and social trends (Carpenter 1993; Naish 1993).

Second, Project 2000 afforded the opportunity to make efficiency savings.
Managerialism in the NHS was rapidly gaining ground following the *Griffiths Report*
(Department of Health and Social Security 1983) and was to be further consolidated
by the 1990 NHS and Community Care Act. The emphasis on cost containment was
strong and, in the context of market competition, issues of human resource management were brought center stage (Paton 1993). As the largest occupational group in a
labor-intensive industry, nursing has always been a prime target for health service planners concerned with reducing expenditure, and government acceptance of Project
2000 was accompanied by an important rider: that nurses agree to a new training for
health support workers which be determined by the National Council for Vocational
Qualifications[4] (Beardshaw and Robinson 1990). The health care assistant (HCA), as
this new support worker came to be called, would undertake a wider range of work
than the traditional auxiliary.

The 'New Nursing' ideology, which infused the Project 2000 recommendations,
reflected the aspirations of certain segments of the occupation to establish a domain
of professional practice that was free from medical control. As a means to this end,
efforts were being made to reintegrate intimate tending and caring activities into the
professional nursing role, work, which, in the past, had been devalued and delegated
to support staff. The introduction of the HCA was clearly in tension with this professional vision and the conviction of the proponents of Project 2000 that all aspects of
nursing should be carried out by qualified staff. As Celia Davies (1995) has observed,
there was no explicit bargain struck at national level that the cost of educational
reform was restructuring, and the question of who should do what in the caring division of labor was not explicitly addressed. Rather, the onus was shifted to the Regional
Health Authorities to produce individual plans for replacement staff and for the numbers of admissions to the new Project 2000 programs. Responsibility for agreeing to

the division of labor between qualified nurses and support workers was left to local determination.

A further key development at this time was the Junior Doctors' Hours Initiative which aimed to improve the working conditions and career opportunities of junior medical staff.[5] Local task forces were set up and given the power to remove educational approval from service providers if standards were not met. *The New Deal* (National Health Service Management Executive 1991) set firm limits on junior doctors' contracted hours (72 hours per week or less in most hospital posts) and working hours (56 hours per week). It called for an increase in the number of career grade posts and suggested new ways of organising junior doctors' work. Of significance for the purposes of this article was the suggestion that key clinical tasks be shared by nurses and midwives.

Nationally, the nursing response to The New Deal was mixed. Many supported role expansion in principle but there was unease about the bracketing of role developments with the Junior Doctors' Hours Initiative. A number suggested that once again doctors were dumping their dirty work on an already overburdened group and that nurses risked becoming minidoctors, subject to medical direction. As we have seen, much of the impetus behind the Project 2000 reforms was the desire to differentiate the nursing contribution from that of medicine, and this entailed a rejection of the old hierarchy of prestige which elevated technical (medical) tasks over bedside (nursing) care. Others reasoned that The Junior Doctors' Hours Initiative offered an opportunity for nursing and argued that a high-profile political initiative commanded more resources and support than professionally driven change (Allen and Hughes 1993).

It was in this context that the UKCC published *The Scope of Professional Practice* (UKCC 1992). In the past, in order to undertake tasks not covered in basic training, nurses had needed extended role certificates which were signed by doctors to indicate they were proficient to practice. Eschewing the hierarchy implicit in the previous system, the new guidelines were based on a professional model in which the onus for defining the boundaries of nursing was shifted to individual practitioners. Nurses were cautioned that they should be competent to work in an extended role and that any boundary changes should not result in unnecessary fragmentation of patient care or lead to the inappropriate delegation of work.

The interactive effect of these developments was to create jurisdictional ambiguity at the medical-nursing and the nurse-support worker boundaries, raising many questions about the future shape of nursing work. My aim in undertaking the research was to capitalise on the natural experiment afforded by these policy developments and study the ways in which these changes in occupational frontiers were being managed by staff in the workplace. The study was framed by an interactionist perspective: occupational jurisdiction was conceptualised as a practical accomplishment.

THE STUDY

The research was carried out between September 1994 and June 1995 at Woodlands, a large district general hospital in the middle of England.[6] At the time it had an annual budget of £60 million, almost 900 beds and about 2,800 staff. It provided general, acute, obstetric, and elderly services to a population of 254,000. Together with two other local hospitals, it had acquired Trust status in 1993.[7]

I carried out field observations on a medical and a surgical ward (three months each) and elsewhere in the organisation through attendance at meetings and in-service study days. As far as it was possible, field notes were recorded contemporaneously in a spiral-bound note-book and a behaviorist, low-inference style was adopted. That is, I recorded verbatim interactions rather than relying on my own interpretations of events. Certain activities were also tape-recorded: meetings, nursing handover, and study days. Data were also generated through fifty-seven tape-recorded, semifocused interviews with ward nurses (n = 29), doctors (n = 8), auxiliaries (n = 5), health care assistants (n = 3), and clinical managers (n = 11)[8] and spontaneous extended conversations. The latter were not tape-recorded but had a different flavor to the briefer discussions held with staff while they worked. I also employed documentary evidence.

Data were analysed using a holistic approach. I compared material from different sources in order to make judgments as to how each piece should be interpreted. I then related individual segments of data to the emergent picture in order to evaluate their meaning and, on the basis of my analysis of these extracts, I reassessed the meaning of the whole. *Folio Views Infobase Production Kit version 3.1* was used to facilitate data handling.

RESEARCH ROLE

Although I am myself a nurse, I did not work as such during the fieldwork, but I did participate in hospital life when it felt appropriate to do so. I wore a white coat in the ward areas like other visitors to the clinical setting. I was overt about my nursing background, but I emphasised and de-emphasised this aspect of my personal biography according to the demands of the fieldwork. My badge was inscribed with the title 'research student.'

An issue frequently raised in the methodological literature (Burgess 1984) is of the relative advantages and disadvantages of researching settings with which one is familiar. Having a background in nursing had a number of advantages. First, I was well versed in nursing and medical speak and so, for the most part, did not have to grapple with understanding a strange language. Second, knowing that I had a background in nursing meant that the study participants perceived me as someone who knew what it was really like, a factor which I felt made respondents more inclined to give candid accounts of their actions. Third, in negotiating access to the wards, I was able to persuade gatekeepers that as a result of my nursing experience I had sufficient native wit to know when to keep a low profile so as not to disrupt the work.

The methodological literature suggests that familiarity with a setting may disadvantage researchers in that they may not be able to recognise cultural patterns other than those things that are conventionally there to be seen. The way in which I endeavored to deal with this was by making detailed field notes of my observations which, as I have indicated, had a behaviorist character. As Burgess (1984) has pointed out, however, the debate concerning the degree of familiarity or strangeness the sociologist may encounter in a cultural setting has been polarised in some of the literature. The assumption seems to be made that situations are either totally familiar or totally strange. This is clearly not the case. As a nurse researching nursing I, like Robinson (1992), was not studying a strange tribe. Yet, I had not practiced as a nurse for some six years and I had never worked at the study site, so there were many things that were strange to me. But, as a nurse studying contemporary nursing issues, I could only play the naive researcher to a limited extent. Many of the interviews I carried out and the conversations that I had resembled a dialogue between two people grappling with the problems facing practitioners in the 1990s. This was particularly the case with many of the senior nurses who, because of the positions they occupied within the organisation, had a special interest in the subject of my research. A more extensive description of the research methodology and the fieldwork process can be found in Allen (1996).

CHANGING THE DIVISION OF LABOR AT WOODLANDS HOSPITAL

During the research period, the formal division of labor between nursing, medical, and support staff in the study site was being reconfigured in response to national policy initiatives. A number of nurse practitioner posts had been founded which involved nurses undertaking work that had previously been the remit of doctors. All these new positions had been developed in the context of the 'Junior Doctors' Hours Initiative.' They covered a range of clinical areas such as urology, rheumatology, IV cannulation, pain control, colposcopy, and general surgery. The New Deal had also acted as the impetus for the more general realignment of the medical-nursing boundary: ward-based nursing staff throughout the organisation were being encouraged to develop the scope of their practice. The principal areas in which nurses were developing their skills were the administration of intravenous antibiotics, venepuncture, ECGs, male urethral catheterisation, and intravenous cannulation.

The boundary between nursing and support staff was also being redrawn with the introduction of the HCA. Formally distinct from the auxiliary, the HCA role embraced certain technical procedures – such as measuring and recording temperature, pulse, and blood pressure; collecting blood from the blood bank; taking patients to theater; removal of IV cannulae; and the removal of urinary catheters – which had previously been the remit of qualified nurses.

It was senior nurses and medical staff employed in clinical management positions who were responsible for taking these changes forward. This was a relatively small number of individuals who coalesced in different ways around a number of issues. The medical managers comprised: the Director of Medicine (who was a member of the Trust executive board) and 11 clinical directors, that is, consultants who managed speciality budgets.[9] The nurse managers included: the Director of Nursing (also a member of the Trust executive board), four nurse managers of clinical directorates, and five specialist nurse managers.

In the UK, nursing has a long history of management hierarchy and nurse managers are often identified as a distinct segment within the occupation. Traditionally, this group has been associated with a 'service' version of nursing work in contradistinction to the professional view (Strong and Robinson 1990). I was somewhat surprised, therefore, to discover that the nurse managers at Woodlands employed a professional discourse and espoused many of the ideals of the New Nursing. Although their vision of nursing was tempered by a fair degree of pragmatism, it was clear that professional issues were very influential in their work. As such, the nurse managers acted as important mediators of the tensions between professional and service versions of nursing work in the study site. The one exception to this overall generalisation was the Quality Manager who, unlike his colleagues, appeared to have embraced much of the rhetoric of managerialism. However, he had minimal involvement in taking role changing forward.

BOUNDARY-WORK

In the following sections, I will analyse the strategies nurse managers employed in negotiating role realignment as examples of boundary-work. Gieryn (1983, 1999) developed this concept to refer to an ideological style employed by scientists in their attempts to create a public image for the discipline. They attributed selected characteristics to the institution of science for the purpose of constructing a social boundary that distinguished it from nonscientific or technical activities. Of course, scientists have access to considerable material and professional opportunities which are not available to nonscientists and thus the interactional work which is done in the social production of occupational boundaries has to be understood as a micro-political process. Gieryn focuses on 'public science,' that is, the kinds of claims which are made for science in public and political arenas. But as Abbott (1988) has pointed out, and Gieryn (1999) himself acknowledges, boundary-work processes are also found in the workplace, where the accomplishment of occupational jurisdiction is a routine feature of everyday practice. In this article, I extend the boundary-work concept to embrace the practices as well as the rhetorical devices nurse managers used in accomplishing demarcation. Moreover, I suggest that it can also be applied to the occupational identity work in which medical and nurse managers engaged in their accounts of role realignment.

It was through these different boundary-work processes that the formal division of labor was negotiated at Woodlands. Like all negotiation processes, however, they were constrained in important ways by key features of the negotiation context. Although the nurse managers felt deeply uncomfortable with many of the developments they were being asked to take forward within the organisation, they felt powerless to resist them.

> Junior doctors' hours are going to reduce anyway whether we like it or not. It's something that Parliament is quite keen to do and it's going to happen [. . .] If your patient needs an aminophylline drip there and then, I think it's inevitable and it's a must that we do do it. (Interview – Nurse Manager)

As we will see, one of the ways in which they appeared to have accommodated themselves to these constraints was by taking control of the initiatives as they arose and using them for professional purposes.

ACCOMPLISHING NURSING'S BOUNDARY WITH MEDICINE

The nurse managers in the research setting were equivocal about the changes in the nursing-medical boundary which were occurring. Although they supported nursing role development, they felt that it should be shaped by the holisitic needs of patients. There was concern that jurisdictional change had become irrevocably linked with the 'Junior Doctors' Hours Initiative' and was therefore being driven by the needs of doctors. Nevertheless, junior doctors' hours had a high political profile and nurse managers reasoned that it was preferable for nurses to expand their scope of practice than to allow another category of worker into the division of labor which would further fragment patient care.[10]

For the most part, the medical managers were happy to devolve certain technical tasks to nursing staff – intravenous antibiotic administration, venepuncture, ECGs, cannulation, and male urinary catheterisation – although a number also felt these were key medical skills which they did not wish doctors to lose. Where an activity came closer to the focal tasks of medicine – such as taking a medical history – they became more ambivalent. Some expressed the view that nursing staff had the skills to undertake this work in a limited sense, providing they worked within clearly defined protocols. Others argued that this entailed nurses making diagnoses which was a responsibility that most doctors (and also nurses) believed should remain with the doctor.

Taking control

Despite their reservations about its linkage with the Junior Doctors' Hours Initiative, it was nurse managers who took charge of the implementation of role development in the study site. This, in itself, may be seen as an example of boundary-work – albeit of a defensive kind – for, as the following extract indicates, it seems that the nurses were galvanised into action by the fear that their medical colleagues would takeover the process.

> There was almost like a splinter group of the medical staff and they were going to be writing the protocols for us which was one of the big pressures for the nursing staff to get their act together and to produce these packages and things because otherwise it would have been imposed on us from the medics. It's been a hell of a struggle getting all the paperwork sorted out but we didn't want someone else setting it up for us. We wanted to do everything ourselves. (Interview – Nurse Manager)

In the light of their powerlessness to challenge government policy, the nurse managers decided it was preferable for them to seize the initiative. They may have had reservations about the overall direction of these developments, but this way they could at least exert some influence over the shape they were to assume in the local setting.

In managing the process of boundary realignment, nurse managers had developed a number of self-directed learning packages which nursing staff had to complete and then sign to indicate that they were competent to practice. At the time of the research, this rather bureaucratic approach appeared at odds with the UKCC guidance on nurses' scope of practice which had abolished the need for extended-role certification. Yet, faced with the prospect of protocols being written by medical staff, the nurses' action can be understood as a further piece of boundary-work. Control of education and training is vital in retaining professional jurisdiction (Abbott 1988; Jamous and Peloille 1970) and historically this has been a major obstacle to nursing's professional project (Dingwall, Rafferty, and Webster 1988; Rafferty 1996). By insisting on taking charge of the education and training of nurses for role development in the study site, the nurse managers were asserting the professional autonomy of nursing and resisting coming under the control of the medical profession.

Establishing expertise

In developing the learning packages to support role expansion, the nurse managers underlined the need for ward staff to have an adequate knowledge base. At one level, this reflected risk management and litigation concerns; at another, it can be seen as further example of demarcatory practice. The following extract is taken from a meeting of senior nurses charged with responsibility for implementing nursing role developments at Woodlands. Two of the senior nurses in the group have expressed concern that the process was in danger of becoming bureaucratised.

> Nurse Manager: I take these points that Simon and Felicity made about it –
> we're being in danger of it becoming a bit cumbersome – but I mean what
> I would want to say is that the fact that the doctors and phlebotomists
> aren't trained how to do it doesn't make it right, does it?
> Nurse Practitioner (Felicity): No.
> Nurse Manager: I mean surely we ought to be putting ourselves in a better
> position than that.
> Ward Manager (Simon): I agree with you. (Meeting – Tape)

By ensuring practitioners had the theoretical knowledge to support changes in their role, nurse managers at Woodlands were attempting to differentiate the nursing contribution from the 'see one, do one, teach one' training of medical staff, and from other workers – such as phlebotomists and operating department assistants – who were also being trained to undertake similar activities. Moreover, as textual representation of nursing knowledge, the learning packages may also be understood as important boundary markers in the social production of nursing jurisdiction in the study site.

The nurses' efforts to establish expertise were ridiculed by senior medical staff, however, who, in undertaking boundary-work of their own, claimed that the detailed knowledge included in the training packages was largely superfluous and unnecessary for the needs of nurses. The following extract is taken from an internal communication to the Director of Medicine by a consultant surgeon.

> re: *Scope of Professional Practice – Flushing of Central Lines* [. . .] I find this document exceedingly complex and probably overcomprehensive for the needs of nursing staff who may be required to flush a central line. In fact, it is so complex that I myself am unable to answer some of the questions required of the nursing staff, and I suspect that the majority of the medical staff within the hospital would also be unable to satisfactorily complete the questions. I feel that if the protocol is to be adopted within the hospital and I myself am unable to comply with it, then I must regard myself as being unsuitable for the insertion, let alone the flushing of central lines. On this basis, I would suggest that I am no longer a suitable person for the insertion of these lines, including of course Hickman and other central lines. I would, therefore, suggest that we no longer use central lines within this hospital. (Document)

This theme was also echoed in the interviews with medical managers.

> [It's] crazy – for what is a practical procedure with some theory behind it, actually putting it into a context where the theory is totally outstripping the practical nature that it's intended for. And nurses are practical people at the end of the day. (Interview – Medical Manager)

> They've produced a manual! [. . .] all they needed was to spend an afternoon in theater. If someone needs two hourly turns, they order her a special bed because there's a tissue viability nurse. (interview – Medical Manager)

As a number of analysts (Abbott 1988; Hughes 1984; Jamous and Peloille 1970) have pointed out, the nature of an activity is not fixed and, in the context of jurisdictional disputes, the definition and meaning of task areas can become the subject of intense conflict. According to Jamous and Peloille (1970), central to this is the indetermination/technicality ratio. This refers to the part played in the production process by skills which can be mastered and communicated in the form of rules in proportion to those skills which, in a given historical context, are attributed to the individual talents of producers. The indeterminate portions of a task area provide a more enduring basis for the maintenance of exclusive control of an occupational domain due to their inaccessibility to the uninitiated. Jamous and Peloille (1970) suggest that one of the ways in which a profession can defend the frontiers of its jurisdiction, when task areas are being taken over by other competing groups, is by reducing the role of their competitors to that of 'technicians' or operatives. The boundary-work of the medical managers can be seen as micro-political processes of precisely this kind, that is, an attempt to recast nurses in the subordinate role of technician in the face of their claims to a more elevated status.

Identity work

The contested nature of these activities at the medical-nursing boundary was also evident in the ways in which the task area was rhetorically constructed in field actors' accounts of boundary realignment. Although I did not interview all the clinical managers, my transcripts are characterised by distinctive discursive repertoires. Medical staff typically downgraded the tasks that were being devolved to nursing, emphasising their repetitive, practical nature and their relative safety.

> It is not difficult to put in a cannula and the more that you do, the better at it you get. (Interview – Medical Manager)

> [A] lot of what the juniors were doing were these repetitive tasks which were no good for their educational training [. . .] nurses are good at doing repetitive tasks (laughs). So you know, to be able to get nurses to do the tasks that were indicated like IV drugs, catheters, [. . .] and taking blood, giving intravenous injections was fine – the so-called drudgery. (Interview – Medical Manager)

Nurse managers' accounts, on the other hand, were permeated with the rhetoric of holism. This was a useful linguistic device through which they were able to bring the professional-client relationship into play so as to construct a higher margin of indeterminancy around the task area and fabricate a distinctive approach to patient care.

> Sarah [Nurse Practitioner] said that [. . .] [The doctors] just want to shove an IV in. They don't think about the patient as a whole. (Field notes)

> [W]e're not developing our skills just to take off the menial jobs from the doctors [. . .] we're doing it because we want to and because it's more holistic individualised patient care. (Interview – Senior Nurse)

> I have a lot of excitement about The Scope because I think [. . .] nurses are in an ideal position to give more holistic care, not tasks. You know you ring the doctor up and it doesn't matter who the doctor is, but he'll come along and do the IVs for you. He might never have seen that patient. But if a nurse has got a relationship and understanding with the patient and she spends a bit of time giving an IV, then there's a lot of communication and relationship building going on there. (Interview – Nurse Manager)

At one level, the field actors' accounts may be understood as evidence of the broader micro-politics at work in the study site over the meaning and value of activities situated at the medical-nursing interface. At another level, however, these data arise in the interview context and so can also be understood in terms of the locally situated identity work they are rhetorically assembled to perform. The concept of identity work is widely used in the literature to refer to the impression of management activities (Goffman 1959), in which individuals engage to accomplish a particular type of personal identity. Snow and Anderson (1987) suggest that the social construction of identity can entail management of physical settings and props, attention to personal appearance (see, for example, Phelan and Hunt 1998), selective association with individuals and/or groups, as well as the narrative construction of particular identities (see, for example, Antaki and Widdicombe 1998; Cohan 1997; Rosenfeld 1999; Snow and Anderson 1987). Hunt and Benford (1994) argue that identity talk is a 'discourse that reflects actors' perceptions of a social order and is based on interpretations of current situations, themselves and others' (492).

By constituting the nature of these devolved activities in such different ways, I suggest that the medical and nursing managers were attempting to construct accounts of shifts in the division of labor which were consistent with their respective occupational identities and their perceptions of the position of nursing and medicine within it. Doctors rhetorically constituted the task area so as to subordinate the nursing contribution to that of a technician, whereas nurses explicitly resisted the charge that they were unwilling recipients of doctors' dirty work and emphasised their distinctive professional contribution to care and the indeterminacy involved in the production process. The interactional work being done here relates to the identification of the nursing and medical managers with their respective clinical occupations and their associated professional rhetoric and, as such, this occupational identity work may be considered a variant of boundary-work.

ACCOMPLISHING NURSING'S BOUNDARY WITH SUPPORT WORKERS

As we have seen, the division of labor between nursing and support staff was also being redrawn in the study site, as the hospital started to employ HCAs. Nurse managers accepted the need for better trained support staff in order to compensate for the loss of student nurses' service contribution following the introduction of Project 2000. They felt that a highly trained support worker would provide for a flexible division of labor and help to avoid the fragmentation of care that Project 2000 was designed to overcome. Nevertheless, working within a fixed budget, nurse managers had elected to staff wards with smaller teams but with a higher ratio of nurses to support staff. Moreover, they were also adamant that the parameters of the HCA role should be under the control of nurses, both in formal policy and in daily clinical practice.

Taking control

It was the nurse managers who, in consultation with the ward sisters, defined the official parameters of the HCA role. A list of activities HCAs were permitted to undertake had been devised which, like the learning packages, functioned as a textual marker of the limits of support workers' occupational license. Yet the extent to which HCAs practiced within these formally defined boundaries was to be determined by staff at the point of service delivery according to the requirements of the ward and the exigencies of the work.

> Nurse Manager: [Y]ou are working in very different areas and your areas have very different needs of you and those needs will vary from time to time and

I can't go along and say to you, 'You will be doing this, this, this, and this'. All I can do is say to you, 'As an organisation [. . .] we have things that have been agreed for you to actually start to undertake.' (Training day – Tape)

This is a very powerful boundary-work strategy for defending nursing jurisdiction because it effectively denies HCAs a clearly defined area of practice. Officially, at least, the role of the HCA is what the registered nurse decides that it is on a given occasion.

Another strategy nurse managers employed in defense of nursing jurisdiction was to exert control over the education and training of HCAs. When Project 2000 was implemented, it was agreed that HCA training was to be taken forward under the auspices of the National Council for Vocational Qualifications (NVQ). At the time of the research, however, there had been little national guidance on the introduction of HCAs and it became apparent that there was local variation in the ways in which the role was being implemented. There was no compulsion for the HCAs to gain NVQ qualifications in the study site – but they had to undertake a 25-day training program provided in-house. This gave the nurse managers control over HCAs' knowledge base and also created an opportunity for them to undertaken boundary-work of other kinds. This was important because, despite their careful policing of boundaries, the senior nurses knew that pressures of work on the wards presented a powerful countervailing force. They recognised that ward nurses were concerned with responding to the vicissitudes of daily practice and had little interest in the wider professional implications of devolution to support staff.

Cautionary tales

The nurse manager responsible for HCA training had a number of well-rehearsed 'atrocity stories' (Bosk 1979; Dingwall 1977) which she employed on training days for support workers and qualified staff which highlighted the strain towards dilution on the wards.

I still get phone calls now saying – I had one not too many weeks ago – 'What else can the health care assistant do' and I said, 'Well what are they doing?' Thinking, 'I don't really want to know.' So she proceeded to tell me – this is a ward manager – proceeded to tell me this, that and the other and she said 'In fact they do everything.' So I thought, 'Ah Ha!. So what is the registered nurse then doing?' (Nurse Manager – HCA training program – Tape)

My field observations revealed these stories to have some substance. Work pressures could result in HCAs undertaking work for which they were not trained or in staff working with inadequate supervision.

Authoring the landscape

The nurse managers also used the training days as opportunities to counteract the strain towards dilution and to shore up occupational frontiers. These were 'orchestrated encounters' (Dingwall 1980) which enabled them to author the organisation (Shotter 1993) by formulating the landscape of enabling-constraints (Giddens 1979, cited by Shotter 1993: 149) and moral positions relevant to HCAs. One of the ways in which they did this was to emphasise the possible legal implications of HCAs crossing the legitimate limits of their jurisdiction.

> Nurse Manager: Now it's very easy for me to stand here and say 'You don't do this, you do that, and do the other,' very easy. But what I'm saying is: 'This organisation will not support you if you go ahead and do these sorts of things.' (training day – tape)

Additionally, in-service training days for qualified nursing staff underlined their professional accountability for HCA practice. At the time of the research, concern with litigation and risk management was strong at all levels of the organisation. This provided senior staff with a powerful discourse on which to draw in their efforts to encourage frontline workers to police the parameters of their practice in the face of contrary pressures from the ward.

On the HCA training program considerable effort also went into differentiating the role of qualified nurses from that of support staff. An entire day of the course was developed to the role of the registered nurse. Although the HCAs questioned its relevance, from the perspective of nurse managers it represented an opportunity to make the nursing contribution visible, representing an important piece of boundary-work. Here is a typical example of the kind of rhetorical devices employed by the nurse manager responsible for HCA training.

> Senior Nurse: Right – you are there to *assist* the registered nurse. You're not there to do the registered nurse's job. You're there to *assist* [. . .] You will not be involved in assessing patients [. . .] You are there to *assist* in the implementation of care. Assessing patients can be anything from admitting a patient to doing a bed-bath and looking at them. As a registered nurse, I can assess the situation there and then. It doesn't matter if it's the beginning of the patient's stay the middle, or the end. I am assessing all the time because that's what I have been trained to do. If you're in a position to assess, then you're in the wrong position. Just let us take the TPR [temperature, pulse, and respirations] situation [. . .] from a registered nurse's point of view there is more to doing a pulse than just counting. I've got to know the rate, the rhythm, the depth of that pulse. By me putting my hands on that patient, I am assessing that patient. I'm assessing all those different things there. If that's what is required, then the registered nurse should be going in there and doing that, but if all that is required is a number then I don't see a problem with you getting in there. Assessment is a very fine line and it makes it very difficult to explain to you what you can and can't do. (training day – tape)

The extract begins with an explicit attempt to differentiate the support worker contribution from that of qualified staff. Notice the way in which the nurse emphasises that the role of HCAs is to assist the registered nurse and the explicit statement that they will not be doing 'the registered nurse's job' which, in this instance, is formulated in terms of 'assessment'. There are also clear parallels with the boundary-work we observed in relation to the nursing-medical interface. For example, the senior nurse's appeal to the indeterminacy of nursing skills – '[a]ssessment is a very fine line and it makes it very difficult to explain to you what you can and can't do' – which she contrasts with the narrow technical role of support staff – 'if all that is needed is a number.' In the same way as the medical staff attempted to diminish the nursing contribution to that of technician, the senior nurse imputes a subordinate role to HCAs: 'If you're in a position to assess, then you're in the wrong position.'

DISCUSSION AND CONCLUSIONS

In this article, I have examined the boundary-work nurse managers employed in accommodating jurisdictional change at the medical-nursing and nursing-support worker interfaces. I have argued that these processes may be understood as micro-political strategies through which work identities and occupational margins are negotiated. I have described the practices through which nurse managers attempted to accomplish professional autonomy by taking charge of the realignment of the medical-nursing interface and the development of training packages for nurses. We also saw how the support worker role was defined in ways which prevented them from developing an area of autonomous practice. Additionally, I have highlighted the rhetorical devices field actors employed in talking their work boundaries and the demarcatory and identity work purposes to which they were oriented. Nurses employed a discourse of holism which differentiated their approach to care from that of medicine, whereas doctors' accounts were linguistically assembled in order to cast nurses in the subordinate role of technician. Nurse managers employed an analogous type of rhetoric in relation to the nurse-support worker interface. HCAs were constituted as mere technicians lacking theoretical knowledge in contrast to the indeterminacy of nursing practice.

The empirical focus of this article is relatively unusual within the tradition of interactionist studies of hospital work because it centers on the social production of work boundaries in organisational arenas other than the 'shop floor.' As Dingwall and Strong (1997) have observed, if one focuses solely on the activities of grassroots personnel, there is a danger of missing the coordinating and disciplining devices which bind their actions together. I have concentrated on what is micro-sociologically interesting in the finegrain of nurse managers' boundary-work and for what they reveal of the interpretative horizons (Gubrium and Holstein 1995) and discursive domains within which they practice. As I have indicated, however, the study also examined the negotiation of work roles at the ward level and it seems appropriate in bringing this article to a close to briefly comment on the relationship between the social production of work boundaries in these two domains.

Like the nurse managers, ward nurses also expressed concern about the general thrust of national policy, yet they accomplished their work with little explicit face-to-face negotiation of jurisdiction or reference to formal organisational rules. Moreover, contrary to the situation in the management arena, there was little evidence of overt boundary disputes at ward level in respect of the changes which were taking place.

One way of understanding these findings is in terms of the extent to which formal role realignment had been preempted at ward level in the informal work practices developed by staff in response to the daily requirements of practice. For example, the social organisation of ward work at Woodlands frequently created space for experienced nurses to exert influence over junior doctors in relation to treatment decisions and led to them informally undertaking certain 'medical tasks' (Allen 1997).

> I do blood forms and things like that even though I know I shouldn't. Because it's an easier life and I know things are going to get done. (Interview – Junior Sister)

Boundary blurring was also a routine feature of the nurse-support worker interface. The organisation had a long history of staff shortages and this had resulted in experienced auxiliaries informally extending the scope of their practice to include many of the activities assigned to the new HCA role. Moreover, nursing care was organised according to routines which resulted in support workers frequently working without supervision.

> HCA: [Y]ou get a lot of pressure – because you're the ones that are actually with the patients, so they [nurses] come to you all the time and asking you if the patient's all right (HCA training day – Tape)

Clearly, this routine breaching of jurisdictional boundaries was not without limits, but it is difficult to assess the extent to which staff oriented to the formal organisational plan as an external constraint on action. Ward personnel certainly shared many of the discursive resources employed by nursing managers. Nurses made reference to support staff having an inadequate knowledge to undertake certain activities, and HCAs, nurses, and doctors all employed a vocabulary of 'risk' in talking about role change. Furthermore, on occasion, staff also employed explicit 'vocabularies of structure' (Meyer and Rowan 1977: 349) in explaining their work practices. Nevertheless, they also had access to alternative discourses which were not shared by nurse managers and which were more frequently used in accounting for their actions. For example, they were more likely to refer to personal skills and experience and invoke the rhetoric of 'a fair wage' in legitimating the edges of their practice than they were the formal organisational rules.

> I would decide individually not as a job, not as a 'Well, she's a D grade staff or she's a health care assistant'; I would take it as who they are and what experience they've got behind them. (interview, junior sister)
> She told me that sister had decided that because the auxiliaries and HCAs removed catheters and IVs, then they might as well amend the care

plans . . . She said . . . 'I don't see why I should take on that sort of responsibility when I'm not paid for it.' (field notes)

One way of conceptualising organisations is as a configuration of interrelated interpretative domains comprised of the 'local knowledge' (Garfinkel 1967; Geertz 1983;
Gubrium 1989, all cited by Miller 1997) that setting members employ in making sense
of their experiences (Miller 1997). These 'normative frameworks' (Gubrium 1988)
furnish discursive resources through which social reality is routinely interpreted and
accomplished. In this study, although members of the same organisation and profession, nurse managers and ward-level staff were clearly located within separate
interpretative domains or 'social worlds' (Strauss 1982). They had disparate interests,
priorities, and concerns; access to different vocabularies of motive; and operated
within different constraints. This led them to accomplish jurisdiction in distinctive
ways: nurse managers were concerned with the social production of formal organisation and related professional issues, whereas ward staff were preoccupied with the
practical accomplishment of caring for the sick.

It may be difficult to explicate the precise nature of the relationship between the
social constitution of jurisdiction in these different domains in the study in question,
but what these data do indicate is that the interactional accomplishment of work
boundaries is profoundly situated. Heimer (1998) has suggested that frontline workers are far more likely to comply with regulatory structures when they are closely
articulated with indigenously developed organisational routines. The degree of fit
between the formal and social organisation of work is therefore crucial. Further sociological research is clearly needed in order to identify the different interpretative
realms in which work roles are routinely produced and the way in which these different normative frameworks are articulated in the doing of demarcation. Only then
can we hope to develop a better understanding of their interrelationships in hospital
workplace settings and beyond.

AUTHOR'S NOTE

The study on which this article draws was supported by a Department of Health Nursing and
Therapists Research Training Award. The views expressed here are my own and do not represent
those of the Department of Health. Thanks are due to Professor Robert Dingwall (School of
Sociology and Social Policy) and Professor Veronica James (School of Nursing and Midwifery
Studies) at the University of Nottingham, who supervised the original research. I am also grateful to Professor Robert Dingwall, Professor Julia Evetts, Rob Benford, and three anonymous
reviewers for their helpful comments on earlier drafts of the manuscript. I would also like to
express my gratitude to the research participants who found time in their busy lives to talk to
me; without their support none of this would have been possible. An earlier version of this article was presented at the BSA Medical Sociological Group Annual Conference, University of
York, September 1998.

NOTES

Journal of Contemporary Ethnography 29 (3): 325–355. Reprinted by permission of Sage Publications.

1 The United Kingdom Central Council for Nursing, Midwifery and Health Visiting (UKCC) is a statutory body responsible for the establishment of standards for training and professional conduct and the protection of the public from unsafe practice. It is charged with the responsibility for maintaining a single register of all practitioners and determining the conditions of entry. It is supported by four national boards of the four countries of the UK: England, Wales, Scotland, and Northern Ireland, who all have responsibility for implementing the policies and rules of the UKCC.

2 Prior to the Project 2000 reforms nurses could undertake a two-year-hospital-based training to become an enrolled nurse or three years to become a registered nurse, although there was a growing number of college-based degree programs. The SEN/RGN distinction in the UK has parallels with the LPN/RN distinction in the U.S.

3 In the past, the need to deliver nursing care with a variable skill mix – qualified staff and learners at different stages of training – had resulted in the development of a system of hierarchical task allocation. This skills hierarchy was implicitly based on a medical model. Junior nurses were allocated all hands-on care activities and senior staff undertook medically derived technical tasks and ward management. New Nursing aimed to replace this with a patient-centered model of care in which all patient-care needs are provided by one nurse, and the value of intimate tending was underlined.

4 This is a generic – non-nursing – accrediting body responsible for a wide range of work-based vocational and technical education.

5 In the UK, junior doctors are those doctors in training – preregistration house officers, senior house officers, registrar and senior registrar. This is roughly equivalent to interns in the U.S.

6 A District General Hospital is a nonteaching hospital which provides a range of services to a local population.

7 Trust hospitals were established in the UK as a result of the 1990 National Health Service and Community Care Act. Hospitals and community units which were able to satisfy specified management criteria were allowed to apply for self-governing status. They remained publicly owned but were, in theory, no longer subject to direct bureaucratic control by the NHS. Services were provided under contract to the National Health Service purchasers in an arms-length relationship (Le Grand 1990).

8 These figures do not add up because one person was interviewed more than once and two auxiliaries were interviewed together.

9 The involvement of doctors in general management is a relatively new feature of health care systems in the UK. Medical dominance (Freidson 1970) has long presented problems for health service governance on both sides of the Atlantic and the introduction of general management into the NHS in the 1980s was in large measure an attempt to control doctors (Strong and Robinson 1990). When attempts to bring doctors under the sphere of influence of general managers brought only limited success, the reverse tactic of involving doctors in management was introduced (Packwood et al. 1991). The extent to which these developments have been successful in incorporating doctors into the new management ethos remains empirically moot.

10 Similar arguments were made in the U.S. in the 1970s. Nurses' initial resistance to the development of the nurse practitioner role was overcome in the face of the threat posed to them by the development of the non-nursing physician's assistant role.

11 I am grateful to Lesley Griffiths for drawing my attention to Shotter's work.

REFERENCES

Abbott, A. 1988. *The system of professions: An essay on the division of expert labor*. Chicago: University of Chicago Press.

Allen, D. 1996. The shape of general hospital nursing: The division of labour at work. Unpublished PhD thesis. University of Nottingham.

Allen, D. 1997. The doctor-nurse boundary: A negotiated order? *Sociology of Health and Illness* 19 (4):498–520.

Allen D., and D. Hughes. 1993. Going for growth. *The Health Service Journal* 103 (5372):33–34.

Anspach, R. R. 1987. Prognostic conflict in life-and-death decisions: The organization as an ecology of knowledge. *Journal of Health and Social Behavior* 28:215–231.

Anspach, R. R. 1993. *Deciding who lives: Fateful choices in the intensive-care nursery*. Los Angeles: University of California Press.

Antaki, C. and S. Widdicombe., eds. 1998. *Identities in talk*. London: Sage Ltd.

Beardshaw, V., and R. Robinson. 1990. *New for old? Prospects for nursing in the 1990s*. London: Kings Fund Institute.

Benson, J. K. 1977a. Organizations: A dialectic view. *Administrative Science Quarterly* 18:5–18.

Benson, J. K. 1977b. Innovation and crisis in organizational analysis. *Sociological Quarterly*. 18: 5–18.

Benson, J. K.. 1978. Reply to Maines. *The Sociological Quarterly* 19:497–501.

Bosk, C. L. 1979. *Forgive and remember: Managing medical mistakes*. Chicago: The University of Chicago Press.

Brown, P. 1989. Psychiatric dirty work revisited: Conflicts in servicing nonpsychiatric agencies. *Journal of Contemporary Ethnography* 18 (2):182–201.

Burgess, R. G. 1984. *Into the field: An introduction to field research*. London and New York: Routledge.

Carpenter, M. 1993. The subordination of nurses in health care: Towards a social divisions approach. In *Gender work and medicine: Women and the medical division of labour*, edited by E. Riska and K. Wegar, 96–130. London: Sage Ltd.

Chambliss, D. 1997. *Beyond caring: Hospitals, nurses and the social organization of ethics*. Chicago: University of Chicago Press.

Cohan, M. 1997. Political identities and political landscapes: Men's narrative work in relation to women's issues. *The Sociological Quarterly* 32 (2):303–319.

Davies, C. 1995. *Gender and the professional predicament in nursing*. Buckingham: Open University Press.

Day, R. A., and J. V. Day. 1977. A review of the current state of negotiated order theory: An appreciation and critique. *Sociological Quarterly* 18:126–142.

Day, R. A., and J. V. Day. 1978. Reply to Maines. *The Sociological Quarterly* 19:499–501.

Department of Health and Social Security. 1983. *Inquiry into NHS management* (The Griffiths Report). London: HMSO.

Department of Health and Social Security. 1987. *Hospital medical staff (Achieving a balance) @ 151 Plan for action*. Health Circular 87, 25. London: HMSO.

Department of Health. 1989. *Working for patients: The health service caring for the 1990s*. London: HMSO.

Dingwall, R. 1977. Atrocity stories and professional relationships. *Sociology of Work and Occupations* 4:317–96.

Dingwall, R. 1980. Orchestrated encounters: A comparative analysis of speech-exchange systems. *Sociology of Health and Illness* 2:151–173.

Dingwall, R., A. M. Rafferty, and C. Webster. 1988. *An introduction to the social history of nursing*. London: Routledge.

Dingwall, R., and P. M. Strong. 1997. The interactional study of organizations: A critique and reformulation. In *Context and method in qualitative research*, edited by G. Miller and R. Dingwall, 139–154. London: Sage Ltd.

Emerson. R., and M. Pollner. 1976. Dirty work designations: Their features and consequences in a psychiatric setting. *Social Problems* 23:243–54.

Evers, H. 1982. Professional practice and patient care: Multidisciplinary teamwork in geriatric wards. *Ageing and Society* 2:57–76.

Friedson, E. 1970. *Medical dominance*. Chicago: Aldine.

Friedson, E. 1976. The division of labor as social interaction. *Social Problems* 23:304–13.

Garfinkel, H. 1967. *Studies in ethnomethodology*. Engelwood Cliffs, NJ: Prentice Hall.

Geerts, C. 1983. *Local knowledge*. New York: Basic Books.

General Medical Council. 1993. T*omorrow's doctors*. London: GMC.

Giddens, A. 1979. *Central problems in social theory: Action, structure and contradiction in social analysis*. London: Macmillan.

Gieryn, T. 1983. 'Boundary-work' and the demarcation of science from non-science: Strains and interests in professional ideologies of scientists. *American Sociological Review* 48:781–895.

Gieryn, T. 1999. *Cultural boundaries of science: Credibility on the line*. Chicago: The University of Chicago Press.

Glaser, B., and A. S. Strauss. 1964. Awareness contexts and social interaction. *American Sociological Review* 29:669–79.

Goffman, E. 1959. *The presentation of self in everyday life*. Harmondsworth, Middlesex: Penguin Books.

Gubrium, J. 1988. *Analyzing field realities*. Beverly Hills, CA: Sage.

Gubrium, J. 1989. Local cultures and service policy. In *The politics of field research*, edited by J. F. Gubrium and D. Silverman, 94–112. London: Sage Ltd.

Gubrium, J., and J. A. Holstein 1995. Biographical work and new ethnography. In *Interpreting experience: The narrative study of lives*, edited by R. E. Josselson and A. Llieblich, 27–44. Thousand Oaks, CA: Sage.

Guillemin, J. H., and L. L. Holmstrom. 1986. *Mixed blessings: Intensive care for newborns*. New York: Oxford University Press.

Heimer, C.A. 1998. The routinization of responsiveness: Regulatory compliance and the construction of organizational routines. *American Bar Foundation Working Paper*: 9801.

Hughes, D. 1980. The ambulance journey as an information generating process. *Sociology of Health and Illness* 2 (2):115–132.

Hughes, D. 1988. When nurse knows best: Some aspects of nurse/doctor interaction in a casualty department. *Sociology of Health and Illness* 10 (1):1–22.

Hughes, E. C. 1984. *The sociological eye*. New Brunswick, NJ: Transaction Books.

Hunt, S. A., and R. D. Benford. 1994. Identity talk in the peace and justice movement. *Journal of Contemporary Ethnography* 22 (4):488–517.

Jamous, H., and B. Peloille. 1970. Changes in the French university-hospital system. In *Professions and professionalization*, edited by J. A. Jackson, 111–154. Cambridge: Cambridge University Press.

Le Grand, J. 1990. *Quasi-markets and social policy*. Bristol: School for Advanced Urban Studies.

Maines, D. R. 1977. Social organization and social structure in symbolic interactionist thought. *Annual Review of Sociology* 3:235–59.

Maines, D. R., and J. C. Charlton. 1985. The negotiated order approach to the analysis of social organization. In *Foundations of interpretative sociology: Original essays in symbolic interaction.* Studies in symbolic interaction, supplement 1, edited by H. A. Faberman and R. S. Perinbanayagam, 271–308. London: JAI.

Mesler, M. A. 1989. Negotiated order and the clinical pharmacist: The ongoing process of structure. *Symbolic Interaction* 12 (1):139–157.

Mesler, M. A. 1991. Boundary encroachment and task delegation: Clinical pharmacists on the medical team. *Sociology of Health and Illness* 13 (3):310–331.

Meyer, J. W., and B. Rowan. 1977. Institutionalized organizations: Formal structure as myth and ceremony. *American Journal of Sociology* 83:340–363.

Miller, G. 1997. Towards ethnographies of institutional discourse: Proposals and suggestions. In *Context and method in qualitative research,* edited by G. Miller and R. Dingwall, 155–171. London: Sage Ltd.

Miller, G., and J. A. Holstein. 1993. Disputing in organizations: Dispute domains and interaction process. *Mid-American Review of Sociology* XVII 2:1–18.

Millman, M. 1976. *The unkindest cut: Life in the backrooms of medicine.* New York: William Morrow.

Naish, J. 1993. Power, politics and peril. In *Project 2000: Reflection and celebration,* edited by B. Dolan, 17–29. London: Scutari Press.

National Health Service Management Executive. 1991. *Junior doctors: The new deal.* London: NHSME.

Packwood, T., J. Keen, and M. Buxton. 1991. *Hospitals in transition: The resource management experiment.* Milton Keynes, UK: Open University Press.

Paton, C. 1993. Devolution and centralism in the National Health Service. *Social Policy and Administration* 27 (2):83–108.

Phelan, M. P., and S. A. Hunt. 1998. Prison gang members' tattoos as identity work: The visual communication of moral careers. *Symbolic Interaction* 21 (3): 277–298.

Porter, S. 1991. A participant observation study of power relations between nurses and doctors in a general hospital. *Journal of Advanced Nursing* 16:728–735.

Rafferty, A. M. 1992. Nursing policy and the nationalization of nursing: The representation of 'crisis' and the 'crisis' of representation. In *Policy issues in nursing,* edited by J. Robinson, A. Gray, and R. Elkan, 63–83. Milton Keynes: Open University Press.

Rafferty, A. M. 1996. *The politics of nursing knowledge.* London: Routledge.

Robinson, J. 1992. Introduction: beginning the study of nursing policy. In *Policy issues in nursing,* edited by J. Robinson, A. Gray, and R. Elkan, 1–8. Milton Keynes: Open University Press.

Rosenfeld, D. 1999. Identity work among lesbian and gay elderly. *Journal of Aging Studies* 13 (2):121–144.

Rosenthal, C., R. S. Marshall, A. S. Macpherson, and S. E. French. 1980. *Nurses, patients and families.* London: Croom Helm.

Roth, J. and D. J. Douglas. 1983. *No appointment necessary: The hospital emergency department in the medical services world.* New York: Irvington.

Shotter, J. 1993. *Conversational realities: Constructing life through language.* London: Sage Ltd.

Snow, D. A. and L. Anderson. 1987. Identity work among the homeless: The verbal construction and avowal of personal identities. *American Journal of Sociology* 92 (6):1336–71.

Strauss, A. L. 1978. *Negotiations: Varieties, contexts, processes and social order.* London: Jossey-Bass.

Strauss. A. L. (1982) Social worlds and their segmentation processes. *Studies in Symbolic Interaction* 5:123–139.

Strauss, A. L., S. Fagerhaugh, and B. Suczet. 1985. *Social organization of medical work.* Chicago: University of Chicago Press.

Strauss, A. L., L. Schatzman, D. Ehrlich, R. Bucher, and M. Sabshin. 1963. The hospital and its negotiated order. In *The hospital in modern society*, edited by E. Friedson, 147–169. New York: Free Press.

Strauss, A. L., L. Schatzman, R. Bucher, D. Ehrlich, and M. Sabshin. 1964. *Psychiatric ideologies and institutions.* London: Free Press.

Strong, P. and J. Robinson. 1990. *The NHS under new management.* Milton Keynes: Open University Press.

Sudnow, D. 1967. *Passing on.* Englewood Cliffs, NJ: Prentice-Hall.

Svensson, R. 1996. The interplay between doctors and nurses – a negotiated order perspective. *Sociology of Health and Illness* 18:379–98.

Taylor, C. 1970. *In horizontal orbit: Hospitals and the cult of efficiency.* New York: Holt, Rhinehart and Winston.

United Kingdom Central Council for Nursing, Midwifery and Health Visiting. 1987. *Project 2000: The final proposals.* London: Author.

United Kingdom Central Council for Nursing, Midwifery and Health Visiting. 1992. *The scope of professional practice.* London: Author.

Zerubavel, E. 1979. *Patterns of time in hospital life.* Chicago: University of Chicago Press.

Chapter 12

Towards a more holistic conceptualisation of caring

M. NOLAN, G. GRANT, J. KEADY

Introduction

There are probably few more emotive and delicate subjects for discussion than the caring that goes on within families – for example, between a parent and a child with a disability or a child caring for an aged frail parent. There are also few more invisible subjects to investigate. This invisibility is a major problem for research because research proceeds upon the principle of visibility. The unarticulated only becomes a visible, workable entity for the researcher after its existence is hypothesised, some instrument is designed to detect its presence and it is fitted into certain categories, compared with other entities and made to do work for the researcher. And classification itself inevitably considers as identical, entities that are, in some respect of less interest to the classifier, quite dissimilar.

In this chapter Mike Nolan, Gordon Grant and John Keady turn their attention to the subject of family caring, and are at pains to deal with it in the most sensitive way. They draw on many years of data they have collected from a variety of family carers in a range of different – and often difficult – circumstances to develop an understanding that does justice to its often elusive character. They argue the need for this work by suggesting that much previous analysis has emphasised instrumental aspects of caring, tending to focus on the practical, 'hands-on' help provided by a carer. Of course, as they acknowledge, some writers have understood and formalised the emotional aspects of caring, some have classified carers according the their degree of immersion in their role as carer, and some, taking a more philosophical perspective, have understood the ability to care as a fundamental human characteristic.

Nolan and his colleagues develop the categories originally derived by Bowers from her work with carers in the 1980s to propose a new understanding of the subtleties of family care-giving. They propose the following categories and, in the extract from their chapter which follows, they give examples of various components in operation:

- anticipatory care
- preventive care
- supervisory care
- instrumental care
- protective care
- preservative care
- (re)constructive care
- reciprocal care

The difficulty of investigating the topic may become clear from their view of family caring as, 'a delicate and dynamic process of negotiation in which the family history and biography interact, resulting in "the development of commitments" over time'. The meaning and significance of any action cannot be separated from the issue of intention. For example, sometimes cared-for persons may be excluded from some discussions in order to protect their sense of independence, but sometimes in order to disempower them. One characteristic of caring, they suggest, involves the subtleties of negotiation aimed at providing help before a request for help needs to be made. In other words Nolan and colleagues realise, to put it simply, that caring cannot be understood in sole relation to what carers do — this certainly would not accord with what carers them- selves say — because much caring does not include overt behaviour.

Interestingly, when the authors turn to look briefly at professional caring, they find even less clarity about its meaning. This in spite of the fact that nursing 'probably lays greatest claim to base itself on an ethos of care'. As with family care-giving, profes- sional care has been seen as multi-dimensional; behavioural, moral, cognitive and emotional, with strong cultural influences on all of these dimensions. They also note a striking resemblance between the outcome of a review of different definitions of professional caring (undertaken by Janice Morse) and the characteristics of family carers. Yet, they argue, the notion that a family care-giver has to be 'competent' to deliver care is rarely addressed.

In the passage that follows, Nolan and colleagues give examples of their categories in action. In some instances they report what appear to be quite gross failures of professional care, as reported by the family members of people who have suffered them. They argue, convincingly, that more in-depth knowledge of the character of family caring on the part of caring professionals may have forestalled some of these failures.

NOLAN, M., G. GRANT AND J. KEADY (1996)

Towards a more holistic conceptualisation of caring*

What is this thing some call caregiving?

(Gubrium 1995: 268)

In the introduction to a special edition of *Qualitative Health Research*, focusing on the topic of 'The Caregiver Relationship', Jaber Gubrium (1995) 'takes stock' of the existing state of knowledge in the field of caregiving. Although succinct, the text is insightful and cogent, posing a number of fundamental questions, the most telling of which is quoted above. For whilst Gubrium acknowledges the extensive literature on caregiving he bemoans the fact that much of what has emerged from several years of study does not capture adequately the nuances of caring but instead 'second-guesses' the lived experience of carers by relying primarily on a causal modelling approach. The way towards a better understanding is, he argues, 'definitely not more of the same'. He signals the need for a critical assessment, not simply another literature review, which attempts a deconstruction of the taken-for-granted language of caregiving, including the term 'caregiving' itself. Others have also taken a similar view (Langer 1993; Opie 1994; Brody 1995), recognising that whilst the terms 'caring' and 'caregiving' have been extensively used, they remain poorly defined (Abrams 1985; Bulmer 1987; Arber and Ginn 1990).

It is the intention of this chapter to outline an alternative perspective on caregiving and to present a reconceptualisation of the differing types of care first described by Bowers (1987, 1988). This revised and extended typology is based on a reanalysis of several years of data collected by the authors from a variety of family carers providing care both to individuals with learning difficulties and to older people with varying forms of physical and/or cognitive frailty. The chapter begins with a brief overview of the ways in which both family and professional caring are currently construed, highlighting in particular the instrumental focus that dominates service ideologies. This is followed by a consideration of how responsibilities are negotiated within 'normal family' life as described by Finch and Mason (1993), providing a backcloth to Bowers's work and our revision of it. The chapter concludes by addressing the implications of an alternative conceptualisation of caring for the planning and delivery of services.

CARING: OFTEN USED, RARELY DEFINED

Although the above question posed by Gubrium appears deceptively simple, providing a comprehensive answer is much more complex. This challenge was identified several years ago by Bulmer (1987), who noted that whilst the meaning of care is intuitively fairly obvious, the types of help, support and protection it connotes are far from clear. Parker (1981), in attempting to disentangle care, draws a distinction between 'care' which can be construed as 'caring about' – as for example in generalised 'concern for' another person, in expressed emotion, or perhaps in financial donations and gift-giving – and 'care' as expressed in 'tending', as seen in more practical 'hands-on' terms. Survey studies typically concentrate on the latter. Green's (1988) national sample survey, for example, categorised the tasks of informal care into personal care, physical help, help with paperwork and finances, 'other practical help', keeping the person company, taking the person out, giving medicine and surveillance. These were used as the basis of the secondary analysis carried out by Parker and Lawton (1994) which, following a cluster analysis, resulted in six mutually exclusive categories of care: personal *and* physical care, personal *not* physical care, physical *not* personal care, other practical help, practical help only and other help. What emerges nevertheless is a largely instrumental model of caring.

Parker and Lawton alluded to other possibilities for developing a typology of caring activity based on the characteristics of the carers or of those being cared for, the nature of the caring activity or some combination of these. They also noted that 'tending' activity can be defined in terms of timing, frequency, urgency, complexity and how long tasks take. Context also provided another set of parameters such as the nature of impairment, the level of responsibility carried by the carer and so on. The primary purpose behind their reanalysis of Green's data, however, was to distance caring from its social or relational context.

Like Parker and Lawton, other writers have noted the lack of a comprehensive model for understanding family care and have attempted to extend how it may be visualised, though what emerges is not dissimilar to Parker's (1981) earlier description. Qureshi (1986) sees caring in two dimensions of practical tending and catering to social and emotional needs. Pearlin *et al.* (1990) suggest that caring is best taken as referring to the affective component whereas the term 'caregiving' more closely describes the behavioural aspects. Bulmer (1987) includes both affective and practical domains but suggests that caring also involves a more generalised concern for the welfare of others. The dual focus suggested by these commentators has perhaps been the most pervasive within British family care studies.

On a more philosophical level, Griffin (1983) contends that caring is a primary mode of being, a fundamental concept in our understanding of what constitutes human nature, a point captured by Benner and Wruebel (1989), who suggest that caring is 'the most basic way of being in the world'. This possibly helps to explain why people have been reported to continue providing care in the absence of affection (Qureshi 1986). Other studies have emphasised a categorisation of care and carers based on a hierarchy of obligations, responsibilities and position in the life-cycle (Ungerson 1987; Qureshi and Walker 1989; Finch and Mason 1993), which may give rise to a set of informal rules by which individuals assume responsibility for the care of other family members.

Some writers have cast their ideas about care within the context of social support, viewing care as no more than an integral part or extension of ordinary interpersonal relationships. Based on how ordinary people construct ideas about the issue, Kahn and Antonucci (1980) for example have defined social support in terms of the three As: namely affect (caring and emotional intimacy), affirmation (provision of information about the rightness or wrongness of one's actions or thoughts) and aid (direct help through money, time and effort). Barrera and Ainlay (1983) discuss six categories of support drawn from a content analysis of reviewed research papers: material aid, behavioural assistance, intimate interaction, guidance, feedback and positive social interaction. Although taking definitional parameters beyond a concern with the instrumental, these studies are still primarily concerned with care as a set of tasks or activities.

Some have taken the analogy between care and a set of tasks or activities a stage further and used the metaphor of labour or work to categorise what carers do. Arber and Ginn (1995) for example cite James (1992), who describes caring in terms of three essential components:

- physical labour
- emotional labour
- organisational/managerial labour.

Arber and Ginn (1995) note that whilst physical labour is the most obvious and visible form of caring, the latter two are likely to be more important to the quality of life of an elderly cared-for person. Others have commented on the 'hard physical labour' component of caring (Bulmer 1987; Lewis and Meredith 1989; Twigg and Atkin 1994) but have also reasserted that caring is about more than just physical work. Lewis and Meredith (1989) consider that caring may also involve loving attention, and that for some carers it constitutes both an activity and a source of identity.

An appreciation of the role of emotional or affective components is clearly central to a more complete understanding of caregiving, although the emotions engendered are often mixed and may comprise such conflicting reactions as love, guilt, compassion and gratitude (Ungerson 1987), stirring both ambiguous and ambivalent feelings (Lewis and Meredith 1988a,b). Twigg and Atkin (1994) add another dimension to this already potent mixture, that relating to a perceived sense of responsibility whereby a carer becomes the 'arbiter of standards'. Indeed these authors go as far as to suggest that such a sense of responsibility may be the 'core feature that underpins all caregiving'. We will pursue this in more detail later, as the notion of carers maintaining and monitoring excellence in care is one that has considerable empirical support. Recognition of this is important, as the perceived ownership of expertise greatly influences the interactions between family and professional carers.

From a different but related perspective others have attempted to delineate various types of *caregiver* as opposed to the components of care itself. Lewis and Meredith (1989) for instance differentiate between carers who adopt a *balanced* mode in which they are able to combine caregiving with other important parts of their lives such as paid employment. They compared this type of carer with those who *integrated* caring into their lives, with caring providing a sense of purpose and of satisfaction. The third category Lewis and Meredith describe is caregivers who become *immersed*, who invest heavily in caregiving and find it extremely difficult to disentangle themselves. According to Lewis and Meredith, the consequences for carers vary depending upon which caregiving position they occupy. The most negative effect is experienced by the immersed carer.

There are considerable conceptual similarities between the categories defined

Table 12.1 Definitions of a carer

Date	Source	Definition
1982	Equal Opportunities Commission	Anyone who looks after or cares for a handicapped person to any extent in their own home or elsewhere.
1984	Social Work Services Development Group	A person who takes prime responsibility in the home care of a person who, because of handicap or illness, needs almost continuous care.
1988	Green	A person looking after or providing some form of regular service for a sick, handicapped or elderly person living in their own or another household.
1990	Braithwaite	People who assume the major responsibility for providing caregiving services on a regular basis to someone who is incapable of providing for him/herself.
1991	Social Services Inspectorate	A person who is not employed to provide the care in question by anybody in the exercise of its function under any enactment. Normally, this will be a person who is looking after another adult in the home who is frail, ill and/or mentally or physically disabled, and where the dependency relationship 'exceeds that implicit in normally dependent relationships' between family members.
1995	British Medical Association	A carer is someone who gives unpaid care to a relative or friend who is dependent because of age, physical or other disability and who would, if not cared for, require support from the state or other means.

above and those outlined by Twigg and Atkin (1994), namely: the *engulfed* carer who subordinates their life to that of the disabled person; the carer who is able to *balance / set boundaries* and the carer who is able to construct a *symbiotic* relationship from which they gain positive benefits. The affective domains of caregiving described earlier by Opie (1994) of commitment, dissociation, obligation and repudiation also have clear parallels with those of Lewis and Meredith (1989) and Twigg and Atkin (1994).

The obvious diversity and complexity of caring has led some observers to the conclusion that the search for a single 'dichotomous' definition that distinguishes a carer from a non-carer is 'over ambitious and probably futile' (Arber and Ginn 1990). Yet all too often such a definition is sought. Table 12.1 presents a number of definitions of a carer that have emerged over the last 15 years. Whilst there is variation in the relative emphasis within these definitions, they are all consistent in that their primary focus is on the instrumental aspects of caring. In terms of service provision it seems that Twigg and Atkin (1994) were correct in their belief that physical dependency is the defining feature of family caregiving. It is just such a view that we seek to counter. However, before proceeding to outline an alternative view of family caring, we want to look at what is meant by professional caring. Such a consideration is necessary if a better understanding of the interface between family and professional care is to emerge.

THE NATURE OF PROFESSIONAL CARE

If there is uncertainty about a definition of the nature of family caring, the meaning and components of professional care are equally unclear. The nursing profession probably lays greatest claim to base itself on an ethos of care; a brief consideration of the extensive literature on this subject brings into sharp relief the areas of similarity and contrast between family and professional caring.

The concept of caring has been the subject of considerable scrutiny within the nursing literature and yet despite extensive usage, its meaning, as with family care, is uncertain (Radsma 1994; Fealy 1995; Kyle 1995; Scott 1995). Radsma (1994) notes the linguistically ambiguous position of caring, suggesting that it can be used as both a noun, as in home care, and a verb, as in caregiving. Mirroring Bulmer (1987), she comments on the intuitive appeal of the concept, reflected in feelings of warmth, respect, nurturance and regard. Interestingly, there is also considerable concern within the nursing literature about the emphasis on the tasks of caring and the relative neglect of the less tangible emotional components (Radsma 1994; Kyle 1995; Scott 1995). As with family caregiving, nursing care is seen as complex, comprising a number of elements. These are defined by Kyle (1995) as behavioural, moral, cognitive and emotional, with each element also being culturally and contextually bound (Fealy 1995; Kyle 1995). Fundamentally, however, the essence of nursing care is the belief that the person who is the recipient of care in some way 'matters' (Nikkonen 1994; Fealy 1995; Scott 1995). 'The widest basis on which one cares for another is that the other is a fellow human being, worthy of dignity and respect. This is crucial to all caring' (Fealy 1995: 136).

Scott (1995) describes good professional care as 'constructive' care, the achievement of which requires both competence in the physical (clinical and technical) aspects *and* humaneness, sensitivity and compassion. This contention provides a most interesting comparison because although there are obvious similarities between the definitions of family and professional care so far considered, the notion that a family carer has in some way to be 'competent' to deliver care is rarely formally addressed – this is an issue that we shall return to at a number of points later in the book.

In synthesising the requirements for acceptable professional care, Kitson (1987) identifies three criteria: respect for the person; an ability and willingness to care; and the possession of the necessary knowledge, skills and attitudes. However, it seems that such criteria are not seen as essential for family care. Qureshi (1986) for example describes how affection is not a necessary condition for family care, although in its absence caring is more difficult. In drawing comparisons between caring for a parent and child care it seems very likely that if a parent was not considered to have affection for her child and was deemed to lack the skills of parenting then considerable concern would be voiced. However, with regard to the care of older people, whilst the absence of affection and/or skills might be noted, it hardly seems to raise the same level of professional concern. It is interesting to speculate as to whether this is a manifestation of ageist attitudes, a desire not to interfere in family life or simply ignoring the issues for fear of the potential consequences in terms of the availability of family care.

Returning to professional caring, Morse *et al.* (1990), in undertaking a synthesis of 35 definitions of caring from the literature, outlined five main perspectives, defining care as either: an affective response; a human trait; a moral imperative; a therapeutic intervention or an interpersonal interaction. The similarities between such dimensions and family caregiving are apparent as, with the exception of care as a 'therapeutic intervention', the other criteria span both professional and family care. Yet, much of what family caregivers do could be seen to constitute a therapeutic intervention. This 'therapeutic' element will become apparent when we describe the satisfactions of caring in Chapter 4. At this point it is sufficient to note that although family carers might not use the term 'therapeutic', this is often their intent. It therefore seems that the differences between professional and family caregiving are not as great as might be thought, apart from the fact that one group is formally trained and usually quite well paid, and the other is not. As Twigg and Atkin (1994) note, recent feminist perspectives on care have much emphasised the notion of payment for family care.

Bond (1992) argues that it is time to 'professionalise' family caring, not in the 'traditional' sense but to the extent that 'the skills used by caregivers are valued in themselves, to be encouraged and improved' (p. 18). The concept of carer 'expertise' (Nolan and Grant 1992a) will be developed in greater detail later in this chapter.

From this brief overview of both family and professional caring, it seems that analytically they are characterised more by what they have in common than by how they differ. Both are seen to consist of a number of like attributes, some visible and obvious, some subtle and invisible. Moreover, there is concern in both the family and professional caring literature that it is the visible, physical components of care that are most recognised, whilst the less tangible but more important aspects are given tacit acknowledgement at best.

FAMILY CARE: WIDENING HORIZONS

A useful starting point in developing a broader conceptualisation of family caring is to look at the way in which responsibilities are negotiated in 'ordinary families' who are not providing care. In unpacking the manner in which help and assistance is organised within such families, Finch and Mason (1993) assert 'with some certainty' that there is no clear consensus about the division of responsibility nor are there universal normative rules. Rather a delicate and dynamic process of negotiation occurs in which the family history and biography interact, resulting in the 'development of commitments' over time. They identify a number of key components to the negotiation process, foremost amongst which are reciprocity and balance. The intention of these activities is to maintain as far as possible family perceptions of independence. To achieve this, negotiations are often tacit and implicit, rather than being open and explicit. Indeed, Finch and Mason (1993: 71) contend that often the potential recipient of help is deliberately excluded from discussions to protect their sense of independence: 'There is an analytic distinction between exclusions which are intended to protect people . . . and those which are intended to disempower.'

It is therefore the context and meaning of such exclusions that are paramount rather than the act itself. In other words it is not the *task* that is important but the *purpose* or *intent* behind it. Similar subtle processes underlie the maintenance of reciprocity and the giving of and asking for help, which is seen to involve much more than 'simply doing the tasks' (p. 93). A delicate balance is achieved between the offer of help and having to ask for it. Most people consider it wrong to expect help as a right, but having to ask for help is also seen as something to be avoided if possible. In situations where the need for help is therefore apparent, offering to provide it before someone has to ask is the most psychologically satisfactory outcome for all parties. This complexity is heightened by the fact that many negotiations occur in advance of any help being required.

Therefore negotiations relate to both real and 'anticipated' situations, especially when older family members are the potential recipients of help. Finch and Mason believe that during such interactions, 'Peoples' identities are being constructed, confirmed and reconstructed' (p. 170).

In trying to identify those factors which influence negotiation it seems that gender, ethnicity, culture or income do not explain support in any straightforward way. Moreover, there are no rules of obligation in terms of rights or duty, but rather guidelines for action, based upon responsibilities that have been created over time. In conclusion Finch and Mason contend that there are no fixed beliefs in the giving and receiving of support, but a negotiated balance in which people strive not to become too dependent and work to maintain at least an element of interdependence.

Though we have presented only an outline of what are quite subtle processes of negotiation and adaptation between parties, we believe that there is much of value that might profitably be applied to family caregiving in the present context. For if family negotiations are based upon the perceived purpose rather than the tasks of care, and gender, ethnicity, culture and income play relatively little part, it is likely that similar factors will pertain to family caregiving.

Certainly the instrumental aspects of care so prominent in the definitions previously considered seem inadequate to capture the above subtleties. It was such a concern that led Bowers (1987) to explore further the meanings and purposes of care as defined by carers themselves. Working on the premise that effective interventions to assist family carers could not be designed until there was a more adequate understanding of the carers' experience, she sought to develop a new typology of intergenerational care.

Data were collected using semi-structured interviews with mainly female adult children caring for their elderly parents suffering from various degrees of dementia. Bowers argued that most previous conceptualisations had defined caring by the nature of the task involved: that is, what carers do. This emphasis did not, however, accord with the accounts given by the carers themselves. This led Bowers to conclude that the process of caregiving is much more complex than these commonly used definitions would indicate, and that much of the stress of caregiving is unrelated to the presence of tasks.

On the basis of her data, Bowers suggested that much of the work of caregiving is 'invisible', in that it does not include overt behaviour and is not apparent to the cared-for person. Bowers considered that caring should be differentiated by purpose rather than task. Developing these arguments further, she outlined five distinct but often overlapping types of care.

First, there is *anticipatory care*, based on anticipated future need, with the key notion being 'just in case'. Anticipatory care can begin many years before any actual help is required and, as such, it is deliberately kept from the individual who is the focus of its attention. However, it can have a profound effect on the carer's life as major life decisions can be influenced by such anticipated future needs.

The second type of care in Bowers's model is termed *preventive care*, the main component of which is monitoring at a distance. As with anticipatory care, this does not usually involve directly observable assistance and therefore the 'cared-for' person may remain largely unaware of its existence. Examples of this type of care are keeping a subtle check that medication regimes are followed, that diets are adequate, and so on.

When such a monitoring role requires more direct intervention, such as assistance with actually taking medication, then Bowers considers that the stage of *supervisory care* has been reached. At this point, the cared-for person is more likely to be aware of the interventions but the carer may still try to minimise such awareness.

None of the above categories of care are accounted for in the definitions previously considered. As the need for direct assistance increases and the carer has to 'do for', then the stage of *instrumental care* has been reached. This is the type of care on which most of the previous research and current interventions have focused. The cared-for person is now largely aware of his/her need for help but carers will often try to maintain an element of reciprocity in their relationship. Bowers argues that carers find this aspect of caring the least stressful.

Underpinning the whole model is the notion of *protective care*, the purpose of which is to maintain the self-esteem of those being cared for. This involves minimising their awareness of their failing abilities and maximising the extent to which they still perceive themselves as independent. According to Bowers, carers see protective care as the most difficult, the most important and the most stressful. Furthermore, it is often in conflict with other aspects of caring, especially the instrumental functions. It can, for example, be very difficult both to do something for someone while, at the same time, maintaining his/her perceptions of his/herself as independent. Consequently, carers would often prefer to ignore certain instrumental tasks in order to preserve protecting caring.

In a later paper describing carers' perceptions of care in a nursing home, Bowers (1988) replaced the notion of protective care with *preservative care*, based on the need to preserve the cared-for person's sense of 'self'. Four broad types of preservative activity were described which were intended to help maintain family connections, and the dignity, hope and sense of control of the person in care. According to Bowers, family carers considered that staff should work collaboratively with carers in order to ensure that the essential elements of preservative care were maintained in the family's absence.

Given and Given (1991) identify the potential of Bowers's typology; they believe that it captures the more complex and sophisticated observations and judgements that define much of family care. However, they suggest that it requires further empirical confirmation. An appraisal of some of the current literature provides additional support for many of Bowers's arguments.

With respect to the notion of anticipating care, Finch and Mason (1993) suggest that anticipating the need for future help is a feature of ordinary family life and that negotiations can take place even if such help is never actually needed. Similarly, in a study explicitly to determine the extent to which daughters anticipate the future care needs of their mothers, Conway-Turner and Karasik (1993) discovered that of their sample of 103 daughters, 99 per cent actively anticipated caring for their mothers, and 68 per cent said they did this either frequently or daily. Such anticipation was not confined to middle-aged daughters with elderly mothers but with daughters still in their twenties, with many of the potential recipients of care being fit and active and in their early to mid-sixties. On the basis of their study Conway-Turner and Karasik suggest that the anticipation of caring responsibilities is a normal part of life, occurring several years before any care may be needed and irrespective of whether the need for care ever materialises.

In terms of preventive and supervisory care, Lewis and Meredith (1988b) outline a caring sequence which, if not identical, is distinctly similar to Bowers's (1987). They note that periods of what they term 'semi-care' and 'part-time full care' precede care proper. In semi-care there is usually little or no need for physical support but daughters 'monitor' the situation 'just in case', a phrase applied by Bowers to anticipatory care. Lewis and Meredith point out that semi-care can go on for several years. They claim that despite its apparently nebulous nature it is in fact very tying. However, it is not explicitly recognised by professionals who therefore do not see carers as requiring support during this period.

Instrumental care is recognised by all authors, but as Bowers (1987, 1988) points out, carers often work hard to maintain an element of reciprocity and interdependence in their relationships. This is consistent with the results of studies by Finch and Mason (1993) and Ellis (1993) who describe how carers and cared-for persons often negotiate a finely tuned set of responsibilities in order to preserve the perceived independence of the older person. Indeed Ellis suggests that the receipt of services is sometimes seen as synonymous with deterioration and therefore help is rejected even if it is required. Likewise Qureshi (1986) argues that some older people may prefer to abandon a goal, such as bathing, rather than see themselves dependent upon others.

All of these studies provide further support for Bowers's (1987) concept of protective care, which is explicitly confirmed in the work of Finch and Mason (1993), who draw the analytic distinction between excluding people from negotiations in order to protect their self-esteem and exclusion which is intended to disempower. The former is entirely consistent with Bowers's category of protective care. Upon first reading Bowers's (1987, 1988) work we were struck with how it accorded with much of our own data collected from a number of studies. However, there also appeared to be a number of limitations which suggested the need for further elaboration, because it was developed:

- with respect to intergenerational care only (as were many of the other studies cited above in support of it);
- specifically with dementia caregivers;
- without adequately accounting for reciprocity within the caregiving relationship, taking only a carer's perspective;
- without reference to a longitudinal perspective, limiting (for example) anticipatory care to the early stages of the caregiving process.

This prompted us to undertake a reconceptualisation of Bowers's typology in order that it could be tested against a more diverse set of caregiving circumstances (Nolan *et al*. 1995a). It is hard to trace the exact evolution of this new typology because it is not the product of a single discrete study but has emerged from several studies conducted over a number of years. On the basis of these studies a subtle dialectic and iterative process occurred, during which Bowers's original work was tested out against both new and previously collected data. Data analysis during the course of one particular study (Keady and Nolan 1993a,b) acted as a stimulus, honing emergent ideas and concepts into a more coherent whole. A tentative refinement of Bowers's typology was the result; this occasioned a return to data from early studies to check the veracity and robustness of the proposed revisions. The limitations of this approach need to be acknowledged as it constitutes only a partial and somewhat inadequate process – most of the data were not collected for the purpose of either developing or testing the typology. Nevertheless, the revised categories proved robust, and the data provided empirical support for the new dimensions as they are currently conceptualised. These are:

- anticipatory care
- preventive care
- supervisory care
- instrumental care
- protective care
- preservative care
- (re)constructive care
- reciprocal care.

As will readily be apparent, Bowers's categories remain at the heart of the typology; but we have redefined anticipatory care whilst retaining both protective and preservative care, rather than replacing protective care with preservative care as Bowers (1988) suggests. Moreover, we have added two new categories: (re) constructive care and reciprocal care. These constitute the broad *types* of care used by family caregivers.

Preventive care, supervisory care and instrumental care remain unchanged and these will not be described in further detail. However, anticipatory care has been extended considerably and the relationship between protective and preservative care has changed; these will be considered in greater depth, as will the new categories of care we have suggested (Nolan *et al.* 1995a).

REDEFINING CARE: A NEW TYPOLOGY

Bowers (1987) saw the key concept underpinning anticipatory care as being 'just in case'. She describes anticipatory care as being invisible (i.e. it is not based on overt behaviour, nor is it recognised by the cared-for person) and as occurring mainly prior to other forms of care being needed. Furthermore, she suggests that anticipatory care is used mainly by children who are not sharing a household with their parents.

This broad conceptualisation is consistent with the other work we have cited, for example semi-care (Lewis and Meredith 1988b) and the studies of Finch and Mason (1993) and Conway-Turner and Karasik (1993). We would suggest, however, that anticipation is a more pervasive and prolonged activity and is of relevance not only *before* but *throughout* the period of caring.

Anticipating some possible future event is not of course restricted to caring, and is probably a universal human activity. Bowers (1987) argues, however, that anticipating the need to care for a relative, whether or not this need actually materialises, can have profound effects on people's lives. To take an extreme example, anticipating the need to care for an ageing parent might be a factor dissuading an only child from emigrating abroad. On the other hand, we would argue that this form of anticipation is not confined to children thinking about caring for their parents and is of relevance in other contexts. Wenger *et al.* (1996) for example suggest that spouses often move to a smaller house, with a smaller garden and nearer to shops or adult children, in anticipation of potentially increased dependency. There are some subtle but important distinctions between anticipatory care as envisaged by Bowers and that described here. Anticipation in Bowers's sense does not usually result in direct action (although clearly it may inhibit certain activity) and is more of a cognitive activity, whereas a move of house is an overt act. Also Bowers contends that anticipation by adult children is not shared with their parents for fear of causing offence. Anticipation in spousal relationships, on the other hand, is more likely to be shared and explicit rather than implicit.

Furthermore, we would suggest that anticipatory care extends throughout the caregiving history but that it changes in nature and form over time. Therefore anticipatory care, which occurs before other forms of care are needed, is most probably largely invisible but this should not be seen as axiomatic. For instance, it is becoming increasingly more common for parents to express their own wishes and preferences for care options should they anticipate future dependency needs. Rather than the notion of 'just in case', which Bowers sees as underpinning anticipatory care, we would see the question 'what would I do if . . . ?', as being more appropriate for this type of anticipatory care. When other more overt forms of care are actually required, we would contend that anticipatory care does not diminish but rather that it changes in character. Therefore, whilst it might still be appropriate to ask the question 'what would I do if . . . ?', an increasingly more relevant question, especially in progressive conditions, is 'what will I do when . . . ?'.

This form of anticipatory care shifts focus away from anticipated *possible* events to anticipated *likely* events. This shift in perception recognises that anticipatory care develops along a continuum. At one end lies possible future caregiving before any overt help is actually needed, whilst at the other end lies a discontinuation of caregiving either because of death of the carer or cared-for person, or alternative care being required. For example, for the elderly parents of disabled children, care of this type tends to focus increasingly on what will happen when the parents die (Richardson and Ritchie 1986; Grant 1989, 1990). Such care is still largely invisible and unknown to the ultimate recipient. Moreover, it is something which older parents have been contemplating throughout the life-cycle from the point at which a diagnosis of disability first came to light. Parents are known to adopt varied and changing strategies to prepare the way for the inevitable: some seek early reassurances from statutory services about continued formal care, others negotiate the transfer of responsibility for care with other siblings, still others find it so traumatising that all they can do is live on a day-to-day basis. Anticipating care in this context is known to be the cause of stress and high levels of anxiety amongst these elderly carers.

We would also contend that in addition to a change in emphasis, anticipatory care may also change in form. We have coined the terms 'speculative anticipation' and 'informed anticipation' to differentiate these (Nolan et al. 1995a).

Speculative anticipation occurs when the carer has little information or advice on which to make a decision or a judgement. In such circumstances the carer is likely to overanticipate or underanticipate possible future demands. Inadequate information has been recognised for some time to be a major deficit in responding to carers' needs (Nolan and Grant 1989), and despite numerous calls for more information to be made available, little seems to have improved (Twigg and Atkin 1994). Adequate information is particularly important at critical transition points, especially at the start of caring (Nolan and Grant 1992b) or at the end of the period of instrumental care (Nolan et al. 1996). Information allows for a balanced perspective to be gained and facilitates the development of more effective coping strategies. For example, Archbold et al. (1992, 1995) have demonstrated that the 'preparedness' of a caregiver at the start of caregiving is a major factor influencing the future burdens of care; however, little thought and attention is given as to how carers acquire their role (Stewart et al. 1993). Even when this occurs at a time of health crisis and hospitalisation, when one might expect support to be available, there is little in the way of systematic professional input to help prepare carers (Nolan and Grant 1992b; Stewart et al. 1993). In such circumstances carers can take on their role with no idea of the level of commitment that is required, either in terms of the intensity or duration of care (Nolan and Grant 1992b; Opie 1994).

In contrast, informed anticipation occurs when the carer has adequate advice, information, and support which allows for informed choice. This is important throughout the caregiving history, but especially in transition points. For example, in

a series of recent studies looking at the admission of older people to some form of res-
idential or nursing home care (Nolan *et al*. 1996), it emerged that carers are
increasingly making decisions on behalf of frail older relatives but are doing so in the
absence of adequate guidance and advice. Moreover, because the carer and cared-for
persons do not usually discuss preferences prior to alternative care being required,
carers have few criteria upon which to choose a home. This compounds an already
stressful period and further heightens existing guilt and anxiety.

However, information alone is insufficient for fully informed anticipation, which can
only occur when decisions are shared and options discussed. This can be illustrated
with a quote taken from an interview with a wife caring for her husband who had
recently suffered a stroke: 'He just clams up and won't express himself and tell me how
he feels and that makes caring all the more difficult. I don't know his worries and fears
for the future which means I can't share mine with him.'

Recognising and acknowledging the importance of anticipatory care has a number
of implications for those working with carers. In particular there is a need to ensure
that sufficient information is available and that carers are adequately prepared for
their role. This should include not only the provision of information but also emotional
support to assist in the formation of realistic perspectives and facilitate informed
choice. However, as Stewart *et al*. (1993) argue, carers usually acquire their knowledge and skills on a trial-and-error basis. This is eloquently but tellingly recounted
in the following excerpt from an interview with a mother whose child has learning
difficulties:

> It was a little GP hospital and there was no doctor there and I was having dif-
> ficulty, so by the time the doctor came to the hospital things were looking
> pretty bad and she was delivered by forceps and apparently, though we've
> never really been able to get this on record, she was damaged with the forceps
> and it tore a membrane in her brain and she had a brain haemorrhage and it's
> left her as handicapped as she is. Though we didn't actually find out the
> extent of the handicap until she was about 2, the first that I really knew
> about it was when the health visitor came to the house and she always kept
> her little hands very stiff and her arms; and being naive, not knowing much
> about babies, I didn't realise that there was anything wrong and I asked the
> health visitor when she came to the house to test her hearing why were her
> hands so stiff and she said 'My dear, spastic children are always like this' and
> that's how we were told that she was having problems . . . We knew nothing
> about her handicap, I just had to learn as the days went by and for a long time
> I lost myself because I just didn't know what had happened, and I didn't
> know really how to handle it and the best way I can describe it is I lost the
> shiny bits in my life, all my sparkle, you know, all my identity and I just
> became this caring machine, feeding, caring, coping and wondering why and
> blaming myself and generally lost my identity for a long time. And every time
> you visited a doctor or a specialist you were told something worse than you
> were told the time before and it became very difficult and it wasn't until my
> younger daughter was born that we realised the full extent of her handicap

because she started doing things at six weeks old that – couldn't do at 5 and then it really hit home so that was a really difficult time.

Over a period of five years, the parents in this case were not adequately informed either about their daughter's handicap, nor her potential for future growth and development. Similar deficits have recently been described with respect to dementia care, with carers often returning to their GPs over several years trying to obtain a diagnosis and subsequent information and advice (Williams *et al*. 1995). This problem is not confined only to dementia caring, as in this example of a wife caring for her husband who has had a stroke:

The GP told me to get all the help I could but he never told me where to get it from or what was available. For years it was like wandering around in the dark. It took me 11 years to get a wheelchair and yet it's the best thing that ever happened to me. If only I'd had it from the start.

The whole issue of preparation for caring and the acquisition of knowledge and skills is considered later when the longitudinal model of caring is described.

PROTECTIVE, PRESERVATIVE AND RECONSTRUCTIVE CARE

These are presented together, because they are considered to have a temporal relationship. Bowers (1987) conceptualised protective care as being primarily concerned with keeping the cared-for person unaware of their failing abilities and increasing dependency. She later substituted the concept of preservative care (Bowers 1988), the purpose being to maintain as much of the person's sense of 'self' as possible. By implication such preservative care denotes 'former self'.

In terms of protective care, we would argue that it is a strategy of relatively limited duration and value. Whilst it may be functional in the short term or in certain circumstances, as with denial (Lazarus 1993), there comes a point when protective care is counterproductive and covering up dependency is neither possible or desirable. This form of care undoubtedly exists and is often motivated by high ideals, such as 'protecting' the cancer patient from their diagnosis. However, although well meaning, it is essentially paternalistic and often not in the best interests of either the carer or cared-for person. The following example of a daughter caring for her mother with Parkinson's disease provides an illustration:

Well, mum is starting to have a few accidents during the night now, you know, wetting the bed. Nothing much, only a few drops but it still leaves a little stain. I don't think she's aware of it though, she's certainly never mentioned it and there doesn't seem to be a problem in the day. So I've not told her I've noticed, she's so particular and would be really embarrassed and upset if she thought this was happening.

Whilst one can see the logic and positive virtues of this approach it still leaves a number of questions unanswered, particularly the identification of potentially treatable causes for the mild incontinence.

Other forms of supposed protection are not so clearly altruistic and, whilst couched in terms of benefit to the cared-for person, are intended to save carers and/or professionals from having to face difficult decisions. For example in the studies of admission to care homes (Nolan *et al.* 1996), instances were identified where an older person had been admitted to care in the belief that this was a temporary measure when in reality the carer and the professional involved saw it as a permanent move. Explanations from carers and professionals were frequently offered, usually in terms of not wanting to upset the older person. It was reasoned that when they settled in they would be told of their relocation. Although it is easy to see how a carer might construe such a perception, the fact that a professional colluded with them is a cause for some concern.

When protective care is no longer possible or desirable, preservative care becomes the preferred or main strategy. Bowers (1988) describes preservative care primarily in terms of preserving the dignity, hope and sense of control of the cared-for person; she developed the concept following a study of admissions to a nursing home. We would argue, however, that it occurs throughout the various stages of the caregiving history and extends beyond preserving dignity and self-esteem to include the preservation of skills, abilities and interests, as in this example of a daughter caring for her mother with severe arthritis:

> She's always been very proud of her skills in the kitchen, especially her baking. So when she moved in with us we thought, 'we need to keep her involved', so she sort of took over that part of the house. But now of course she's getting much worse and not only can't she walk but she can't do much with her hands. So making pastry is out of the question. She's still bright as a button though, so she's become the resident expert on cooking who we turn to for advice and the like.

The value of such care is quite apparent but we would contend that it is only functional to a certain point. One of the main adaptive tasks in chronic illness or disability is to develop new but equally valued roles to replace former ones (Charmaz 1983, 1987). Brandstädter (1995) contends that the maintenance of self-esteem amongst older people can be achieved by balancing assimilative and accommodative activities. Assimilative strategies are aimed at maintaining former abilities and interests for as long as possible, whereas accommodative strategies seek to build new abilities and interests when old ones can no longer be sustained. Brändstadter reviewed several years of research conducted by himself and his colleagues which provides convincing evidence that self-esteem and psychological health in older age are optimised by those individuals who balance accommodative and assimilative strategies and develop realistic perceptions of their capabilities. Within this context it is easy to appreciate how a rigid adherence to preservative care (which has clear conceptual similarities with assimilative activity) is not necessary in the long-term interest of either carer or

cared-for person. It is here that (re)constructive care begins to figure more promi-
nently.

The purpose of (re)constructive care is to build upon the past in order to develop
new and valued roles. We have named it *(re)constructive* care in recognition of the differences that are apparent in certain caring relationships. Parents of children with
learning difficulties, for example, are more likely to engage in *constructive* care in
order to build an identity and a set of roles for their child. On the other hand, carers
of either spouses or parents are more likely to engage in *reconstructive* care where the
purpose is to rebuild an identity on the foundations of past histories and biographies.
As noted before, parents of children with learning difficulties strive to construct a
future for them, as in this instance of a mother caring for her 21-year-old daughter.

> Well I think it's up to me and her Dad in a way to make things right for her.
> We have to do our best to make sure that what happens to her in the future
> is the best that we can possibly do for her. I don't want to see her stuck along
> with 200 or 300 other people in a large building where they're trying to cope
> with all these different disabilities and perhaps she'll be there from 9 till 5 for
> the next 40 years. I don't want that for her . . . So we have to look at the
> options and see just what is the best for her and I want people to be positive.
> I don't want them to see the handicap first. I want them to look at her and
> think: Gosh, she's lovely, she's happy, let's try, let's face the challenge, let's be
> more positive. Just don't write her off because they might need to pick her
> up and put her on the toilet so many times a day or somebody might have to
> give up ten minutes to feed her during the lunch time. I don't want that.

The message here is quite clear: the need to 'construct' an acceptable future is
pressing. Such considerations apply equally well in other caring relationships but the
emphasis, if not the purpose, is different. This is illustrated in an interview undertaken
with a woman caring for her partner who had recently had a major stroke which left
him with a degree of dysphasia and considerable residual motor deficits. Her partner
was a newly retired bank manager who had been an extremely active person in both
a professional and personal capacity, including charity work, hill-walking and amateur
dramatics/operatics. Shortly before the stroke they had moved to the country with an
active retirement in mind. The stroke had wreaked havoc with their well-laid plans.
The interviewee spoke tellingly and eloquently about their efforts to rebuild a future
and to substitute interests. Because active participation in dramatics was perceived to
be unlikely, she struggled to develop skills in appreciation and active listening. Whilst
this was difficult, she was of the opinion that good progress was being made. She was
extremely disappointed, however, that those professionals who were involved seemed
unable to see beyond her partner's physical defects. Indeed when one of the authors
was interviewing the sister of the respite unit that her partner attended, he was
described as 'a depressed little dysphasia'.

This sort of insensitivity, although not conveyed quite so forcibly to the carer herself, was nevertheless apparent to her and was a cause of considerable concern. As a
consequence she was considering withdrawing from the respite service despite

desperately needing the break. Although an extreme example, this illustrates the legacy of an overemphasis on physical functioning and dependency, both as an indicator of the need for support and as the perceived outcome of successful rehabilitation. A less dramatic although still telling example, is recounted by Ellis (1993) when she describes how an assessment of need of an elderly woman focused on the functional aspects, totally ignoring her love of painting which provided a major source of pleasure. Ellis describes a number of other insights into the way that professional assessment of need seems to run counter to the perspectives of disabled people themselves. This often undermines rather than sustains their efforts at (re)constructing an identity.

The metaconcept uniting the various components of our typology is what we term 'reciprocal care'. The major limitation of Bowers's model is its failure to account for the reciprocal element of care. Given the context in which it was developed, this is understandable, as the opportunities for reciprocity in dementia, especially the later stages, are probably more limited than in any other condition. But ignoring the reciprocal element in a caregiving relationship is not uncommon. Kitson (1987) suggests that the recipient of care is the more passive partner who more or less complies with the decisions made by the carer.

This statement also seems to imply that the cared-for person has an extremely limited role to play in decision-making. This may be true in certain cases but, as a generalisation, it is untenable. Kitson (1987) later qualifies this by stating that dependence lasts only until the recipient is able to resume responsibility for their own welfare. This may not always be possible in chronic or progressive conditions. Whilst direct exchange of the same type and level of care *is* extremely unlikely, the supposition that there is no form of reciprocity in caring is based *only* on the notion of the exchange of instrumental care. We would suggest that care can be reciprocal on a number of levels. Indeed, the growing evidence on the satisfaction of carers (Clifford 1990; Grant and Nolan 1993; Nolan and Keady 1993) clearly indicates that there are diffuse and subtle reciprocities in the majority of caregiving relationships. Even at high levels of dependency, forms of reciprocal helping at the financial, material and psychological levels has been reported in some studies (Grant 1986, 1990). There is nothing new of course in asserting that reciprocity is important in caring, as various studies attest (Abrams 1985; Qureshi 1986; Bulmer 1987; Lewis and Meredith 1988a,b; Qureshi and Walker 1989; Ellis 1993; Finch and Mason 1993). We believe, however, that the role of satisfaction in caring has been neglected, possibly due to the theoretical stance adopted by many studies. Although we will deal with the satisfactions of caring in some detail in Chapter 4, we state here our belief that reciprocity and satisfaction should be seen as the norm in most caregiving relationships and that these can be sustained even in the face of objectively adverse circumstances. Indeed, the absence of reciprocity and satisfaction should act as a warning sign indicating the need for additional support and possibly the search for alternative caring arrangements.

The types of care we have described above are not of course mutually exclusive, and in presenting them in the way we have we are conscious of creating an overly neat and orderly perception. Clearly many types of care can and do occur simultaneously, and the manner in which protective, preservative and reconstructive care slip into one another is subtle and often insidious. We repeat our intention that the typology and subsequent models to be outlined are not meant to be viewed as literal representations of reality but as alternatives to the current dominant instrumental viewpoint. Certainly carers would not label their activities and purposes as protective or reconstructive care or indeed any of the other categories we have employed. However, we believe that they do *deliberately* use certain strategies to achieve the types of outcomes described above, albeit with considerable variation depending upon the nature of the caregiving relationship and the stage of the caregiving trajectory. Of course instrumental aspects of care are a central component and must not be overlooked. However, we believe that typologies that focus exclusively or primarily on such aspects not only fail to capture the subtleties and meanings of care but, given their link to service delivery, have the potential to do carers a considerable disservice. If applied in an uncritical and unthinking manner they can deny access to support to the potentially most stressed carers (Levesque *et al.* 1995).

APPLYING THE TYPOLOGY: IMPLICATIONS FOR SERVICE DELIVERY

Despite the lack of a coherent strategy for the delivery of services to carers, a number of actual and potential interventions are nevertheless available. We believe that the extent to which such support is deemed acceptable and successful from a carers' perspective depends in no small measure on the degree to which it is sensitive both to the caregiving trajectory and the caring strategies that are employed. For example, Bowers (1987) points out that services which threaten carers' efforts at protective care are likely to be rejected. Other authors have made similar observations on the need for professionals to work actively with carers, taking due account of the carers' knowledge and expertise (Lewis and Meredith 1989; Braithwaite 1990; Nolan and Grant 1992a; Harper *et al.* 1993; Schultz *et al.* 1993; Greene and Coleman 1995; Montgomery 1995).

We suggest that interventions can be viewed along a continuum ranging from *facilitative* to *obstructive*, with the position on this continuum being mediated by the extent to which service providers actively engage carers as partners in the intervention process, taking particular account of the carers' expertise and caregiving strategies. This is different to Twigg and Atkins's (1994) notion of a carer as a co-worker, because unlike the co-worker the intention of a partnership is not primarily to maintain the carer in their role. Rather it is to facilitate the best outcome for both carer and cared-for person. In the majority of cases this will mean a continuation of the caring relationship; but working with carers as partners also means recognising that in certain circumstances a search for alternative forms of care is the most appropriate strategy.

Facilitative interventions denote an overt, planned and relatively systematic input, augmented by instant access to additional help in cases of urgent need. A prerequisite for effective facilitative support is that it complements the type of care provided by the caregiver. This requires a sensitivity and awareness of the caregiving dynamic and of the expertise of the carer. For carers new to their role there may be a need to provide information, advice and training so that they are adequately prepared and feel competent to provide good care (Archbold *et al.* 1992, 1995; Nolan and Grant 1992b; Stewart *et al.* 1993). It also means that in certain circumstances family members should not be expected to adopt a caregiving role in the first place. As Qureshi and Walker (1989) argue, family care can be amongst the best and the worst of human encounters – forcing someone into the caring role is likely to result in 'potentially disastrous close physical and emotional relationships'. Yet this is often what occurs when reluctant family members are pressured to take on the role of carer, particularly at the time of hospital discharge (Nolan and Grant 1992b). Nolan and Grant noted that hospital consultants based their decisions about future care almost exclusively on physical dependency, whereas potential carers placed far more emphasis on the nature and quality of their previous relationships.

The potential for conflicting perceptions between consultant and carer readily became apparent. Carers who *wished* to take a *very frail* relative home were often advised not to, whilst others (particularly children) were *expected* to take a *relatively able* parent home despite the fact that they might not wish to. For children who voiced doubts about their ability and willingness to care for a parent, there often appeared to be little choice in the matter. One carer described how she had been asked to come and see the consultant and then 'given a good telling off', after which she felt obligated. Despite the relatively good functional ability of the mother in this case and the fact that she did not live with her daughter, the situation soon became very fraught: 'I knew as soon as I started that things could only go from bad to worse. We'd never been very close anyway but I was surprised how, in just a couple of days, I could grow to almost hate my mother.' Given the above reaction it is certainly questionable if all people should be expected to care, and the availability of a relative must not be taken to mean that such an individual should automatically assume the role of carer. Within the present climate of ever more rapid hospital discharge, the time available for both carers and cared-for persons to make important decisions about future care options is diminishing. It seems increasingly likely that growing numbers of carers will adopt the role without adequate thought, advice and preparation.

On the other hand, experienced carers often have considerable expertise of their own; facilitative interventions are sensitive to this and recognise that such knowledge should actively be drawn upon. A failure to do so can result in frustration and annoyance, as with this mother caring for her daughter with learning difficulties:

> Sometimes it can be very annoying because if you've had three hours sleep at night and you get this young woman come in straight out of college or straight out of training and she says: 'Well I think you're doing this wrong and you're doing that wrong' and you just want to sit there and let everything fold in around you with a Valium sandwich. That can be very, very annoying.

However, another excerpt from the same interview illustrates how even experienced carers value an outside perspective, as it can often help to sort out the 'wood from the trees':

> They can distance themselves, they can look from the outside in. They can see things that perhaps I'm too close to and they can make suggestions and I think: Oh yes, we'll try that, perhaps this will work, whereas my role is so intense with – I have to think, I have to anticipate, I have to be one step ahead a lot of the time, I have to be physically able to do the lifting and the caring and the general physical activities that need to keep her occupied during the day, so I am very intensively involved. So sometimes you need to be able to step back and have someone from the outside look in and just give you a general overview of the situation and say: 'Well you've tried this. Now try it this way and see if this will work', and I find that can be positive sometimes.

It is important to note that facilitation is not a function of the *amount* of help or support given. The key determinant is that services are planned in conjunction with the carer and cared-for person to complement their needs. Such services are, unfortunately, not the norm.

Contributory interventions are based on a more *ad hoc*, unplanned and less systematic basis but nevertheless still more or less complement the primary caregiver's role. However, in contrast to facilitative interventions this complementarity has not been achieved by a process of genuine negotiation. Rather, it has arisen in a serendipitous manner, occurring more by chance and good fortune than reasoned judgement. Services, especially those provided by the statutory agencies, which actually complement the primary carer's role, more usually do so on this basis.

Efforts to support the primary caregiver which are neither facilitative nor contributory serve little or no useful purpose. Indeed, they are likely to do more harm than good. Unfortunately, all too often, formal services fall into this category by failing to take account of the caregiver's needs and dominant type of care.

We have termed such services either *inhibitory* or *obstructive* (Nolan et al. 1995a), both of which run the risk of being rejected by carers. Inhibitory services are usually not rejected out of hand as, on balance, the benefits are seen to outweigh the costs. However, such services are often accepted reluctantly and carers experience guilt at using them. Respite care provides a good example. It has been suggested that most elderly users of respite care 'tolerate' the admission at best (Nolan and Grant 1992a), finding the experience one of boredom and inactivity. In such circumstances, their self-esteem and morale may fall. However, as carers need the break, they still accept the respite care but feel guilty at doing so. Such a service, whilst maintaining the caring relationship, can inhibit carers' efforts to engage in preservative, reconstructive and reciprocal care.

This is illustrated by the following case history taken from a study of day care provision (Nolan and Cunliffe 1991). During one of the interviews a husband caring for his wife with dementia told of his experience of a respite service. The carer in question carried out all his wife's personal care whilst she was at home and took particular pains to ensure that his wife's hair was well washed and set in a certain way. The style he chose was his wife's favourite and the one that he felt she would have chosen for herself had she been able to. When his wife went in for respite care, he explained this to the staff involved. He was therefore disappointed and distressed to see that, when he visited his wife, her hair had been set in a different style. Whilst he appreciated the fact that the staff were attending to his wife's personal hygiene needs, their efforts were negated by their failure to heed the advice he had given them. Although he still used the service in question as no alternative was available, he was less than happy about doing so.

Obstructive interventions, rather than inhibiting the carer's efforts, are perceived as a direct effort to block them. This is again illustrated by a case study taken from a study of respite care (Nolan and Grant 1992a). One interviewee, an elderly woman caring for her husband with dementia, experienced difficulties with his wandering behaviour. However, she never sedated him but had developed an effective way of dealing with the problem. She attributed her husband's wandering to the fact that he had been a prisoner of war in the Second World War and had made repeated escape attempts. She rationalised that when he wandered he was going back to that period and often quite desperate attempts to get out of the house were an effort to 'escape'. To forestall this, she would notice the signs of his increasing agitation and let him 'escape'. She normally found that once he had gone a few steps out of the house that he could easily be distracted and would return home quite happily.

She had accepted the initial offer of respite care only reluctantly. On the first admission she had tried to explain her way of dealing with her husband's agitation and wandering to the sister. She was told that, as 'experts', the unit had ways of dealing with wandering patients (it was not a specialist EMI unit). Not wanting to argue, she accepted this. She returned on her visit to find her husband heavily sedated with his mouth full of half-chewed food. She took him home immediately and vowed never to let him go for respite care again.

Twigg and Atkin (1994) suggest that one of the core features that underpin caregiving is the role as the 'arbiter of standards' – the continuum of interventions we have outlined above illustrates this process. Carers consider the appropriateness and relevance of services with regard to their own caregiving strategies and the degree to which professionals acknowledge the carer's expertise. At the extremes of the continuum, services are either welcomed or rejected, whereas for the two intervening positions a delicate balancing act occurs. The need for a break or help is measured against the guilt carers experience and the perceived benefits/disbenefits for the cared-for person. Motenko (1988) described a conceptually similar process in studying the reactions of husbands to their wives' use of respite care. He noted that husbands took pride in what they did as carers and considered themselves to have a store of knowledge and expertise. They required respite workers to exhibit the same qualities and attributes as themselves and only temporarily relinquished care of their wives to workers who met their standards. On the basis of his study Motenko argued that the perceived quality of a service is more important than the quantity.

In relation to social work practice, Fisher (1990: 244) too believes that carers should be seen as experts, 'experts in their own caring arrangements, in communicating with a dependent relative, in balancing competing demands, in interweaving practical and emotional care and in surviving'.

Taraborrelli (1993) argues that the expertise of family carers frequently surprises formal carers and must be better acknowledged. Taking a similar line of reasoning, a number of authors have called for the creation of closer partnerships between carers and professionals (Nolan and Grant 1992a; Ellis 1993; Hughes 1993; Harvath *et al.* 1994). This will require that professionals are prepared to learn from caregivers (Hasselkus 1988; Nolan *et al.* 1994), who often have a strong desire to 'teach' staff how to care. Recognition of the different but complementary skills and knowledge possessed by family and professional carers is therefore essential (Hasselkus 1988; Pitkeathley 1990; Nolan and Grant 1992a; Harvath *et al.* 1994). As Ellis (1993) notes, this will require a considerable reorientation of current professional practice and attitudes. Most fundamentally of all this must include a shift away from the preoccupation with the instrumental and physical aspects of care. Such components cannot and should not be ignored, but as Schultz *et al.* (1993: 5) argue, interventions based solely or primarily on the tasks of care have very little impact 'precisely because they fail to address the inner world of the carer and related major concerns such as loss and grief, guilt, anger and resentment'.

We opened this chapter with a question posed by Gubrium (1995), 'What is this thing some call caregiving?'. In attempting to provide a more complete (although still partial) answer we have outlined an extended typology of care based around carers' purposes and intentions rather than the tasks they perform. Implications for service delivery have also been addressed. In the next chapter we narrow the focus somewhat and consider how carers cope with the varying demands they face.

NOTES

* *Understanding Family Care*. Milton Keynes, Open University Press. pp. 28–51. Reproduced with permission of the Open University Press.

REFERENCES

Abrams, P. (1985) (Edited by Bulmer, M.) Policies to promote informal care: some reflections on voluntary action, neighbourhood involvement and neighbourhood care. *Ageing and Society*, 5: 1–18.

Arber, S. and Ginn, J. (1995) Gender differences in informal caring. *Health and Social Care in the Community*, 3: 19–31.

Archbold, P., Stewart, B. J., Greenlick, M. R. and Harvath, T. A. (1992) The clinical assessment of mutuality and preparedness in family caregivers of frail older people, in S. G. Funk, E. M. T. Tornquist, S. T. Champagne and R. A. Weise (eds) *Key Aspects of Elder Care: Managing Falls, Incontinence and Cognitive Impairment*. New York: Springer.

Archbold, P. G., Steward, B. J., Miller, L. L., Harvath, T. A., Greenlick, M. R., Van Buren, L., Kirschling, J. M., Valanis, B. G., Brody, K. K., Schook, J. E. and Hagan, J. M. (1995) The PREP system of nursing interventions: a pilot test with families caring for older members, *Research in Nursing Health*, 18: 1–16.

Barrera, M. and Ainlay, S. L. (1983) The structure of social support: a conceptual and empirical analysis, *American Journal of Community Psychology*, 11: 133–43.

Benner, P. and Wruebel, J. (1989) *The Primacy of Caring: Stress and Coping in Health and Illness*. Menlo Park, CA: Addison Wesley.

Bond, J. (1992) The politics of caregiving: the professionalisation of informal care, *Ageing and Society*, 12: 5–21.

Bond, S. and Bond, J. (1992) *Evaluating Continuing Care Accommodation: an Overview of Nursing Staff Survey, Report no. 60*. University of Newcastle-upon-Tyne: Centre for Health Services Research.

Bowers, B. J. (1987) Inter-generational caregiving: adult caregivers and their ageing parents, *Advances in Nursing Science*, 9(2): 20–31.

Bowers, B. J. (1988) Family perceptions of care in a nursing home, *The Gerontologist*, 28(3): 361–7.

Braithwaite, V. A. (1990) *Bound to Care*. Sydney: Allen and Unwin.

Brandstädter, J. (1995) Maintaining a sense of control and self-esteem in later life: protective mechanisms. Paper presented at III European Congress of Gerontology, Amsterdam, 30 August–2 September 1995.

Brody, E. M. (1995) Prospects for family caregiving: response to change, continuity and diversity, in R. A. Kane and J. D. Penrod (eds) *Family Caregiving in an Ageing Society*. Thousand Oaks, CA: Sage.

Bulmer, M. (1987) *The Social Basis of Community Care*. London: Allen and Unwin.

Charmaz, K. (1983) Loss of self: a fundamental form of suffering in the chronically ill, *Sociology of Health and Illness*, 5(2): 168–95.

Charmaz, K. (1987) Struggling for self: identity levels of the chronically ill, *Research in the Sociology of Health Care*, 6: 283–321.

Clifford, D. (1990) *The Social Costs and Rewards of Care*. Aldershot: Avebury.

Conway-Turner, K. and Karasik, R. (1993) Adult daughters' anticipation of caregiving responsibilities, *Journal of Women and Aging*, 5(2): 99–114.

Ellis, K. (1993) *Squaring the Circle: User and Carer Participation in Needs Assessment*. York: Joseph Rowntree Foundation.

Fealy, G. M. (1995) Professional caring: the moral dimension, *Journal of Advanced Nursing*, 22(6): 135–40.

Finch, J. and Mason J. (1993) *Negotiating Family Responsibilities*. London: Routledge.

Fisher, M. (1990) Care management and social work: working with carers, *Practice*, 4(4): 242–52.

Given, B. A. and Given, C. W. (1991) Family caregivers for the elderly, in J. Fitzpatrick, R. Tauton and A. Jacox (eds) *Annual Review of Nursing Research*, vol. 9. New York: Springer.

Grant, G. (1986) Older carers, interdependence and the care of mentally handicapped adults, *Ageing and Society*, 6, 333–51.

Grant, G. (1989) Letting go: decision-making among family carers of people with a mental handicap, *Australia and New Zealand Journal of Developmental Disabilities*, 15(3 & 4): 189–200.

Grant, G. (1990) Elderly parents with handicapped children: anticipating the future, *Journal of Aging Studies*, 4(4): 359–74.

Grant, G. and Nolan, M. (1993) Informal carers: sources and concomitants of satisfaction, *Health and Social Care in the Community*, 1(3): 147–59.

Green, H. (1988) *Informal Carers*. General Household Survey 1985 series. GHS No. 15, supplement 16. London: OPCS Social Survey Division.

Greene, V. L. and Coleman, P. D. (1995) Direct services for family caregivers: next steps for public policy, in R. A. Kane and J. D. Penrod (eds) *Family Caregiving in an Ageing Society: Policy Perspectives*. Thousand Oaks, CA: Sage.

Griffin, A. P. (1983) A philosophical analysis of caring in nursing, *Journal of Advanced Nursing*, 8: 189–295.

Gubrium, J. (1995) Taking stock, *Qualitative Health Research*, 5(3): 267–9.

Harper, D. J., Manasse, P. R., James, O. and Newton, D. T. (1993) Intervening to reduce distress in caregivers of impaired elderly people: a preliminary evaluation, *International Journal of Geriatric Psychiatry*, 8: 139–45.

Harvath, T. A. (1994) Interpretation and management of dementia-related behaviour problems, *Clinical Nursing Research*, 3(1): 7–26.

Hasselkus, B. R. (1988) Meaning in family caregiving: perspectives on caregiver/professional relationships, *The Gerontologist*, 28(5): 686–91.

Hughes, B. (1993) A model for the comprehensive assessment of older people and their carers, *British Journal of Social Work*, 23: 345–80.

James, N. (1992) Care = organisation + physical labour + emotional labour, *Sociology of Health Illness*, 14(4): 488–509.

Kahn, R. and Antonucci, T. C. (1980) Convoys over the life course: attachment, roles and social support, in P. B. Baltes and O. Brim (eds) *Life Span Development and Behaviour*. Lexington, MA: Lexington Books.

Keady, J. and Nolan, M. R. (1993a) Coping with dementia: understanding and responding to the needs of informal carers. Paper given at the Royal College of Nursing Research Conference, University of Glasgow, April 1993.

Keady, J. and Nolan, M. R. (1993b) Coping with dementia: towards a comprehensive assessment of the needs of informal carers. Paper given at International Conference on Mental Illness in Old Age. Institute of Human Ageing, Liverpool, June 1993.

Kitson, A. (1987) A comparative analysis of lay caring and professional (nursing) caring relationships, *International Journal of Nursing Studies*, 24(2): 155–65.

Kyle, T. U. (1995) The concept of caring: a literature review, *Journal of Advanced Nursing*, 21(3): 506–14.

Langer, S. R. (1993) Ways of managing the experience of caregiving for elderly relatives, *Western Journal of Nursing Research*, 15(5): 582–94.

Lazarus, R. S. (1993) Coping theory and research: past, recent and future, *Psychosomatic Medicine*, 55: 234–47.

Levesque, L., Cossette, J. and Laurin, L. (1995) A multidimensional examination of the psychological and social well-being of caregivers of a demented relative, *Research on Ageing*, 17(3): 322–60.

Lewis, J. and Meredith, B. (1988a) *Daughters Who Care: Daughters Caring for Mothers at Home*. London: Routledge and Kegan Paul.

Lewis, J. and Meredith, B. (1988b) Daughters caring for mothers, *Ageing and Society*, 8(1): 1–21.

Lewis, J. and Meredith, B. (1989) Contested territory in informal care, in M. Jeffreys (ed.) *Growing Old in the Twentieth Century*. London: Routledge.

Montgomery, R. J. V. (1995) Examining respite care: promises and limitations, in R. A. Kane and J. D. Penrod (eds) *Family Caregiving in an Ageing Society: Policy Perspectives*. Thousand Oaks, CA: Sage.

Morse, J. M., Solberg, S. M., Neander, W. L., Bottroff, J. L. and Johnson, J. L. (1990) Concepts of caring and caring as a concept, *Advances in Nursing Sciences*, 13(1): 1–14.

Motenko, A. K. (1988) Respite care and pride in caregiving: the experience of six older men caring for their disabled wives, in S. Reinharz and G. Rowles (eds) *Qualitative Gerontology*. New York: Springer.

Nikkonen, M. (1994) Caring from the point of view of a Finnish mental health nurse, *Journal of Advanced Nursing*, 19: 1185–95.

Nolan, M. R. and Cunliffe, C. (1991) A study of EMI day services in Gwynedd. Unpublished study conducted for Gwynedd Health Authority, Bangor.

Nolan, M. R. and Grant, G. (1989) Addressing the needs of informal carers: a neglected area of nurses practice, *Journal of Advanced Nursing*, 14: 950–61.

Nolan, M. R. and Grant, G. (1992a) *Regular Respite: an Evaluation of a Hospital Rota Bed Scheme for Elderly People*. London: Age Concern.

Nolan, M. R. and Grant, G. (1992b) Helping new carers of the frail elderly patient: the challenge for nurses in acute care settings, *Journal of Clinical Nursing*, 1: 303–7.

Nolan, M. R. and Keady, J. (1993) Every cloud has a silver lining: exploring the dimensions of carer satisfaction. British Society of Gerontology Annual Conference on the Experience of Older People – Solidarity Across the Generations, UEA, Norwich, 17–19 September.

Nolan, M. R. and Scott, G. (1993) Audit: an exploration of some tensions and paradoxical expectations, *Journal of Advanced Nursing*, 18: 759–66.

Nolan, M. R., Grant, G., Caldock, K. and Keady, J. (1994) *A Framework for Assessing the Needs of Family Carers: a Multi-disciplinary Guide*. Stoke-on-Trent: BASE Publications.

Nolan, M. R., Keady, J. and Grant, G. (1995a) Developing a typology of family care: implications for nurse and other service providers, *Journal of Advanced Nursing*, 21: 256–65.

Nolan, M. R., Walker, G., Nolan, J., Williams, S., Poland, F., Curan, M. and Kent, B. C. (1996) Entry to care: positive choice or fait accompli? Developing a more proactive nursing response to the needs of older people and their carers, *Journal of Advanced Nursing*, 24: 265–74.

Opie, A. (1994) The instability of the caring body: gender and caregivers of confused older people, *Qualitative Health Research*, 4(1): 31–50.

Parker, G. and Lawton, D. (1994) *Different Types of Care, Different Types of Carer: Evidence from the General Household Survey*. London: HMSO.

Parker, R. (1981) Tending and social policy, in E. M. Goldberg and S. Hatch (eds) *A New Look at the Personal Social Services*. London: Policy Studies Institute.

Pearlin, L. I., Mullan, J. T., Semple, S. J. and Skaff, M. M. (1990) Caregiving and the stress process: an overview of concepts and their measures, *The Gerontologist*, 30(5): 583–94.

Pitkeathley, J. (1990) Painful conflicts, *Community Care (Inside)*, 22 February: i–ii.

Qureshi, H. (1986) Responses to dependency: reciprocity, affect and power in family relationships, in C. Phillipson, M. Bernard and R. Strang (eds) *Dependency and Interdependency in Old Age: Theoretical Perspectives and Policy Alternatives*. London: Croom Helm.

Qureshi, H. and Walker, A. (1989) *The Caring Relationship: Elderly People and Their Families*. Basingstoke: Macmillan.

Radsma, J. (1994) Caring and nursing: a dilemma, *Journal of Advanced Nursing*, 20(3): 444–9.

Richardson, A. and Ritchie, J. (1986) *Better for the Break: Parents' Views about Adults with a Handicap Leaving the Parental Home*. London: King Edward Hospital Fund for London.

Schultz, C. L., Smyrnios, K. X., Grbich, C. F. and Schultz, N. C. (1993) Caring for family caregivers in Australia: a model of psychoeducational support, *Ageing and Society*, 13: 1–25.

Scott, P. A. (1995) Care, attention and imaginative identification in nursing practice, *Journal of Advanced Nursing*, 21(6): 1196–1200.

Stewart, B. J., Archbold, P. G., Harvath, T. A. and Kkongho, N. O. (1993) Role acquisition in family caregivers of older people who have been discharged from hospital, in S. G. Funk, E. H. Tornquist, M. T. Champagne and R. A. Weise (eds) *Key Aspects of Caring for the Chronically Ill: Hospital and Home*. New York: Springer.

Taraborrelli, P. (1993) Exemplar A: becoming a carer, in N. Gilbert (ed.) *Researching Social Life*. London: Sage.

Twigg, J. and Atkin, K. (1994) *Carers Perceived: Policy and Practice in Informal Care.* Buckingham: Open University Press.

Ungerson, C. (1987) *Policy is Personal: Sex, Gender and Informal Care.* London: Tavistock.

Wenger, G. C. (1996) Social network research in gerontology: how did we get there and where do we go next? in V. Minichiello, N. Chappell, A. Walker and H. Kendig (eds) *Sociology of Ageing*. Melbourne: International Sociological Association.

Williams, O., Keady, J. and Nolan, M. (1995) Younger onset Alzheimer's disease: learning from the experience of one spouse carer, *Journal of Clinical Nursing*, 4(1): 31–6.

PART THREE

Clinical effectiveness

Chapter 13

Controlled trial of psychiatric nurse therapists in primary care

ISAAC MARKS

Introduction

It is clear that nurses have never held a monopoly on nursing research, nor could or should they. Indeed the same argument would apply to any professional group. It is gratifying however that nursing has attracted attention from researchers beyond its ranks. And in some cases there may be advantages in doing so in politically sensitive areas where, regardless of rigour, such involvement conveys a sense of neutrality and independence. Mental health has long been regarded as a Cinderella and perhaps, as a result, more open to therapeutic experimentation. Psychiatry has been in the forefront of developing advanced practice roles for nurses, arguably long before they were invented in other sectors. Originating as a pragmatic response to the paucity of primary care doctors and growing policy preference for community care in the 1970s, it was clear that doctors alone would never be able to provide the contribution and cover necessary to underpin the promising new service. Behaviour therapy developed in the 1960s and came increasingly to be recognised as a viable therapeutic option, but one whose delivery was compromised by the lack of a suitably trained workforce. Motivated by his experience earlier in South Africa with barefoot doctors, Isaac Marks, then a lecturer in psychiatry at the Institute of Psychiatry, became a pioneer of the nurse therapist movement in the UK. This was not an isolated development, but built on previous studies demonstrating that patients of GPs, physicians and psychiatrists, managed by advanced clinical nurses, 'did as well' as patients managed by other professionals. A full economic evaluation had been published previously.

The study we have included here extended over 4 years, from 1978 to 1982, and involved three nurse therapists with 3300 patients drawn from 20 general practitioner lists each with 47 000 patients. A psychiatrist was the blind assessor. Interventions included therapy for phobic, obsessive/compulsive, habit disorders and sexual dysfunction. Patients who were willing to participate were reviewed by a nurse following referral by the GP. 'Outcomes' were assessed on a variety of rating scales related to main problem fear, global phobia, anxiety and depression scales, work adjustment, social and private leisure. Attrition in attendees following 254 referrals through screening for suitability and refusals reduced the numbers entered into the trial to 92 for randomisation. The mean duration of the problem for which therapy was sought was 7 years, compared with 10 in similar out-patient departments.

This method involved exploring three questions; how effective is a nurse therapist with suitable patients? 'Suitable' patients were assigned randomly to behavioural treatments by a nurse therapist working within a general practice, or to routine non-behavioural management by a nurse therapist. The second question explored whether there was a viable role for a nurse therapist as part of a primary care team. This was ascertained by data collected from informal sources from the primary care team and the nurse therapist. The third question related to estimating the proportion of patients who attended surgery who were 'suitable' for behavioural treatment. This was addressed by examining consecutive patients who attended, and offering a general psychiatric consultation service in two practices.

Phobic and obsessive/compulsive patients had significantly better outcomes up to a one-year follow-up after receiving behavioural psychotherapy from a nurse therapist rather than routine treatment from a general practitioner. At the end of the year, control patients who had not improved had cross-over behavioural treatment from the nurse and improved. Those who dropped out or refused therapy demonstrated no significant gain. Moreover, patients preferred being treated in the primary care setting rather than the hospital, avoiding the stigma of being labelled as psychiatric. Locating nursing services in primary care was not only deemed viable, but may have saved more resources than it consumed. Even taking clinical outcomes, such as reduction in anxiety, into account, the cost of employing a nurse therapist was offset by reduction in time off work and lower rate of reliance on health care resources by patients. Other opportunistic benefits were obtained from the presence of the nurse and extension of the role into other areas of work. Finally, the duration of the clinical problem was 30% less for these patients compared with similar cohort of hospital patients. While psychiatric nurses were playing an increasingly important clinical role in the therapeutic management of psychiatric patients, there had been little management and rigorous evaluation of the impact of this. This was the first controlled study of psychiatric nurses caring for patients who attend the GP surgery, and a pioneering development in community psychiatric care.

MARKS, I. (1985)

Controlled trial of psychiatric nurse therapists in primary care*

INTRODUCTION

The results of research from several countries and settings have shown that when the patients of general practitioners, physicians, and psychiatrists are managed by advanced clinical nurses they do at least as well as patients who are managed by other professionals.[1] Although psychiatric nurses play an increasingly salient clinical part, no controlled study has been made of the work of such nurses in primary care in the United Kingdom. Impressive controlled findings were reported for the follow up of discharged patients with neurosis by community psychiatric nurses who were based in a hospital,[2] and psychiatric nurse therapists have been monitored mainly in uncontrolled hospital settings.

A controlled inquiry was therefore undertaken of behavioural psychotherapy given by nurse therapists in primary care. This is a preliminary report of the outcome. A full account will appear elsewhere.[1] It is the first controlled study of psychiatric nurses caring for patients who attend the surgery of a general practitioner rather than a hospital.

METHOD

Three questions were asked in the study: (i) How effective is a nurse therapist with suitable patients? This was answered by assigning suitable patients with neurosis at random to behavioural treatment by a nurse therapist who worked in a general practice or to routine non-behavioural management by the general practitioner. The latter patients were controls and were offered (crossover) behavioural treatment from the nurse at the end of a year if they did not improve. (ii) Is there a viable role for a nurse therapist as part of a primary care team? This was answered from informal data collected from the primary care team and the nurse therapist. (iii) What proportion of patients who attend surgery has disorders suitable for behavioural treatment? This was answered by examining consecutive patients who attended and also by offering a general psychiatric consultation service in two practices. The answer to a fourth question about controlled cost-benefit analysis of the outcome has been reported in full.[3]

A full time nurse therapist gave the behavioural psychotherapy. Over the four years of the study (1978–82) there were three therapists working consecutively for 13, four, and 27 months respectively. A psychiatrist was the blind assessor.

Initially one health centre (five general practitioners) and one group practice (five general practitioners) participated in the study (totalling 26,000 patients). A further group of three general practitioners (3,300 patients) was added six months later and another group of seven general practitioners (18,500 patients) at the end of year 1, making a total of 20 general practitioners with lists of 47,800 patients for years 2 and 3.

The general practitioners were briefed about criteria for the suitability of patients for behavioural psychotherapy, asked to refer suitable patients, and given a research referral form. Patients who were willing to participate were offered an assessment interview with the nurse therapist at the health centre or surgery, and a relative was also seen when possible.

The nurse therapist was based with the primary care team and carried out behavioural psychotherapy with suitable patients in the surgery, in the patient's home, or in other settings where the patient's problem would manifest. If the patient drew at random behavioural treatment this began immediately, and the nurse and patient made additional ratings at the end of treatment and six months after entering the trial. Behavioural treatment was tailored to the individual along the lines described elsewhere.[4-6] It included exposure for phobics (21 patients completed therapy) and obsessive-convulsives (4), self regulation for habit disorders (3), and sexual skills training for a patient with sexual dysfunction. Patients had a mean of six treatment sessions (mean of seven treatment hours), a therapeutic investment that was slightly less than that needed during a training programme for nurse therapists.

Patients who drew the control condition were asked to continue to deal with their difficulties as previously under the usual care of their general practitioner. The general practitioner was notified and asked to give the patient for the next year the routine treatment under the National Health Service that he or she would have given anyway had the nurse therapist not been available. Control patients were rerated at three and six months.

At the end of a year in the trial all patients were asked to attend the health centre or surgery for a routine follow up interview by the nurse and psychiatrist. At the start of the interview patients were reminded of the need for the psychiatrist to remain blind, and no mention was made of whether patients had received treatment in the preceding 12 months. After the one year ratings were completed by the patient, nurse, and psychiatrist, control patients who had not improved were offered behavioural treatment by the nurse.

MEASURES

(a) Problem and work/leisure ratings were made by patient, nurse, and psychiatrist on reliable standardised scales. (b) Problem related targets were rated only for patients treated by the nurse, by the patient and the nurse, again on reliable, standardised scales. (c) The fear questionnaire was self rated and provided a broader measure of phobias and anxiety-depression. It has been used extensively in previous studies.[7]

SELECTION OF PATIENTS

The selection criteria were the same as those used for patients with neurosis who were being assessed for behavioural psychotherapy in the outpatient department.[4] All patients (except for one being seen at home) had the initial 30 to 60 minute selection interview conducted by the nurse in the health centre or the surgery of the doctor who referred the patient. The psychiatrist observed this interview of the first 136 patients and asked clarifying questions if necessary. The nurse and psychiatrist then independently rated the patient and recorded their diagnoses, suitability for treatment, and recommendations, after which the psychiatrist withdrew. The patient completed his other ratings; the nurse made the random assignment and then told the patient of the decision about treatment. Patients were referred back to their general practitioners if unsuitable or if they refused to enter the trial.

Referrals – Of 254 patients who were referred, 34 failed to attend for interview, leaving 220 who were assessed. Of these 220, 104 were unsuitable for behavioural psychotherapy. Of the 116 suitable patients, 24 refused to enter the trial. The remaining 92 were randomly allocated (balanced for diagnosis and numbers) to the control waiting list and to immediate treatment conditions (46 in each). Three general practitioners referred proportionately more patients for the trial and for general psychiatric consultation.

No shows – Thirty four (13%) out of 254 referrals failed to attend two appointments for the initial selection interview. This is less than the 18% 'no show' rate of outpatients seen for the nurse therapist training course at the Maudsley.

Refusers – Twenty four (20%) of the 116 suitable patients refused to enter the trial, a refusal rate similar to that in the Maudsley nurse therapist training course. Refusers did not differ appreciably from acceptors for mean scores on the general health questionnaire, the behavioural questionnaire, or on behavioural handicap and problem severity.

Demographic features and duration of problem of referred patients – The mean age of the patients who were accepted into the trial was 35 years, the same as that of patients who were unsuitable for referral. Both groups had twice as many women as men – the usual sex ratio for patients with neurosis. The patients who were entered into the trial and the unsuitable patients did not differ appreciably in their mean scores for the four tests mentioned above.

The mean duration of the problem was seven years compared with 10 years in similar outpatients who received behavioural therapy at the Maudsley. Primary care patients thus presented earlier, though their problems were nevertheless chronic.

Allocation and fate of patients – Patients were randomly allocated to behavioural treatment to be given immediately by the nurse (46 patients) or the control condition of routine support from the general practitioner for a year (46 patients). Of the former group of patients, 29 (63%) completed treatment, which lasted fewer than three months on average, and follow up to one year after entry into the trial. Of the control patients, 37 (80%) remained in the trial to its end. By the end of that year seven control patients had improved, and the remaining 30 were offered behavioural treatment from the nurse. Fewer control patients completed the behavioural treatment given in the crossover phase (46%) than did those who had it immediately (63%). Of the control patients, 20% dropped out during their year (or six months) in routine care; a further 30% refused subsequent crossover treatment, but only 7% dropped out after it began.

Diagnostic categories – Sixty seven of the 92 patients who were randomly allocated

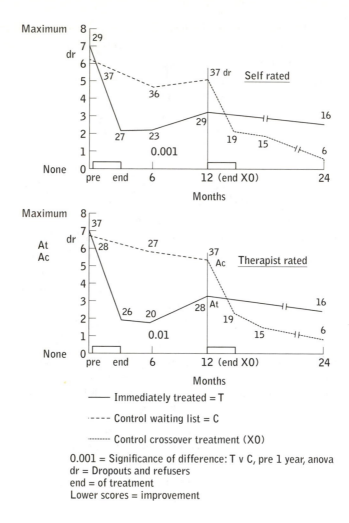

Figure 13.1 Outcome for all patients: main problem. At = assessor ratings for patients who were immediately treated; Ac = assessor ratings for the control patients

were phobics: 37 agoraphobics (19 treated by the nurse, 18 control), 18 specific phobics, and 12 social phobics. The remaining patients included eight obsessive-compulsives, seven with sexual dysfunction, and 10 with habit disorder.

Completers v non-completers (dropped out before six sessions) – The completers and the non-completers of the trial year had a similar duration of their problem and similar initial severity.

RESULTS

The first 139 patients referred were asked to indicate where they would be happy to attend for treatment – at home, the general practitioner's surgery, or the outpatient department of a psychiatric hospital. Patients clearly preferred being seen at the general practitioner's surgery: 96% were agreeable to being treated in the general practitioner's surgery, 84% at home, but only 55% in outpatient departments.

At the selection interview the ratings of the nurse and the psychiatrist correlated highly (p = 0.001): 0.79 primary diagnosis (n = 136); 0.83 suitability for behavioural psychotherapy (n = 136); 0.96 reason for unsuitability (n = 76); 0.93 degree of unsuitability (n = 76); 0.95 method of management (n = 136); 0.58 estimated time needed; and 0.66 estimated number of sessions needed for behavioural treatment (n = 76). This high agreement between the nurse therapist and the psychiatrist about the diagnosis and the management of patients with behavioural disorders in primary care is closely similar to that in psychiatric outpatient departments.[4]

The ratings on entry to the trial and one year later were pooled to compute inter-rater reliability of patient, nurse, and psychiatrist. All interrater correlations were significant well beyond the 0.001 level, those for problem, target, and work ratings varying from 0.81 to 0.97, and ratings of social and private leisure from 0.70 to 0.86. Interrater reliability was thus satisfactory.

CLINICAL OUTCOME

Treatment: nurse v general practitioner – Figures 13.1 and 13.2 show the mean scores for problem and work ratings: the significance (anova) of the differences between the two groups in their improvement from entry into the trial to one year later appear above the horizontal axis of each graph. *At* and *Ac* in the lower half of Figure 13.2 indicate the blind psychiatrist's rating for the patients who were immediately treated and for the control groups respectively and *dr* denotes the rating for dropouts who could be followed up. The full details of the outcome are reported elsewhere.[1]

A year after entry into the trial the patients who had received behavioural psychotherapy from the nurse therapist had improved significantly more than the control patients who had remained on routine treatment from the general practitioner for a year. This superiority was found on main problem, fear, questionnaire on global phobia and anxiety-depression, work adjustment, and social and private leisure (p<0.001–<0.05). All three raters agreed on the superiority of treatment by the nurse. Six months after entry into the trial the same pattern had emerged on the same variables.

Improvement within each group separately – Patients who received behavioural psychotherapy immediately from the nurse had a highly significant improvement (*t* tests) on all 17 variables rated at the end of treatment, and they maintained this improvement on all 22 variables rated at one year follow up. By contrast, during their year control patients improved significantly on only seven of 18 rated variables, and at a lower level of significance. Thereafter, control patients who had not improved were then offered behavioural crossover treatment by the nurse (seven of the 37 had by then improved so that they did not require treatment). By the completion of this treatment these patients improved significantly on 16 of 17 variables rated, mainly at the 0.001 level. On most variables the improvement of control patients during behavioural crossover treatment was significantly greater (*t* test) than that during their preceding year on the waiting list.

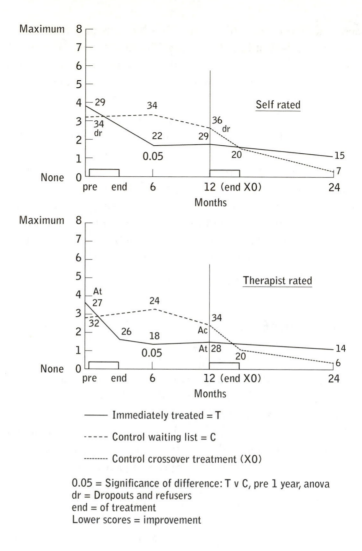

Figure 13.2   Outcome for all patients: work. At = assessor ratings for patients who were immediately treated; Ac = assessor for the control patients.

For the minority of patients who had dropped out or refused treatment who could be rated, the means are seen at the points *dr* in Figure 13.1. These dropouts did not improve – the outcome at one year was like that of control patients.

Psychiatric morbidity – Of the 12 item general health questionnaire 39% of consecutive attenders during a screening week scored three or more out of a possible total of 12, which is comparable with that in two other studies in which the questionnaire was used in primary care.[8, 9] The general practitioners detected psychiatric problems ('conspicuous psychiatric morbidity') in 15% of patients who consulted them during the same screening week, compared with the 14% found in two studies[10, 11] but much lower than the 31% in another study.[12]

'Behavioural' morbidity proved difficult to estimate. The general practitioners varied

greatly in their referral rates, and over the three years they referred 116 patients who were suitable for the trial. Some suitable cases were referred elsewhere, however, and it became evident that many patients were missed when a psychiatrist offered a psychiatric consultation service in two practices. In one practice 15% of patients seen for general psychiatric consultation were sufficiently handicapped to be suitable for systematic behavioural psychotherapy in the research trial, and a further 12% were less severe and needed behavioural counselling. In the second practice 19% had problems suitable for behavioural management. The density of referrals was sufficient to sustain a nurse therapist working with a population of about 25,000 patients registered with 10 general practitioners.

DISCUSSION

In up to one year of follow up patients who were treated by nurses improved significantly more than did control patients. Control patients showed few gains during the year of routine care from the general practitioner but improved significantly when they subsequently had behavioural psychotherapy from the nurse. Those who refused and dropped out and could be followed up did not make useful gains. Most had phobic or obsessive-compulsive disorders. The results are in line with those of other controlled studies, suggesting the value of providing a behaviourally oriented clinical psychology service in a health centre.[13]

There was much additional evidence to support the value of psychiatric nurse therapists working at the general practitioner's surgery. Firstly, there was high agreement between the nurse and the psychiatrist concerning the diagnosis, the suitability for behavioural psychotherapy, and the management of referred patients. This replicated previous similar findings.[4] Little is gained by using a psychiatrist (or, presumably, a psychologist) rather than a nurse therapist to select patients for behavioural therapy in primary care or hospital.

Secondly, patients obviously preferred to be treated at home or in the surgery rather than in psychiatric outpatients departments, thus being seen nearer their homes, in familiar surroundings, and in the environment where their problems manifest, and avoiding the stigma of a 'psychiatric' label.

Thirdly, two cost-benefit analyses, one controlled[3] and another uncontrolled,[14] suggested that, even disregarding 'intangible' benefits, such as lessened fear and anxiety, the cost of employing a nurse was more than offset by tangible economic gains after treatment from the patients having less time off work and fewer expenses and lower use of health care resources. In the long term it may cost the community less to provide nurse therapists for such patients.

Fourthly, two unmeasured benefits emerged. Some patients who were excluded from the research trial because of its stringent criteria nevertheless seemed to gain from brief behavioural counselling given by the nurse at the assessment interview – for example, exposure homework instructions for phobics or sexual counselling for patients with sexual dysfunction. The general practitioners also sought the nurse's advice about general psychiatric patients as well as about behavioural psychotherapy, thus extending the nurse's role towards that of a community psychiatric nurse.

Fifthly, the mean duration of the problem for primary care patients in this study was 30% less than that in a comparable cohort of hospital patients. Working in primary care shortens the chain of referral so that problems may be spotted and resolved earlier.

Sixthly, a higher proportion of patients who were suitable for behavioural psychotherapy was referred over successive years. General practitioners and other primary care professionals learnt from the nurse therapist how to spot suitable cases and also how to give behavioural advice. (During the study several patients with sexual dysfunction were referred to clinics where their chances of getting appropriate behavioural treatment were small.) Informed general practitioners may also be less likely to prescribe psychotropic medication that may be unnecessary and have undesirable side effects. Most of the general practitioners wanted the nurse therapist to continue in their practice after the study was over. The funding of such placements, however, is a problem.

Finally, employing nurse therapists in primary care might lead to fewer referrals to busy psychiatric hospitals, and with suitable training nurses may be able to extend 'behavioural medicine' into managing common problems in general practice such as hypertension, coronary heart disease, insomnia, and the rehabilitation of physical handicap.

There are two possible snags: one is a potentially higher dropout rate of patients in primary care than in outpatient departments – this needs further study; the other is the lower density of referrals. This requires the nurse therapist to work with at least two groups of general practitioners, which leads to more travelling than if the nurse worked in one hospital only and leaves less clinical time. This occurs with community psychiatric nurses and other carers.[15] An attachment to two groups of general practitioners serving about 25,000 patients might be optimum.

CONCLUSION

The value of the work of advanced clinical nurses is underlined by recent controlled research into their effects on patients with neurosis either when community psychiatric nurses follow the patients up after discharge under the care of a psychiatric outpatient team,[2] or, as in this study, when nurse therapists take patients as direct referrals from general practitioners while working with the primary care team. Both studies indicate the worthwhile gains that may ensue to patients and to the community from psychiatric nurses assuming a greater role in the care of patients with neurosis.

A grant from the Department of Health and Social Security supported the research. I thank the nurses who were consecutively concerned as therapists, Martin Brown, Malcolm Day, and Peter Lindley, and the psychiatrist, Helena Waters for their sterling work; David Bainton, Mary Dastgir, Richard France, David Goldberg, Susan Hamer, Bob McDonald, Erville Millar, Joyce Prince, and John Tait for valuable comments on the research at various stages; and the general practitioners whose generous help made this project possible, Drs S Barnes, C Benn, A Brocks, C Challacombe, W Chandler, S Ebrahim, B Essex, C Gillespie, H Graver, C Haigh, R Higgs, N Jackson, D Kirby, J Lee, A Marus, T Mendelsohn, P Randeria, R M Rowland, P Schofield, T Welton, and the late Dr P Freeman.

NOTES

British Medical Journal 290: 1181–1184. Reprinted with permission of the BMJ Publishing Group.

1 Marks IM. *A controlled trial of psychiatric nurse therapists in primary care*. London: Royal College of Nursing (in press).

2 Paykel ES, Griffith JH. *Community psychiatric nursing for neurotic patients*. London: Royal College of Nursing, 1983.

3 Ginsberg G, Marks IM, Waters H. Cost-benefit analysis of a controlled trial of nurse therapy for neuroses in primary care. *Psychol Med* 1984; 14:683–90.

4 Marks IM, Hallam RS, Connolly J, Philpott R. *Nursing in behavioural psychotherapy*. London: Royal College of Nursing, 1977.

5 Bird J, Marks IM, Lindley P. Nurse therapists in psychiatry: developments, controversies and implications. *Br J. Psychiatry* 1979; 135:321–9.

6 Marks IM. *Cure and care of neuroses*. New York: John Wiley, 1981.

7 Marks IM, Matthews AM. Brief standard self-rating for phobic patients. *Behav Res Ther* 1979; 17:263–7.

8 Goldberg DP, Blackwell B. Psychiatric illness in general practice. A detailed study using a new method of case identification. *Br Med J* 1970; i:439–43.

9 Johnstone, A Goldberg D. Psychiatric screening in general practice. A controlled trial. *Lancet* 1976; i:605–8.

10 Chancellor A, Mant A, Andrews G. The general practitioner's identification and management of emotional disorders. *Aust Fam Physician* 1977; 6:1137–43.

11 Goldberg D, Kay C, Thompson L. Psychiatric morbidity in general practice and the community. *Pychol Med* 1976; 6:565–9.

12 Marks JN, Goldberg DP, Hillier VF. Determinants of the ability of general practitioners to detect psychiatric illness. *Psychol Med* 1979; 9:337–53.

13 Robson MH, France R, Bland M. Clinical psychologist in primary care: controlled clinical and economic evaluation. *Br Med J* 1984; 288:1805–8.

14 Ginsberg G, Marks IM; Costs and benefits of behavioural psychotherapy: a pilot study of neurotics treated by nurse-therapists. *Psychol Med* 1977; 7:685–700.

15 Sladden S. *Psychiatric nursing in the community*. Edinburgh: Churchill Livingstone, 1979.

Chapter 14

A randomised clinical trial of early hospital discharge and home follow-up of very-low-birth-weight infants

DOROTHY BROOTEN, SAVITRI KUMAR, LINDA P. BROWN, PRISCILLA BUTTS, STEVEN A. FINKLER, SUSAN BAKEWELL-SACHS, ANN GIBBONS, MARIA DELIVORIA-PAPADOPOULOS

Introduction

Neonatal intensive care is one of the most expensive forms of hospital care. Yet follow-up care has been sparse or nonexistent. The impact on parents and families is significant. Within the first year, very-low-birthweight infants are four times more likely to be rehospitalised, their post-neonatal death rate is five times greater. Elevated risks of failure to thrive, chronic lung disease, anaemia, seizures, developmental and parenting problems are evident in this group. Socio-economically, a higher proportion of very-low-birthweight infants are born to poor young mothers with meagre resources to provide adequate care after discharge. Significantly, evidence of prolonged hospi-talisation had confirmed that babies were more at risk of infection and associated with failure to thrive, child abuse and parental feelings of inadequacy. Although reductions in mortality and morbidity had been attributed to neonatal intensive care units, research had suggested that environmental stresses such as harsh lights and noise levels may have a permanent impact upon an infant's sensory functions such as hear-ing, vision and motor co-ordination. There were therefore sound clinical and economic reasons for considering early discharge as a therapeutic and cost-effective option. This pioneering study was one of the first to suggest that early discharge from neonatal intensive care units could be associated with positive outcomes for low-birthweight babies. It was also one of the first to confirm the economic and clinical effectiveness of Masters-prepared advanced practice nurses enabled to work to an expert agenda.

The strengths of the study are several. First, the context in which this research was being conducted needs to be taken into account. The paucity of home care in the USA for this group of patients, and their families both clinically and economically, makes this an important service development and contribution. Although some research had been conducted in other medical specialties to enhance care and decrease costs, this was a new departure in the field of neonatology. Second, the client group was one at risk, disadvantaged socio-economically and hitherto excluded from such outreach efforts. Previous studies had confined themselves to middle class families, and there was little precedent to build on. Third, it was a clear sphere of nursing practice in which the efficacy of advanced education of specialist nurses could be evaluated. Fourth, economic evaluation was built in rather than bolted onto the study. Fifth, it challenged the prevailing orthodoxy of discharge policy which held that early discharge in adults was associated with negative rather than positive outcomes.

The intervention consisted of contact across the care trajectory: a pre-discharge screening of skills and knowledge of medications, a 1-week post-discharge visit to co-ordinate and assess the environment for care, and further visits at 9, 12 and 18 months. Telephone contact was initiated with parents within the first 2 weeks, up to 3 times per week after discharge with an on-call service. Contact for the first 8 weeks was weekly. The nurse specialist contacted one or both parents soon after the birth and at least once a week during the infant's hospitalisation to promote parents' interaction with the infant, assess parents' concerns about the infant, teach them how to handle and soothe the infant, promote sleep, prevent infection and perform various minor technical tasks such as temperature-taking. Interestingly the frequency of telephone contact initiated by parents far exceeded expectations. Little was made of this in the study, but it points to the potential of this resource being rolled out in telephone triage services such as NHS Direct within the UK. One of the most impressive features of the study is that achievements were possible in a sample where 42% had less than highschool education, 69% were unmarried and had a reported annual income of less than $75,000, 11% had no telephone and 72% had to rely upon the police or public transport in an emergency – all indices of social deprivation. The nurse was the critical link in the chain of care, providing much-needed continuity to this poor, often transient population.

Those in the early-discharge group were discharged before they reached the routine weight, provided they met a standard set of conditions. For such families, instruction, counselling, home visits and daily on-call availability of a hospital-based specialist for 18 months were provided. Infants in the early-discharge group were discharged some 11 days earlier, weighed 200 g less and were 2 weeks younger at discharge than controls. The hospital and physician costs of care were respectively 27% and 22% less for the early-discharge group. When the costs of home follow-up were accounted for, there was still a significant saving. No differences were detected between groups in numbers of rehospitalisations, acute care visits or measures of mental and physical growth. Early discharge of very-low-birthweight infants with follow-up home care by a nurse specialist was regarded as safe and cost effective.

This study challenged the received wisdom in a number of ways. It countered convention and demonstrated that, early discharge, unlike that for adults, could be beneficial for neonates. Funders, peer reviewers and the research community in the first instance had to be convinced that the risks and viability of such an approach would pay off in a politically sensitive field. Government endorsement, as well as that associated with the prestigious Robert Wood Johnson Foundation, benchmark quality through peer review. It is a tribute to the courage and commitment of all that this vision was realised and carried through to fruition. The study was one of the first to demonstrate the value of Advanced Practice Nurses working to an expert agenda. It has since provided a model of research that has helped to set the standards for achievement; cross-disciplinary collaboration and publication in a prestigious mainstream peer-reviewed journal. Each of these contributes to building credibility and political capital for nursing, and demonstrates the utility of the study in forming part of the solution to apparently intractable social problems.

BROOTEN, D., S KUMAR, L.P. BROWN, P. BUTTS, S.A. FINKLER, S. BAKEWELL-SACHS, A. GIBBONS, M. DELIVORIA-PAPADOPOULOS (1986)

A randomised clinical trial of early hospital discharge and home follow-up of very-low-birth-weight infants*

More than 230,000 low-birth-weight infants are born annually in the United States, and more than 36,000 of these infants weigh less than 1500 g.[1–6] In addition, the proportion of live births made up by infants weighing less than 1500 g has changed little in the past several decades.[7,8] Although advances in neonatal intensive care have been credited with reducing mortality and morbidity in this group,[9–11] recent studies suggest that the environment for the neonatal intensive care unit – with its bright lights and high noise levels – may have a permanent adverse effect on an infant's hearing, vision, and motor coordination.[12–14] Prolonged hospitalisation increases the infant's chances of contracting infections and has been associated with failure to thrive, child abuse, and parental feelings of inadequacy.[15–18] Hospital care for these infants is one of the most expensive of all types of hospitalisation.[19,20] Despite initial hospital expenditures averaging up to $167,000 for very-low-birth-weight infants,[21] formalised home care services are almost completely lacking after these infants are discharged. This lack of services is particularly troubling since this group is at high risk for failure to thrive, problems associated with chronic lung disease, anemia, seizures, and developmental delays, as well as parenting problems.[22] In the first year of life, the rate of rehospitalisation for very-low-birth-weight infants is four times the rate for normal-birth-weight infants (≥ 2500 g) and their post-neonatal death rate is five times as high.[10] Compounding these problems, a disproportionate number of very-low-birth-weight infants are born to poor, young mothers with questionable resources to provide adequate care after discharge.[23]

Although home visits by nurses have been used in a variety of medical specialties to improve care and decrease health care costs, the efficacy of visits by perinatal nurse specialists to very-low-birth-weight infants after discharge has not been documented. This clinical trial was undertaken to examine whether it is safe and economical to discharge very-low-birth-weight infants (≤ 1500 g) early if they meet certain conditions and to subsidise home care services with any savings that result from shorter hospitalisations.

METHODS

Infants with birth weights of 1500 g or less who were born at the Hospital of the University of Pennsylvania between October 1982 and December 1984 were randomly assigned to one of two groups, after their parents gave informed consent to their participation in the study. Infants in the control group were discharged according to routine nursery policy, which required that the infant be clinically well, feeding well and weigh approximately 2200 g. Although parents received support and instructions from nursery nurses about their infant and his or her care after discharge, no routine home follow-up care by nurses was provided for this group.

Infants in the early-discharge group were discharged before they weighed 2200 g so long as they met the following criteria: (1) they were clinically well and able to feed by nipple every four hours; (2) they were able to maintain their body temperature in an open crib in room air; (3) no evidence of serious apnea or bradycardia was found in a 12-hour recording of the infant's heart rate and respiration; (4) the mother or other caretaker demonstrated satisfactory care-taking skills; and (5) the physical home environment and facilities for the care of the infant were adequate.

Infants and families in the early-discharge group received home follow-up care provided by a nurse. Since specialty practice in the care of these high-risk infants and their families formally occurs at the master's-degree level in nursing, one full-time nurse and two part-time relief nurses with master's degrees in perinatal and neonatal nursing were hired to provide follow-up care to the families. A nurse specialist contacted one or both parents soon after the infant's birth and at least once a week during the infant's hospitalisation to promote the parents' interaction with the infant; to evaluate the parents' perceptions and concerns about the infant; to teach parents to bathe, handle, and soothe the infant, to take his or her temperature, and to prevent infection; and to provide information about the infant's sleeping patterns, differences in infant temperature, reportable signs and symptoms, and times for routine medical care. Weekly contact with parents helped to establish a rapport between parents and the nurse specialist and provided continuity for the parents as the infant was transferred from the intensive care unit to the intermediate care unit and then home.

Before discharge, parents were required to demonstrate satisfactorily the basic care-taking skills described above and a basic knowledge of any medications or special procedures required in the infant's care. Approximately one week before discharge, the nurse specialist made a home visit to coordinate planning for the discharge and to evaluate the adequacy of heat in the home, the safety of the environment, and the adequacy of facilities for the care of the newborn. When problems were encountered, the nurse specialist consulted with physicians, hospital social-service personnel, and others in the community.

After the infant was discharged, the nurse made home visits during the first week and at 1, 9, 12, and 18 months. The visits included a physical examination of the infant, developmental screening, confirmation of appointments for medical follow-up care, an assessment of the parents' coping ability and care-taking skills and support systems, and instructions and counseling regarding infant care and infant stimulation, if needed. The nurse was in contact with the parents by telephone at least three times a week for the first two weeks after discharge and weekly thereafter for eight weeks. The nurse specialist was on call from 8:00 a.m. to 10:00 p.m. Monday through Friday and from 8:00 a.m. to noon on weekends, to respond to parents' concerns and special problems. Medical backup for the nurse was provided by neonatologists at the hospital. Long-term medical follow-up care for infants in both groups was provided either by the hospital's high-risk follow-up clinic or by private pediatricians.

Infants with life-threatening congenital anomalies, grade 4 intraventricular hemorrhage, extensive surgical intervention, oxygen dependence for a period of more than 10 weeks, or a combination of these factors were excluded from the study.

Sample

Of 136 infants eligible for enrollment at birth, 57 were not included in the study because of death (6 infants), the complications described above as reasons for exclusion (34), family complications (7), or their parents' refusal to participate (10). The sample included 72 mothers and 79 infants: 36 mothers and 39 infants (3 sets of twins) in the early-discharge group, and 36 mothers and 40 infants (4 sets of twins) in the control group (Table 14.1). There were no statistically significant differences between the groups in terms of the mother's age, educational level, marital status, race, or number of children; the family structure; the availability of a telephone in the home; the type of transportation available in an emergency; the family's reported annual income; the type of health insurance; or the number of children under five years of age (a variable associated with increased infection rates among low-birth-weight infants after discharge). Although no data on living conditions were gathered on the control group, inadequate heating, food, and formula were problems during follow-up for 11 percent of the families in the early-discharge group.

There were no statistically significant differences between the groups in terms of the infants' mean birth weight, gestational age, appropriateness of size for gestational age, number of days of ventilation, or number of days spent in the intensive care nursery. Seventy infants were of appropriate size for gestational age at birth, whereas nine infants were small for gestational age (four in the early-discharge group and five in the control group). Ninety-seven percent of the infants had complicating conditions while they were hospitalised; these included respiratory distress syndrome (30 in the early-discharge group and 35 in the control group); necrotising enterocolitis (2 in each group); surgery (1 in each group); and jaundice requiring phototherapy (37 in the early-discharge group and 39 in the control group).

Twenty-five infants (32 percent) were discharged with apnea monitors (14 in the early-discharge group and 11 in the control group). Fifty-nine infants (75 percent) were discharged with medications such as theophylline or vitamin E to be administered at home by their parents (28 in the early-discharge group and 31 in the control group). Because of the time limits of the study, 12 infants, 6 in each group, were followed for less than 18 months.

Table 14.1   Characteristics of very-low-birth-weight infants and their families

Characteristic	Early-discharge group	Control group
Mother		
Number	36	36
Mean age ± SD (range)	24+7 yr	23±6 yr
	(16–44)	12–38)
Education level		
Less than high school	42%	30.5%
High school	28%	39.0%
More than high school	30%	30.5%
Marital status		
Married	31%	33%
Unmarried	69%	67%
Race		
Black	83%	78%
White	17%	22%
Family		
Hospital insurance		
Medicaid	75%	56%
Private	25%	44%
Income		
<$5,000	34%	26%
$5,001–9,999	43%	32%
$10,000–49,000	17%	26%
>$50,000	6%	16%
Infants		
Number	39	40
Mean birth weight ±SD (range)	1187±198 g	1148± 203 g
	(740–1490)	(710–1500)
Mean gestational age at	30±2 wk	30±2 wk
birth ±SD (range)	(26–37)	(26–37)

Statistical analysis

All data are expressed as means ±SD. The significance of differences was determined by unpaired t-tests.

RESULTS

Infants in the early-discharge group were discharged from the hospital a mean of 11.2 days earlier, weighed 200 g less, and were approximately two weeks younger at discharge than the infants in the control group (Table 14.2). The difference in the average length of hospital stay between the groups was statistically significant (P<0.05).

Table 14.2   Characteristics of very-low-birth-weight infants at discharge and during follow-up

Characteristic	Early-discharge group (N = 39)	Control group (N = 40)
Mean days of hospitalisation	46.5±12.5*	57.7±17*
±SD (range)	(20–79)	(21–94)
Mean weight at discharge	2072±131 g	2280±179 g
±SD (range)	(1880–2500)	(1980–2650)
Mean gestational age at discharge	36±2 wk	38±2 wk
±SD (range)	(34–39)	(34–44)
No. of infants rehospitalised		
Within 14 days	4	5
Within 18 months	10	10
No. of infants with acute care visits	29	36
No. of acute care visits	163	186
No. of infants with failure to thrive	0	1
No. of infants reported abused	2	4
No. of infants in foster care	0	2

*The difference in the two means is statistically significant ($P<0.05$).

There were no statistically significant differences between the groups in terms of the number of rehospitalisations, the number of acute care visits, the incidence of failure to thrive, reported child abuse, or foster placement during the 18-month follow-up period. The two cases of reported child abuse in the early-discharge group were in families that did not comply with requirements for medical follow-up during the child's second year of life. Infants in two of the four families in the control group in which child abuse was reported were physically abused and required foster care. One infant in the early-discharge group died of sudden infant death syndrome during the first year of follow-up. There were no deaths in the control group.

There were no statistically significant differences between the groups in the development quotient of infants as measured by the Bayley scale of infant development. Two infants, one in each group, had developmental quotients below 80. Seven infants (four in the early-discharge group and three in the control group) were at or below the fifth percentile in physical growth (weight and length) at the end of the follow-up period. Of these seven infants, one was a twin and two had been small for gestational age at birth. These three infants were in the experimental group.

Despite the nurse's maintaining frequent telephone contact with the parents in the early-discharge group, according to the study protocol, parents initiated more than 300 telephone calls to the nurse during the follow-up period. Seventy-four percent of the calls were made within the first six months after discharge. Parents' concerns were classified into five major areas and ranked according to frequency. The five areas were newborn health problems (30 percent), concerns about routine care of the newborn (25 percent), giving information (22 percent), requesting information (13 percent), and maternal concerns (10 percent). Newborn health problems included questions regarding apnea monitoring, respiratory infections, gastrointestinal problems, fevers, hernias, medicines, skin rashes, injuries, ear infections, and nonspecific symptoms.

Concerns about routine newborn care included questions or problems with feeding, elimination, hearing, sleep, hygiene, immunisation, and development. Giving information included reports by the parents of the infant's condition, providing new telephone numbers for parents, and canceling or making appointments for home visits by the nurse or for follow-up clinic. Requests for information included questions about tests and equipment, requests for physicians' telephone numbers and referrals to community agencies and parent support groups. Maternal concerns included questions about the resumption of sexual activities, frustrations about living conditions, scheduling clinic appointments, and problems with monitor companies. The number and type of telephone calls initiated by parents did not differ according to the type of medical insurance held by the parents.

Total charges for the initial hospitalisation for the 79 infants were $4,974,710, consisting of $4,450,910 in hospital charges and $523,800 for physicians' fees (Table 14.3). The average hospital charge was $56,341 and the average physician's charge was $6,803 for each infant. The difference in the mean hospital charge between the early-discharge group ($47,520) and the control group ($64,940) was $17,420; this difference was statistically significant (P<0.01). The difference in the mean physician's charge between the early-discharge group ($5,933) and the control group ($7,649)

Table 14.3 Costs of care for very-low-birth-weight infants

	Early-discharge group	Control group
Charges for initial hospitalisation ($)		
No. of infants	39	40
Total	1,853,297	2,597,613
Mean	47,520*	64,940*
Range	21,729–106,409	23,619–131,882
SD	19,856	31,545
Charges for physician's services ($)		
No. of infants	38†	39†
Total	225,465	298,335
Mean	5,933††	7,649††
Range	2,275–10,625	3,125–15,725
SD	2,164	3,169
Costs related to nurse specialist's services ($)		
No. of families	36	0
Total cost of nurse specialist's time	19,264	–
Mean cost of nurse specialist's time	535	–
Total telephone charges	966	–
Mean telephone charges	27	–
Total travel costs	500	–
Mean travel costs	14	–

* The difference between the two means is statistically significant (P<0.01) by a one-tailed test.

† Physician's charge data were unavailable for one infant in each group.

†† The difference between the two means is statistically significant (P<0.01) by a one-tailed test.

was $1,716 which was also significant (P<0.01). The mean hospital charge for the early-discharge group was 26.8 percent less than that for the control group. The mean physician's charge was 22.4 percent less than that for the control group. The mean combined hospital and physician's charges for the early-discharge group were $19,136, or 26.4 percent less than for the control group.

The difference between the groups cannot all be counted as savings, since the costs of the nurse specialist's services must be included for the early-discharge group. The parents of the infants discharged early were not charged for the nurse's services, so no charge data exist. Therefore, the actual cost of providing this care was used for this part of the analysis. The cost of the time spent by the nurse in direct care of the infants and families was considered, as well as telephone time, time spent on home visits, travel time to and from home visits, and administrative time. Telephone charges and travel costs were included in the analysis.

The total cost of the home follow-up care for 33 infants for 18 months and 6 infants for 6 months was $20,730 (Table 14.3). This is a mean cost of $576 per infant and consists of the following: the cost of the time spent by the nurse specialist with families before discharge (a mean of $137 per family), the time spent by the nurse specialist with families after discharge ($398 per family), $27 for telephone calls, and $14 in travel costs for home visits. All the families in the early-discharge group lived within 45 miles (72 km) of the hospital.

DISCUSSION

Programs of early hospital discharge for low-birth-weight infants can potentially decrease iatrogenic illness and hospital-acquired infections, enhance parent–infant interaction, and decrease hospital costs for care. With the introduction of diagnosis-related groups and prospective payment systems, such programs are an economic necessity. However, such programs are scarce in the United States, and the majority of them have dealt with healthy infants with higher birth weights and greater gestational age than the infants in our study, and most of the infants have been born to middle-class families.[24–28] Moreover, few of these programs provide the much-needed assistance in caring for the infant during the important transition period in the home, after hospital discharge.

On the basis of our findings, we conclude that early discharge of very-low-birth-weight infants according to the standards used in this study is safe, feasible, and cost effective and provides continuity of care. The hospital-based approach has several advantages: it provides continuity of care by having a nurse with specialised knowledge and skills in caring for these families and infants provide the direct care; it includes the nurse as an integral part of the hospital staff and community network, with backup available from physicians familiar with the past progress of the infant; and it makes the services of the nurse available to the families seven days a week through a telephone service. The continued home monitoring of the infant's physical status, the parents' ability to cope, their compliance with specialised medical procedures, and their use of any equipment required for high-risk infants discharged early mean that home follow-up care must be provided by nurses who have specialised in high-risk neonatal care. The need for this kind of follow-up care can only increase as smaller infants with many complex health problems survive and as the complexity of their home care increases.

Using the study methods described above, we found that infants in the early-discharge group were able to be discharged 11.2 days earlier than controls (46.5 vs 57.7 days). These figures compare with nationally reported means of 63 and 57 days of hospitalisation[10, 29] for infants with birth weights under 1500 g. The early-discharge group in our study had a mean birth weight of only 1187 g.

The safety of early discharge using this approach is supported by the similar numbers of rehospitalisations and acute care visits for infants in the early-discharge and control groups, which are also comparable to nationally reported figures.[29, 30] Furthermore, there were no infants with failure to thrive because of parental neglect, there was no reported physical abuse of infants, and there were no foster placements among the infants in the early-discharge group who were followed by the nurse specialist. These outcomes were achieved in a sample in which 42 percent of the mothers had less than a high-school education, 69 percent were unmarried, 75 percent were insured by Medicaid, 69 percent had a reported annual income of less than $7,500, 11 percent had no telephone, and 72 percent had to rely on the police or public transportation in an emergency.

In addition to its safety, this type of hospital-based home follow-up care for high-risk infants is feasible and cost effective. Even with the largely poor, often transient, mothers in the early-discharge group, loss of high-risk infants to medical follow-up was not a problem in this study. Because of the continuity of care provided by the nurse, her ability to handle the problems of high-risk infants and their parents' concerns, and her availability seven days a week, all but one family in the early-discharge group remained in the study until its completion. That one family moved to another part of the country. Moreover, the direct cost of the nurse specialist's services was very low, especially as compared with the charges for hospitalisation and physicians' services for these infants. The mean savings in hospital and physician's charges for the early-discharge group totaled $19,136, or 26.4 percent of the average charge for the control group, minus the added cost of the nurse specialist ($576). This yielded a net savings of $18,560 per infant, or 25.6 percent of the charges for the control group.

Since data on actual charges were used for physicians' and hospital fees, whereas data on costs were used to determine the offsetting expenses related to the services provided by the nurse specialist, the costs calculated for the two groups of infants were not fully comparable. However, $576 is only 0.8 percent of the combined mean hospital and physician's fees for the control group. If the nurse services were charged at 50 percent more or even at double their direct cost, they would still constitute only 1.2 percent of 1.6 percent of that amount, respectively. Thus, even if the charge for these services were $1,152 (i.e. $576 × 2), the savings would far outweigh these charges.

These figures should be compared with the hospital and physician charges for the early-discharge group, which were 26.4 percent lower than those for the control group. The results of this study suggest that potential for substantial savings in health care costs if our approach were followed nationwide. If only half the 36,000 very-low-birth-weight infants born in the United States each year were discharged early according to the protocol we tested, the annual savings could be as much as $334 million (\$19,136 − \$576 × 18,000). It should be noted that the data on the cost of hospital and physician's care were based on actual charges, not on costs. From the perspective of private insurers and self-paying patients, that is a reasonable approach. However, it may overstate the potential savings to society if charges exceed costs − as they do in some, but not necessarily all, cases. If the hospital and physician's charges were 25 percent, 50 percent, 75 percent, or 100 percent more than the costs of delivering the services, then the potential cost savings from early discharge of half the very-low-birth-weight infants born each year would be \$265 million, \$219 million, \$186 million, or \$162 million, respectively. Thus, even estimating conservatively that half the very-low-birth-weight infants could be discharged early and assuming that charges for all items were double the actual costs, the total savings nationwide could be as much as \$162 million annually.

Earlier discharge of low-birth-weight infants provides numerous potential benefits. These benefits may be offset, however, if high-risk infants are discharged early, and impose increased and highly stressful responsibilities for monitoring and care on their parents. This is particularly true if the parents lack the benefit of supportive programs and continuous contact with persons who are knowledgeable about and familiar with the problems and care of their infants since birth. A need for this type of support and continuity of care was suggested in our study by the number and types of calls the parents made to the nurse, the number of infants who required home apnea monitoring and medication, the number of families that remained in the study, and subsequently, the number of infants who continued to receive medical follow-up.

As prospective payment systems expand, it may well be financially beneficial for hospitals themselves to institute programs such as the one described here. For a hospital the value of such a service lies in the improved, extended service it can provide to families of high-risk infants, especially in view of the demonstrated need for such a program and its usefulness to families. Society also stands to benefit in many ways that cannot be quantified − in the support provided to families through the difficult period after discharge, and the potential reduction in child abuse and foster placement, for example, as well as in reduced health care costs.

NOTES

* *New England Journal of Medicine* 315 (15): 934–9. Reprinted with permission of the Massachusetts Medical Society.
1 National Center for Health Statistics. Monthly vital statistics report, 1975. Vol. 25. No. 10. Washington, D.C.: Department of Health, Education, and Welfare, 1976. (DHEW publication no. (HRA) 77–1120.)
2 *Idem.* Monthly vital statistics report, 1976. Vo. 26. No. 12. Washington, D.C.: Department of Health, Education, and Welfare, 1978. (DHEW publication no. (HRA) 78–1120.)
3 *Idem.* Monthly vital statistics report, 1977. Vol. 27. No. 11. Washington, D.C.: Department of Health, Education, and Welfare, 1979. (DHEW publication no. (HRA) 79–1120.)
4 *Idem.* Monthly vital statistics report, 1978. Vol. 29. No. 1. Washington, D.C.: Department of Health, Education, and Welfare, 1980. (DHEW publication no. (PHS) 80–1120.)
5 *Idem.* Monthly vital statistics report, 1979. Vol. 28. No. 13. Washington, D.C.: Department of Health, Education, and Welfare, 1980. (DHHS publication no. (PHS) 81–1120.)

6   *Idem*. Monthly vital statistics report, 1981. Vol. 30. No. 12. Washington, D.C.: Department of Health, Education, and Welfare, 1982. (DHHS publication no. (PHS) 82–1120.)

7   Lee K-S, Paneth N, Gartner LM, Pearlman MA, Gruss L. Neonatal mortality: an analysis of the recent improvement in the United States. Am J Public Health 1980; 70:15–21.

8   Cohen R, Stevenson D. Prenatal care for VLBW infants. Perinatol Neonatol 1983; 7:13–16.

9   Buckwald S, Zorn WA, Egan EA. Mortality and follow-up data for neonates weighing 500 to 800 g at birth. Am J Dis Child 1984; 138:779–82.

10 McCormick MC. The contribution of low birth weight to infant mortality and childhood morbidity. N Engl J Med 1985; 312:82–90.

11 Saigal S, Rosenbaum P, Stoskopf B, Milner R. Follow-up of infants 501 to 1,500 gm birth weight delivered to residents of a geographically defined region with perinatal intensive care facilities. J Pediatr 1982; 100:606–13.

12 Gottfried AW, Wallace-Lande P, Sherman-Brown S, King J, Coen C, Hodgman JE. Physical and social environment of newborn infants in special care units. Science 1981; 214:673–5.

13 Bess FH, Peek BF, Chapman JJ. Further observations on noise levels in infant incubators. Pediatrics 1979; 63:100–6.

14 Glass P, Avery GB, Subramanian KNS, Keys MP, Sostek AM, Friendly DS. Effect of bright light in the hospital nursery on the incidence of retinopathy of prematurity. N Engl J Med 1985; 313:401–4.

15 Desmond MM, Vordeman A, Salinas M. The family and premature infant after neonatal intensive care. Texas Med 1980; 76(1):60–3.

16 Hayes J. Premature infant development: the relationship of neonatal stimulation, birth condition and home environment. Pediatr Nurs 1980: 6(Nov–Dec):33–36.

17 Jeffcoate JA, Humphrey ME, Lloyd JK. Disturbance in parent-child relationship following preterm delivery. Dev Med Child Neurol 1979; 21:344–52.

18 Larson CP. Efficacy of prenatal and postpartum home visits on child health and development. Pediatrics 1980; 66:191–7.

19 Schroeder SA, Showstack JA, Roberts HE. Frequency and clinical description of high-cost patients in 17 acute-care hospitals. N Engl J Med 1979; 300:1306–9.

20 Kaufman SL, Shepard DS. Costs of neonatal intensive care by day of stay. Inquiry 1982; 19:167–78.

21 Walker D-JB, Feldman A, Vohr BR, Oh W. Cost-benefit analysis of neonatal intensive care for infants weighing less than 1,000 grams at birth. Pediatrics 1984; 74:20–5.

22 Hurt H. Continuing care of the high-risk infant. Clin Perinatol 1984; 11:3–17.

23 National Center for Health Statistics. Factors associated with low birth-weight. Washington, D.C.: Department of Health, Education, and Welfare. (DHEW publication no. (PHS) 80–1915.)

24 Bauer CH, Tinklepaugh W. Low birth weight babies in the hospital: a survey of recent changes in their care, with special emphasis on early discharge. Clin Pediatr 1971; 10:467–9.

25 Berg RB, Salisbury AJ. Discharging infants of low birth weight: reconsidaration of current practice. Am J Dis Child 1971; 122:414–17.

26 Britton HL, Britton JR. Efficacy of early newborn discharge in a middle-class population. Am J Dis Child 1984; 138:1041–6.

27 Dillard RG, Korones SB. Lower discharge weight and shortened nursery stay for low-birth-weight infants. N Engl J Med 1973; 288:131–3.

28 Hurt H, Gealt L, Johnson M, Wurtz M, Brodsky N. Home visiting nurses are beneficial in care of intensive care nursery graduates. Pediatr Res 1985; 19(4:Part 2):239A. abstract.

29 Hack M, DeMonterice D, Merkatz IR, Jones P, Fanaroff AA. Rehospitalisation of the very-low-birth-weight infant: a continuum of perinatal and environmental morbidity. Am J Dis Child 1981; 135:263–5.

30 McCormick MC, Shapiro S, Starfield BH. Rehospitalisation in the first year of life for high-risk survivors. Pediatrics 1980; 66:991–9.

Chapter 15

Comprehensive discharge planning and home follow-up of hospitalised elders

MARY NAYLOR, DOROTHY BROOTEN, ROBERTA CAMPBELL, BARBARA S. JACOBSEN, MATHY D. MEZEY, MARK V. PAULY, J. SANFORD SCHWARTZ

Introduction

It is tempting to take the establishment of advanced practice roles for granted, given their current proliferation. But the evidence base underpinning such roles has been hard won. The threat they posed to the medical profession and the legitimacy crisis this created has led to the generation of evidence valued by medicine. The present study therefore not only utilised a randomised controlled trial design, but also involved physicians as co-investigators. Advanced practice roles began in the USA as a pragmatic response to the maldistribution of doctors in rural and other under-served areas. The Vietnam War, feminism and economics have all been significant drivers of reform. Even so, achieving legal and regulatory change has been slow, and the struggle to do so hard fought. Gradually scepticism, even opposition in medical and policy circles has given way to reluctant recognition of value and effectiveness. But the battle has not been won. Advanced practice roles began by focusing mainly on under-served populations. Since then they have moved more into the mainstream. Research has played a key role in setting the direction and dynamic of the debate. The high-profile nature of the debate within the USA, Australia and latterly the UK has meant that studies have had to withstand strong criticism and demonstrate robustness in both economic and clinical effectiveness terms. Attracting funding for such studies has been challenging. The USA has been fortunate in being able to call upon the support of the Federally funded National Institute for Nursing Research within the esteemed National Institutes for Health as a sponsor.

The study has a number of other features that add to its credibility. Not only did it utilise a randomised controlled trial design, but built in an economic evaluation component through collaborative links between a successful business and nursing school. Publication within a high-impact journal in the USA locates the study within the mainstream of research and the prestigious pedigree of peer review. In doing so it demonstrates the value of nursing to influential target audiences. It enhances its credibility by quantifying the difference that planned nursing intervention can make to reducing risk in a vulnerable population as well as calculating the costs of care.

Precedents for the study however were few. The pressure on hospitals to reduce length of stay and the discharge of elderly patients with complex health problems, combined with the dramatic growth of home care schemes, has generated a research agenda in elderly care. Comprehensive discharge planning by advanced practice nurses has been trialled in elderly care, with specific health care problems showing short-term reductions in readmissions. But the benefits of more intensive follow-up of hospitalised elderly with complex care needs had not been studied. The aim of the present study was to examine the effectiveness of advanced-practice-nurse-centred discharge planning and home follow-up for the elderly at risk of hospital readmission, managed according to a comprehensive protocol. The intervention consisted of a comprehensive discharge planning follow-up protocol designed specifically for elderly patients at risk of poor outcomes, implemented by advanced practice nurses. What it demonstrated was that fewer intervention group patients had multiple readmissions and had fewer hospital days per patient. In addition the time between discharge and readmission was greater with costs of care being less.

The difference in outcomes was attributed to the highly honed assessment skills of the advanced practice nurses. This landmark study testifies to the value of shrewd clinical judgement exercised in close conjunction with carers, doctors and other team members. Interventions focused on medication management, symptom management, diet, activity, sleep, medical follow-up and enhancing the emotional status of the patient and care-givers. These were achieved by home visits, telephone availability, interviews and outreach activity. Outcome data were collected by a research assistant blind to study groups and hypotheses.

A further key message from this research was the preparation that the advanced practice (in the intervention group) and veteran nurses (VNs) (in the control group) had received. Advanced practice nurses (APN) were Masters-prepared in gerontological nursing in contrast to VNs who were Bachelor-prepared generalists. Preliminary analysis of APNs' case studies suggested that joint decision-making with physicians resulted in more timely interventions in the home, preventing negative outcomes. Patterns of work and activity for VNs on the other hand are regulated by reimbursement schedules. The flexibility and freedom that APNs have to exercise judgement specify the frequency and focus of the intervention to cater for individual patients and care-givers, are crucial. Such findings confirm those of previous research, that APNs can make a quantifiable difference to care. They chime with studies adopting a comparable methodological approach, but in a different population, women in a high-risk pregnancy and low-birthweight infants, also included in the present volume. But more than that, they demonstrate that the practice environment can be shaped by nursing expertise and that higher levels of autonomy can be good for patients, nurses, and even doctors.

NAYLOR, M., D. BROOTEN, R. CAMPBELL,
B.S. JACOBSEN, M.D. MEZEY, M.V. PAULY
AND J.S. SCHWARTZ (1999)

Comprehensive discharge planning and home follow-up of hospitalised elders: a randomised clinical trial*

Context   Comprehensive discharge planning by advanced practice nurses has demonstrated short-term reductions in readmissions of elderly patients, but the benefits of more intensive follow-up of hospitalised elders at risk for poor outcomes after discharge has not been studied.

Objective   To examine the effectiveness of an advanced practice nurse-centered discharge planning and home follow-up intervention for elders at risk for hospital readmissions.

Design   Randomised clinical trial with follow-up at 2, 6, 12, and 24 weeks after index hospital discharge.

Setting   Two urban, academically affiliated hospitals in Philadelphia, Pa.

Participants   Eligible patients were 65 years or older, hospitalised between August 1992 and March 1996, and had 1 of several medical and surgical reasons for admission.

Intervention   Intervention group patients received a comprehensive discharge planning and home follow-up protocol designed specifically for elders at risk for poor outcomes after discharge and implemented by advanced practice nurses.

Main Outcome Measures   Readmissions, time to first readmission, acute care visits after discharge, costs, functional status, depression, and patient satisfaction.

Results   A total of 363 patients (186 in the control group and 177 in the intervention group) were enrolled in the study; 70% of intervention and 74% of control subjects completed the trial. Mean age of sample was 75 years; 50% were men and 45% were black. By week 24 after the index hospital discharge, control group patients were more likely than intervention group patients to be readmitted at least once (37.1% vs 20.3%; $P<.001$). Fewer intervention group patients had multiple readmissions (6.2% vs 14.5%; $P = .01$) and the intervention group had fewer hospital days per patient (1.53 vs 4.09 days; $P<.001$). Time to first readmission was increased in the intervention group ($P<.001$). At 24 weeks after discharge, total Medicare reimbursements for health services were about $1.2 million in the control group vs about $0.6 million in the intervention group ($P<.001$). There were no significant group differences in post-discharge acute care visits, functional status, depression, or patient satisfaction.

Conclusions   An advanced practice nurse-centered discharge planning and home care intervention for at-risk hospitalised elders reduced readmissions, lengthened the time between discharge and readmission, and decreased the costs of providing health care. Thus, the intervention demonstrated great potential in promoting positive outcomes for hospitalised elders at high risk for rehospitalisation while reducing costs.

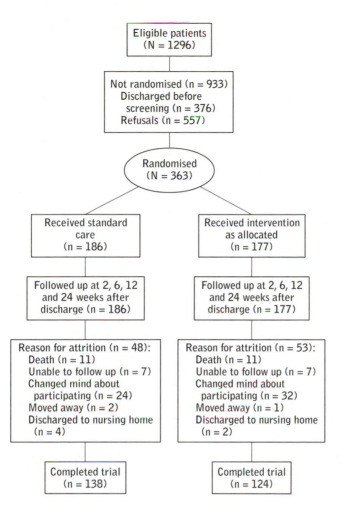

Figure 15.1   Patient flow diagram

The continued growth of diagnosis related groups (DRGs) and capitated reimburse-ment for inpatient care have increased pressures on hospitals to reduce length of stay. Consequently, elders with complex health needs are being discharged from hospitals earlier.[1–3] Home health services and families have served as safety nets for many of these patients. However, the rapid and dramatic growth of home health care has recently resulted in decreased access to services.[4–6] Potential consequences for elders with serious health problems include readmissions and nursing home placement.[7–11]

Recent studies have evaluated innovative interventions to facilitate the transition of older adults from hospital to home.[12–17] Most of these efforts focused on elders hos-pitalised with specific health problems, such as congestive heart failure (CHF).[12–14, 17] A randomised trial[17] that we completed in 1992 demonstrated short-term reductions in readmissions and decreased costs of care for hospitalised elders with medical cardiac

conditions managed according to a comprehensive discharge planning protocol implemented by advanced practice nurses (APNs). Findings suggested that elders at risk for
poor outcomes after discharge might benefit from more intensive home follow-up.

The objective of this randomised clinical trial was to examine the effectiveness of
an APN-centered comprehensive discharge planning and home follow-up protocol for
elders hospitalised with 1 of several common medical and surgical reasons for admission. Based on our earlier research, we hypothesised that this intervention would
improve patient health outcomes and reduce service utilisation and health care costs
compared with usual hospital and home care.

METHODS

Study sample

The study was conducted at the Hospital of the University of Pennsylvania and the
Presbyterian Medical Center of the University of Pennsylvania Health System and was
approved by the institutional review boards at both institutions. All subjects screened
for study participation were aged 65 years or older and were admitted from their
homes to either hospital between August 1992 and March 1996 with 1 of the following diagnoses: CHF, angina, myocardial infarction, respiratory tract infection, coronary
artery bypass graft, cardiac valve replacement, major small and large bowel procedure,
and orthopedic procedures of lower extremities. These diagnoses were among the top
10 reasons for Medicare beneficiary hospitalisation in 1992.[18] The DRGs were assigned
at hospital admission and validated at discharge.

Eligible patients had to speak English, be alert and oriented when admitted, be able
to be contacted by telephone after discharge, and reside in the geographic service area.
Patients also had to meet at least 1 of the following criteria associated with poor postdischarge outcomes in our earlier study:[17] age 80 years or older; inadequate support
system; multiple, active, chronic health problems; history of depression; moderate-to-
severe functional impairment; multiple hospitalisations during prior 6 months;
hospitalisation in the past 30 days; fair to poor self-rating of health; or history of non-
adherence to the therapeutic regimen.

Of the 1296 patients screened, 28% were enrolled, a percentage consistent with
randomised clinical trials involving similar populations.[13, 19] The 72% not enrolled
comprised those discharged before screening (29%) and refusals (43%) (Figure 15.1).
Enrollees and refusals were similar in race ($P = .99$) and sex ($P = .25$). Mean ages differed by 2 years (75.4 years for enrollees vs 77.3 years for refusals, $P<.001$).

Study design

Patients were enrolled in the study within 48 hours of hospital admission by research assistants (RAs) blinded to study groups and hypotheses. After screening patients for eligibility
and obtaining informed consent, RAs notified the project manager who assigned patients
to study groups using a computer-generated algorithm. The project manager contacted

APNs if patients were assigned to the intervention group. Baseline data on both groups (ie, sociodemographic and health status characteristics, functional status, and depression) were collected at enrollment by RAs using standardised instruments (Table 15.1).

Table 15.1 Sociodemographic and health characteristics of elderly patients (N = 363)*

Characteristic	Intervention (n = 177)	Control (n = 186)	P value
Age, y	75.5 ± 6.3	75.3 ± 6.0	.75
Sex			
Men	54	46	.14
Race			
Black	44	46	.76
White	56	54	
Education			
<High school	51	44	.15
≥High school	49	56	
Not employed	85	86	.75
Social support			
Spouse	44	43	
Other relative and/or friend	27	26	.93
None	29	31	
Income, $			
<10,000	42	42	
10,000–19,000	32	28	.56
≥20,000	26	30	
Medicaid	11	9	.61
Diagnosis related group†			
Angina/myocardial infarction	16	15	
Congestive heart failure	30	30	
Respiratory	8	9	
Valve replacement	11	9	.97
Coronary artery bypass graft	22	25	
Bowel	4	5	
Orthopedic	8	8	
Type of admission			
Elective	42	40	
Emergency	46	44	.75
Transfer	13	16	
Index length of stay, total (range), d	1587 (2–54) [9.2 ± 6.7]	1670 (1–60) [9.1 ± 6.7]	.80
Subjective health rating[24] by patient on admission			
Excellent or good	42	45	.63
Fair or poor	58	55	

Table 15.1 *Continued*

Characteristic	Intervention (n = 177)	Control (n = 186)	P value
Short Portable Mental Status Questionnaire[25]‡	9.4 ± 0.9	9.3 ± 1.0	.42
Center for Epidemiologic Studies Depression Scale[23]§	12.1 ± 10.0	10.7 ± 9.8	.26
Physician visits within the past 6 mo	5.5 ± 4.1	6.3 ± 5.6	.79
Hospital admissions within the past 6 mo	0.9 ± 1.1	1.0 ± 1.1	.25
Hospital discharges within the past 30 d	0.36 ± 0.6	0.44 ± 0.7	.17
No. of health conditions§§	5.3 ± 1.8	5.3 ± 1.8	.92
No. of daily medications¶	5.3 ± 2.7	5.2 ± 2.7	.82
Functional status based on the Enforced Social Dependency Scale[22]≠			
Personal	14.5 ± 6.1	14.6 ± 6.0	.90
Social	7.9 ± 2.6	8.0 ± 2.8	.78
Total	22.4 ± 8.1	22.6 ± 8.4	.86

*   Values are expressed as percentage or mean ± SD unless otherwise indicated.
†   Diagnosis related group numbers are: angina/myocardial infarction, 121, 122, 124, and 140; congestive heart failure 127; respiratory, 79, 88, 89, and 96; valve replacement 104 and 105; coronary artery bypass graft, 106 and 107; bowel 148; and orthopedic, 209 and 210.
‡   Values below 6 on a zero to 10 scale equal cognitive impairment.
§   Values below 16 on a zero to 60 scale equal not depressed.
§§ Active health problems requiring therapy as reported by patients and documented in the medical record.
¶   Applies to prescription drugs only.
≠   Higher scores on a 10 to 51 scale equal disability.

Control group

Control group patients received discharge planning that was routine for adult patients at study hospitals. If referred, control group patients received standard home care consistent with Medicare regulations.

Intervention group

The intervention extended from hospital admission through 4 weeks after discharge. The APNs assumed responsibility for discharge planning while the patient was hospitalised and substituted for the visiting nurse (VN) during the first 4 weeks after the index hospital discharge. Over the course of the study, the protocol was implemented by 5 part-time, master's-prepared, gerontological APNs with a mean of 6.5 years (range 2–9 years) postdegree experience in hospital and/or home care of older adults.

Intervention group patients and their caregivers, if available, received a standardised comprehensive discharge planning and home follow-up protocol designed specifically for elders at high risk for poor postdischarge outcomes. The protocol guided patient assessment and management and specified a minimum set of APN visits. However, an important component of the intervention was the ability of the APN, in collaboration with the patient's physician, to individualise patient management within the bounds of the protocol.

The protocol was implemented as follows: initial APN visit within 48 hours of hospital admission; APN visits at least every 48 hours during the index hospitalisation; at least 2 home APN visits (1 within 48 hours after discharge, a second 7–10 days after discharge); additional APN visits based on patients' needs with no limit on number; APN telephone availability 7 days per week (8 AM to 10 PM on weekdays and 8 AM to noon on weekends); and at least weekly APN initiated telephone contact with patients or caregivers.

Hospital visits

The APNs used data generated from instruments of established validity and reliability (Table 15.1) and their clinical skills to identify patients' and caregivers' discharge needs. Assessment focused on nature and severity of health problems; age-related changes; physical functional, cognitive, and emotional health status; and discharge goals. Caregiver assessment also included social support,[20] knowledge and skills, strain,[21] and need for formal support. Based on this information, APNs collaborated with the patient, physician, caregiver, and other team members in designing an individualised discharge plan. The APN implemented the plan through direct clinical care, patient and caregiver education, validation of learning, and coordination of needed home services. The APNs attempted to schedule hospital meetings with caregivers present. Within 24 hours of discharge, physicians wrote discharge orders and APNs scheduled the initial home visit.

Home visits, telephone availability, and outreach

The APNs completed physical and environmental assessments and targeted efforts at increasing patients' and caregivers' ability to manage unresolved health problems. Based on individual needs, APN interventions focused on medications, symptom management, diet, activity, sleep, medical follow-up, and the emotional status of patients and caregivers. A variety of strategies reinforced teaching including written instructions and medication schedules. Through home visits and telephone follow-up, APNs addressed questions or concerns from patients, caregivers, or health team members; monitored patients' progress; and collaborated with physicians to make adjustments in therapies and obtain referrals for needed services.

Discharge summaries

At completion of the intervention, APNs sent written summaries to patients, caregivers, physicians, and other providers to whom APNs had referred patients, detailing the plans, goal progression, and ongoing concerns.

Outcome measures

Outcome measures included hospital readmissions related to any cause, recurrence or exacerbation of the index hospitalisation DRG, comorbid conditions, or new health problems. The primary intervention efficacy test was defined on the basis of time to first readmission for any reason. Secondary outcomes were cumulative days of rehospitalisation, mean readmission length of stay, number of unscheduled acute care visits after discharge, estimated cost of postindex hospitalisation health services, functional status, depression, and patient satisfaction. Outcome data were collected by RAs blinded to study groups and hypotheses.

Standardised telephone interviews with patients at 2, 6, 12, and 24 weeks after index hospital discharge identified patients' readmissions to any hospital and unscheduled acute care visits to physicians, clinics, and emergency departments. Data on functional status (measured by the Enforced Social Dependency Scale),[22] depression (assessed using the Center for Epidemiologic Studies Depression Scale),[23] and patient satisfaction (measured by an investigator-developed instrument) were also collected during these interviews.

Data on the number, timing, reasons, and charges for readmissions, unscheduled acute care visits, and home visits by VNs or APNs (intervention group only), allied health professionals, and assistive personnel were abstracted from patients' records (inpatient, outpatient, and home care) and bills and recorded on standardised data collection forms. Reasons for readmissions were validated in writing by patients' physicians. The RAs categorised the reasons using discharge diagnoses as index-related (discharge diagnosis same as index hospitalisation); comorbid (discharge diagnosis 1 of comorbid conditions identified at index hospitalisation); or new health problem (not related to index diagnosis or comorbid condition during index admission). Estimated resource costs were generated using standardised Medicare reimbursements. Costs of pharmaceuticals, over-the-counter drugs, assistive devices, other supplies, and indirect costs (eg, productivity losses by patients and caregivers) were not included.

Statistical analysis

For patients who did not complete the entire 24-week postindex hospitalisation study period (death or withdrawal), data collected between randomisation and withdrawal were used in the analyses, performed according to the intention-to-treat principle, and censored at time of death or withdrawal.

Baseline data for intervention and control groups were compared using χ^2 tests for categorical variables, t tests for normally distributed continuous variables, and the Wilcoxon rank sum test for abnormally distributed variables. Based on a prior clinical trail,[17] we estimated that in each of the 2 study groups, 125 patients had to complete the study to detect a 50% reduction in hospital admission rates (2-sided α, .05 and power, 0.80, based on a control group readmission rate of 0.30).[26]

Descriptive comparisons between groups used χ^2 tests for the proportions of patients readmitted, t tests or Wilcoxon rank sum tests for number of readmissions, total days of hospitalisation, mean readmission length of stay, number of acute care visits, and reimbursements for postdischarge health services. Multivariate analysis of variance tested for measures of functional status, depression, and patient satisfaction.

Kaplan-Meier survival curves[27] were used to compare control and intervention groups to account for unequal follow-up times for the primary end point of time to first readmission for any reason and the secondary outcomes of time to first index-related readmission and time to first readmission or death. Crude testing of the primary hypothesis that the 2 cumulative readmission-free rate curves were identical was performed using a log-rank statistic.[28] Potentially confounding variables were adjusted using proportional hazards regression,[29] providing an adjusted hospital read-mission rate ratio (incidence density ratios) along with 95% confidence intervals (CIs). A final multivariate model included covariates retaining their bivariate signifi-cance ($P<.05$) along with intervention group to obtain adjusted significance levels and adjusted risk estimates with 95% CIs. Variables were removed in a stepwise manner. Intervention group interactions with significant index diagnoses were assessed by adding appropriate terms to the model.

Group differences in both charges and actual Medicare reimbursements for post-index hospitalisation health services were examined. The more conservative reimbursement results are reported. Although reimbursements are not the same as costs, they are a reasonable proxy and provide reasonably unbiased estimates of rela-tive differences in cost between intervention and control groups. The index hospital reimbursement included the costs of discharge planning services provided by regis-tered nurses, social workers, and discharge planners. Since the APN hospital visits in this intervention substituted for standard discharge planning, no additional costs were assigned to this phase of the intervention. The cost of APN services after discharge was estimated by assessing APN intervention-related effort (from detailed logs) and apply-ing Medicare reimbursement rates. In the primary analysis, postdischarge APN and VN services were assigned the same rate since this reflected Medicare's reimbursement during the study period. Sensitivity analyses were conducted using higher estimates for APN services (actual APN reimbursement plus 20%), reflecting their increased skill and training relative to VNs, and representative annual salary for APNs plus benefits was weighted by percentage of effort attributable to the intervention.

RESULTS

Study patients

A total of 363 patients were enrolled in the study (Table 15.1). The 2 study groups were similar in all sociodemographic and baseline health characteristics, including index hospitalisation DRG, type of admission, and length of stay. Mean age of the entire sample was 75 years, 50% were men, and 45% were black.

The attrition rate from the intervention group (including deaths) was 30% (53/177) compared with 26% (48/186) for the control group ($P = .26$). Of the 363 enrolled patients, 22 (6%) died by 24 weeks after discharge, with 11 deaths in each of the 2 study groups (Figure 15.1). Most of the deaths occurred during the index hospitalisation or in the first 6 weeks after discharge (4% of control, 5% intervention). An additional 4% in each of the study groups withdrew because of inability to complete follow-up interviews (change in health status such as stroke or cognitive decline). The remaining withdrawals (16% control, 20% intervention; $P = 64$) occurred because patients changed their minds about participating (13% control, 18% intervention; $P = .28$); moved away (1% control, 1% intervention); or were discharged to a nursing home (2% control, 1% intervention). Intervention group withdrawals were slightly higher because a few patients in this group decided, after enrolling, to maintain existing VN relationships and services.

Study follow-up did not differ significantly between control and intervention groups (18.1 weeks vs 19.1 weeks; $P = .41$). The 28% attrition rate was consistent with rates reported in other randomised clinical trials with a similar patient population.[17, 19, 30] The 262 patients who completed the study and the 101 persons in the attrition group did not significantly differ in sociodemographic variables and severity of illness measures (eg, number of comorbid conditions).

Readmissions

Control group patients were more likely than intervention group patients to be readmitted at least once (Table 15.2; 37.1% vs 20.3%; $P<.001$; relative risk, 1.8; 95% CI, 1.3–2.6). The 16.8% absolute reduction in hospital readmissions at 24 weeks represented a 45% relative reduction in control group readmission rate. More control group patients had multiple readmissions during the 24-week period than intervention group patients (14.5% vs 6.2%; $P = .01$; relative risk, 2.3; 95% CI, 1.2–4.6).

The intervention resulted in fewer total hospital readmissions at 24 weeks after index hospitalisation discharge (107 controls vs 49 intervention; rank sum test, $P<.001$). The reduction in readmissions was significant during both the first 6 weeks after discharge ($P<.001$) and the 6-week to 24-week period ($P = .02$).

Of the 156 readmissions, 60.3% were related to the index hospitalisation, 22.4% to comorbid conditions, and 17.3% to new health problems. There were fewer readmissions related to the index hospitalisation in the intervention group compared with the control group (30 vs 64; $P = .005$). There were trends toward reduced intervention group readmissions due to comorbid conditions (10 vs 25; $P = .06$) and new health problems (9 vs 18; $P = .10$).

At 24 weeks, control group patients experienced 760 days of hospitalisation, compared with 270 days in the intervention group ($P<.001$). Hospital days per patient were higher in the control group compared with the intervention group (4.09 vs 1.53; rank sum test, $P<.001$ [with or without adjustment for follow-up time]). The mean

Table 15.2   Readmissions and hospital days within 24 weeks of discharge from index hospitalisation

	Intervention (n = 177)	Control (n = 186)	Arithmetic difference	P value*
No. (%) of patients readmitted				
≤1 time	36 (20.3)	69 (37.1)	−16.80%	<.01
≥2 times	11 (6.2)	27 (14.5)	−8.30%	.01
No. of readmissions				
Index-related	30	64	−34	.005
Comorbidity-related	10	25	−15	.06
New health problem	9	18	−9	.10
Total	49	107	−58	<.001
Time of readmissions, No.				
Discharge to 6 wk	17	47	−30	<.001
6 to 24 wk	32	60	−28	.02
Time spent in hospital, d				
All	270	760	−490	
Per patient, mean ± SD	1.53 ± 3.69	4.09 ± 8.35	−2.56	<.001
Median	0	0		
25th Percentile	0	0		
50th Percentile	0	0		
75th Percentile	0	4		
Per readmitted patient, mean ± SD†	7.50 ± 4.7 (n = 36)	10.1 ± 10.6 (n = 69)	−3.51	<.001
Median	6.5	7		
25th Percentile	4	4		
50th Percentile	6.5	7		
75th Percentile	10.75	14.5		

* Wilcoxon rank sum tests used to compare the distribution of per patient rates for number of readmissions and hospital days; χ^2 for proportion of patients readmitted.
† The intervention group had 36 subjects and the control group had 69 subjects.

length of stay for readmitted patients in the control group (n = 69) was higher than the intervention group (n = 36), (11.0 ± 10.6 days vs 7.5 ± 4.8 days; P<.001).

Time to first readmission for any reason was increased in the intervention group (log-rank χ^2_1 = 11.1, P<.001) (Figure 15.2). Twenty-five percent of control patients were readmitted within 48 days after index hospital discharge (95% CI, 34–63 days), whereas 25% of intervention patients were readmitted within 133 days (lower 95% confidence limit, 78 days; upper 95% confidence limit, not estimable). The effect of the intervention on time to first readmission for any reason remained significant (P<.001, Table 15.3) after adjusting for simultaneously significant variables including self-reported health status, number of hospitalisations in the previous 6 months, living arrangements, and diagnosis of CHF. The time to index diagnosis-related readmissions

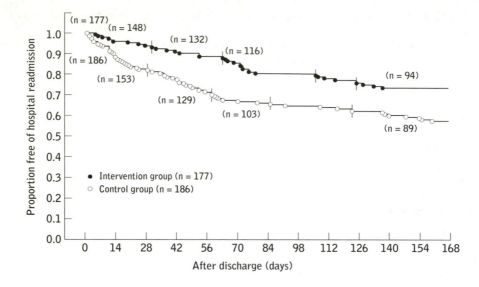

Figure 15.2 Time to first hospital readmission for any reason.
The relative readmission rates comparing the control group with the intervention group are 1.96 (95% confidence interval [CI], 1.31–2.92) for the crude rate and 2.03 (95% C1, 1.34–3.08) for the adjusted rate. The survival curve distance is $P<.001$ (calculated with the log-rank test).

Table 15.3 Time to first hospital readmission by patient characteristics (Multivariate Cox Proportional Hazards Model)

Variable	Incidence density ratio	95% confidence interval	P value
Control group vs intervention group	2.03	1.33–3.08	<.001
Fair or poor self-rating vs good or excellent self-rating	2.18	1.38–3.45	<.001
No. of prior hospitalisations within the past 6 mo	1.29	1.09–1.52	<.002
Living with relative or friend vs spouse	0.59	0.37–0.94	.03
Living with relative or friend vs alone	0.50	0.29–0.84	.009
Congestive heart failure vs other diagnosis related groups	1.64	1.07–2.50	.02

similarly was increased in the intervention group (log-rank $\chi^2_1 = 4.97$, $P = .03$).

Statistical evidence was weak that the relative efficacy differed between patients with and without CHF ($\chi^2_1 = 2.47$, $P = .11$). The crude rates for any readmission per year among control and intervention patients without CHF diagnosis were 1.17 (41 events/35.2 years) and 0.42 (16 events/38 years), respectively, for a crude relative rate of 2.8. Among CHF patients, the crude control and intervention group admission rates per year were 1.93 (25 events/13 years) and 1.48 (19 events/12.8 years),

Table 15.4 Acute care visits, home visits, and reimbursements (costs) for health services after discharge for 24 weeks

Health service	Intervention (n = 177)* Visits†	Costs, $	Control (n = 186)* Visits†	Costs, $	P values Visits	Costs
Acute care visits						
Physician's office	1.5 ± 2.2	24,937	1.6 ± 2.2	27,121	.59	.82
Emergency department‡	0.1 ± 0.5	9,138	0.2 ± 0.4	10,600	.21	.78
Home visits						
Nurses						
Visiting	3.1 ± 7.2	40,097	7.1 ± 12.0	101,049	.05	.05
Advanced practice	4.5 ± 4.3§	61,600	0	0	<.001	<.001
Advanced practice and visiting	7.6 ± 9.4	101,697	7.1 ± 12.0	101,049	.65	.73
Physical therapists	3.5 ± 8.8	44,819	3.1 ± 8.3	40,803	.32	.62
Occupational therapists	0.1 ± 0.9	912	0.2 ± 1.4	2,722	.95	.33
Speech therapists	0.03 ± 05	474	0	0	.31	.32
Social workers	0.03 ± 0.3	676	0.07 ± 0.4	1,252	.23	.40
Home health aides	3.7 ± 11.8	32,725	3.6 ± 12.5	31,163	.46	.78
Total visits and costs	16.6 ± 22.9	215,378	15.9 ± 25.9	214,710	.77	.72
Median	8		4			
25th percentile	3		0			
50th percentile	8		4			
75th percentile	24.5		23.3			

* Visits and costs are aggregate values. Costs were standardised for unequal follow-up by converting to costs per week in the study before significance testing.
† Values are measured as mean ± SD.
‡ Includes only those that did not result in hospital admissions.
§ Mean (SD) number of advanced practice nurses' in-hospital visits, 4.0 (3.2).

respectively, for a crude relative ration of 1.30. In clinical terms, however, the interventions' relative efficacy was significantly larger for patients without CHF compared with patients with CHF (rate ratio, 1.6 vs 2.7).

Relative efficacy did not depend on study site for time to any first admission ($P = .82$). When a secondary end point defining deaths as an event rather than being censored was examined, time until first readmission for any reason remained increased in the intervention group (rate ratio, 1.6; 95% CI, 1.1–2.3; $P = .01$).

Other patient and health services outcomes

Intervention and control groups were similar in mean functional status ($P = .33$), depression scores ($P = .20$), and patient satisfaction ($P = .92$). At 24 weeks, mean functional status scores in both groups were slightly improved over baseline (21.5 to 19.2) as were mean depression scores (10.7 to 6.6). Mean patient satisfaction scores showed little change over time; both groups remained highly satisfied with care.

At 24 weeks after discharge, the control and intervention groups did not significantly differ in the mean number of unscheduled acute care visits to physicians or emergency departments, or home visits by VNs or APNs, allied health professionals, or home health aides (Table 15.4). The pattern of home visits by nurses immediately after index hospital discharge differed between study groups. Only 44% of the control groups received at least 1 home visit by VNs during the first 2 weeks after discharge. Consistent with the study protocol, all of the intervention group received at least 1 APN visit. Of the 69 control patients rehospitalised at least once, 51% received VN visits during the immediate postdischarge period.

Economic impact

At 24 weeks, total and per-patient imputed reimbursements for postindex acute health services in the control group were approximately twice as much as that of the intervention group ($1,238,928 vs $642,595 [$P<.001$] and $6,661 vs $3,630 [$P<.001$]; Table 15.5). Intervention group cost savings were driven by the control group's substantially greater total DRG reimbursements for all hospital readmissions at 24 weeks after discharge ($1,024,218 vs $427,217; $P<.001$). Substitution of charges, adjusted charges, and weighted APN average annual salary and benefits for reimbursements as measures of resource use further increased the estimated differences between groups. Total reimbursements for other postdischarge acute care visits were not significantly different between study groups (Table 15.4; $P = .72$).

Table 15.5   Reimbursements (costs) for readmissions, acute care visits, and home visits for 24 weeks after discharge

| Health service | Aggregate costs, $* | | P value |
	Intervention (n = 177)	Control (n = 186)	
Readmissions			
Index-related	249,436	596,741	<.004
Comorbidities	110,198	250,720	.10
New problems	67,583	176,757	.09
Total readmissions	427,217	1,024,218	<.001
Acute care visits (physician's office, emergency department)	34,075	37,721	.74
Home visits			
Nurses	101,697	101,049	.72
Other visits	79,606	75,940	.70
Totals	642,595	1,238,928	<.001
Per patient	3,630	6,661	<.001

*Cost values were standardised for unequal follow-up by converting to costs per week in the study before significance testing.

COMMENT

This study demonstrated that a comprehensive discharge planning and home follow-up intervention designed specifically for elders at high risk for poor posthospital discharge outcomes and implemented by gerontological APNs reduced hospital readmissions, lengthened the time to first readmission, and decreased cost of care. Improved patient outcomes and health care savings have also been demonstrated when a similar approach to care was tested with women with high-risk pregnancies and low-birth-weight infants.[31–33]

By 24 weeks after the index hospital discharge, 37% of the control group had been rehospitalised compared with 20% of the intervention group. Although non-randomised studies[12, 34, 35] have demonstrated greater reductions in rehospitalisation rates for adult cardiac patients, only 1 randomised clinical trial, limited to patients with congestive heart failure, demonstrated a similar absolute readmission rate reduction.[13] In contrast to this study that included rehospitalisations to any hospital, other studies have examined only readmissions to study hospitals[34] or did not specify if readmissions to hospitals other than study hospitals were included.[13, 35]

Study findings are especially important given the current attention to new models of patient care management. In contrast to the typical disease management model that focuses on all patients hospitalised with a specific primary condition, such as heart failure, this intervention targeted elders hospitalised with common medical and surgical conditions. We believe that the focus of the clinical intervention on the combined effects of primary health problems, comorbid conditions, and other health and social issues common in this patient population, rather than on the management of a single disease, was a major factor in its success.

Other factors may have contributed to these observed outcomes. The target study population, elders at high risk for poor outcomes after hospital discharge, was not limited to those who met current Medicare home-care eligibility requirements. Approximately one third of control patients who did not receive a visit from a VN immediately after the index discharge were rehospitalised. The factors that influence health professionals' decision making regarding which patients are referred for home care is an important area for further study. Home visits alone, however, do not explain the differences in this study. One in 2 control patients visited by VNs immediately after the index hospital discharge were rehospitalised compared with 1 in 5 intervention patients visited by APNs.

While the protocol tested in this study was derived from current research, the framework that guided APNs' decision making was individualised care. In contrast to most VNs who are bachelor's-prepared generalists, the APNs who implemented this protocol were master's-prepared specialists in gerontological nursing. This intervention benefited from APNs' clinical acumen as well as their expertise in communicating, collaborating, and coordinating care with physicians and other health care professionals. For example, a preliminary analysis of APNs' case studies suggests that joint clinical decision making with physicians resulted in timelier interventions in the home and prevented negative outcomes.

Unlike home care nurses, whose visit pattern is constrained by reimbursement and other barriers, APNs used their judgment to define the frequency, intensity, and focus of contacts needed to meet patient and caregiver needs. Consequently, the time and focus of services provided by the APNs varied.

Functional status was not improved with this intervention, a finding consistent with published data from other discharge planning and home care studies in recent years.[30, 36] Reductions in rehospitalisations and cost in the absence of differences in functional status may indicate that the APN-based intervention achieved its benefit by enhancing the capacity of high-risk elders to better cope with their multiple medical problems and disabilities.[37] Mean scores at all data collection points revealed little evidence of depressive symptoms in this study sample.[24] The skewed distribution of patient satisfaction scores suggests the need for more sensitive items.

At 6 months, the intervention generated estimated savings in Medicare reimbursements for all postindex hospital discharge services of almost $600,000 for the 177 intevention group beneficiaries, a mean per-patient savings of approximately $3,000. Thus, the intervention was dominant from an economic perspective — improved outcomes were achieved at reduced cost. Virtually all of the savings resulted from reductions in rehospitalisations, with use of nonhospital postdischarge health services similar in intervention and control groups. When extrapolated to the number of older adults hospitalised each year with similar conditions, the potential patient benefits and savings to the Medicare system resulting from this intervention are substantial.

In conclusion, an APN-centered discharge planning and home care intervention for at-risk, hospitalised elders reduced readmissions, lengthened the time between discharge and readmission, and decreased the costs of providing health care. This intervention has great potential in promoting positive outcomes for this challenging group of elders while reducing costs.

FUNDING/SUPPORT

Funding was provided by the National Institute for Nursing Research of the National Institutes of Health, Bethesda, Md, grant RO1-NR02095. Dr Naylor was the principal investigator.

ACKNOWLEDGMENTS

We are grateful to the APNs for their extraordinary commitment in accomplishing the goals of this study. Special recognition is given to Janice Foust, PhD, RN, and Catherine Wollman, MSN, CRNP, who were involved throughout the entire study period. We also thank Greg Maislin, MS, MA, principal biostatistician, Biomedical Statistical Consulting, Wynnewood, Pa, for his guidance. The support provided by a group of dedicated research assistants is deeply appreciated. Finally, we thank Caroline Stephens, Chris Tweedy, Gina Marziani, MSEd, and Kathryn Bowles, PhD, for their assistance in the completion of the manuscript.

NOTES

Journal of the American Medical Association 281 (7): 613–20. Reprinted with permission of the American Medical Association.

1 Graves EJ, National Center for Health Statistics, National Hospital Discharge Survey: annual summary, 1993. *Vital Health Stat 13*. 1995; 121: 1–63.

2 Titler MG, Pettit DM. Discharge readiness assessment. *J Cardiovasc Nurs*. 1995; 9:64–74.

3 Mamon J, Steinwachs DM, Fahey M, Bone LR, Oktay J, Klein L. Impact of hospital discharge planning on meeting patient needs after returning home. *Health Serv Res*. 1992; 2:155–175.

4 Health Care Financing Administration, Office of Financial and Human Resources. Data from the Division of the Budget. Available at: http://www.hcfa.gov/stats/hstats96/blustat2.htm. Accessed August 5, 1997.

5 Dey AN, for the National Center for Health Statistics. Characteristics of elderly home health care users: data from the 1993 National Home and Hospice Care Survey. *Vital Health Stat 272*. In press.

6 Experton BL, Branch BL, Ozminkowski RJ, Mellon-Lacey DM. The impact of payor/provider type on health care use and expenditures among the frail elderly. *Am J Public Health*. 1997; 87:210–216.

7 Ashton CM, Kuykendall DH, Johnson ML, Wray NP, Wu L. The association between the quality of inpatient care and early readmission. *Ann Intern Med*. 1995; 122:415–421.

8 Oddone EZ, Weinberger M, Horner M, et al. Classifying general medicine readmissions: are they preventable? *J Gen Intern Med*. 1996; 11:597–605.

9 Frankl SE, Breeling JL, Goldman L. Preventability of emergent hospital readmission. *Am J Med*. 1991; 90:667–674.

10 Kane RL, Finch M, Blewett L, Chen Q, Burns R, Moskowitz M. Use of post-hospital care by Medicare patients. *J Am Geriatr Soc*. 1996; 44:242–250.

11 Morrow-Howell N, Proctor E. Discharge destinations of Medicare patients receiving discharge planning: who goes where? *Med Care*. 1994; 32:486–497.

12 West JA, Miller NH, Parker KM, et al. A comprehensive management system for heart failure improves clinical outcomes and reduces medical resource utilisation. *Am J Cardiol*. 1997; 79:58–63.

13 Rich MW, Beckham V, Wittenberg C, Levin CL, Freedland KE, Carney RM. A multidisciplinary intervention to prevent the readmission of elderly patients with congestive heart failure. *N Engl J Med*. 1995; 333:1190–1195.

14 Kornowski R, Zeeli D, Averbuch M, et al. Intensive home care surveillance prevents hospitalisation and improves morbidity rates among elderly patients with severe congestive heart failure. *Am Heart J*. 1995; 129: 762–766.

15 Weinberger M, Oddone EZ, Henderson WG. Does increased access to primary care reduce hospital readmissions? *N Engl J Med*. 1996; 334:1441–1447.

16 Stuck AE, Aronow HU, Steiner A, et al. A trial of in-home comprehensive discharge assessments for elderly people living in the community. *N Engl J Med*. 1995; 333:1184–1189.

17 Naylor M, Brooten D, Jones R, Lavizzo-Mourey R, Mezey M, Pauly M. Comprehensive discharge planning for the hospitalised elderly: a randomised clinical trial. *Ann Intern Med*. 1994; 120:999–1006.

18 *The DRG Handbook: Comparative Clinical and Financial Standards (1996)*. Baltimore, Md: Health Care Investment Authority, Cleveland, Ohio: Ernst and Young.

19 Landefeld CS, Palmer RM, Kresevic DM, Fortinsky RH, Kowal J. A randomised trial of care in a hospital medical unit especially designed to improve the functional outcomes of acutely ill older patients. *N Engl J Med*. 1995; 332:1338–1344.

20 Pearlin LI, Mullan JT, Semple SJ, Skaff MM. Caregiving and the stress process: an overview of concepts and their measures. *Gerontologist*. 1990; 38:583–594.

21 Robinson BC. Validation of a caregiver strain index. *J Gerontol*. 1983; 38:344–348.

22 Moinpour C, McCorkle R, Saunders J. Measuring functional status. In: Frank-Stromborg M, ed. *Instruments for Clinical Nursing Research*. Boston, Mass: Jones & Bartlett; 1992: 285–401.

23 Radloff LS. The CES-D scale: a self-report depression scale for research in the general population. *Appl Psychological Meas*. 1977; 1:385–401.

24 Maddox GL. Self-assessment of health status: a longitudinal study of selected elderly subjects. *J Chronic Dis*. 1964; 17:449–460.

25 Pfeiffer E. A short portable mental status questionnaire for the assessment of organic brain deficit in elderly patients. *J Am Geriatr Soc*. 1975; 23:433–441.

26 Elashoff JD. *NQuery Advisor, Version 2.0: User's Guide*. Los Angeles, Calif: Dixon Assoc; 1997.

27 Kaplan EL, Meier P. Nonparametric estimation from incomplete observations. *J Am Stat Assoc*. 1958; 53:457–481.

28 Lee ET. *Statistical Methods for Survival Data Analysis*. 2nd ed. New York, NY: John Wiley & Sons Inc; 1992.

29 Cox DR. Regression models with life-tables (with discussion). *J R Stat Soc*. 1972; 66:188–190.

30 Cummings JE, Hughes SL, Weaver FM, et al. Cost-effectiveness of Veterans Administration hospital-based home care. *Arch Intern Med*. 1990; 150:1274–1280.

31 Brooten D, Kumar S, Brown L, et al. A randomised clinical trial of early discharge and home follow-up of very low birthweight infants. *N Engl J Med*. 1986; 315:934–939.

32 Brooten D, Roncoli M, Finkler S, Arnold L, Cohen A, Mennuti M. A randomised clinical trial of early hospital discharge and nurse specialist home followup of women and unplanned cesarean birth. *Obstet Gynecol*. 1994; 84:832–838.

33 Brooten D, Naylor M, York R, et al. Effects of nurse specialists transitional care on patient outcomes and costs: results of five randomised trials. *Am J Managed Care*. 1995; 1:35–41.

34 Smith LE, Fabbri SA, Pai R, Haywood JT. Symptomatic improvement and reduced hospitalisation for patients attending a cardiomyopathy clinic. *Clin Cardiol*. 1997; 20:949–954.

35 Fonarow GC, Stevenson LW, Walden JA, et al. Impact of a comprehensive heart failure management program on hospital readmissions and functional status in patients with advanced heart failure. *J Am Coll Cardiol*. 1997; 30:725–732.

36 Townsend J, Piper M, Frank AO, Dyer S, North WR, Mead TW. Reduction in hospital re-admission stay of elderly patients by a community based hospital discharge scheme: a randomised controlled trial. *BMJ*. 1988; 297:544–547.

37 Institute of Medicine. *Health Outcomes for Older People: Questions for the Coming Decade*. Feasley J, Ed. Washington, DC: National Academy Press, 1996.

Chapter 16

An evaluation of health visitors' visits to elderly women

KAREN A. LUKER

Introduction

Health visiting has been plagued by problems in developing an evidence base for its practice, making it vulnerable to radical restructuring, even elimination, of services. This is not a new problem, as Karen Luker demonstrates. Part of the intention of the *Developments in Nursing Research* series published in the early 1980s, from which this chapter is taken, was to 'promote nursing progress and knowledge'. In the second volume of such studies, the editor, Jenny Wilson-Barnet, comments that after two decades of nurses researching predominantly administrative and educational topics, it was high time to tackle the possibly methodologically more challenging subject of measuring the impact of nursing interventions.

In her chapter, Luker challenges the claim by many health visitors that the effects of their work are too subtle, intangible or elusive to be evaluated adequately. Measuring the process in terms of outcome and effectiveness has been claimed to be impractical. Moreover its domestic location often renders it invisible to others. Luker rejects these as lame and illogical excuses for inaction. For, if the service is so diffuse, there seems little point in providing it in the first place. And where research has been conducted it has tended to focus on the dependent aspects of the health visitor's role, assisting the doctor in screening programmes rather than on the independent surveillance functions. The need to provide an evidence base is strengthened by the demand the service makes on resources with a growing elderly population and the potential benefits to be gained from screening this population for disability. Indeed, government recommendations for health visitors to increase their contact with the elderly create a moral as well as policy imperative to do so. So if health visitors are providing a valuable service its impact needs to be evaluated.

Having said that, the methodological challenges of doing so are many. Preventive activities, by their very nature, are long-term, requiring some shorter-term intervention to be identified. Second, deterioration in health may well occur as a result of the ageing process. An experimental study design however provides one way of over-coming some of these drawbacks. A cross-over design was deployed, involving 230 female patients aged 70 years or over, living alone with no mental impairment and not in receipt of health visiting. Patients were randomised to either an experimen-tal or control group prior to assessment and introduced to the study via a letter from their general practitioner (GP). Agreement to participate in the study also involved completing an assessment form and the identification of actual and poten-tial health problems. Patients in the experimental group received focused health visiting from a research assistant once a month for four months, the control group received 'usual nursing services' which in this case meant none. The first post-test was conducted at two months, followed by cross-over intervention, the second post-test following at a further two-month interval. Problems were recorded in a systematic way after each visit, using a problem-oriented schedule which included a plan of action targeted to each patient. The research assistant noted any change in status. At four months, the first post-test was conducted, using the Life Satisfaction Index. Changes in status were noted and patients were asked their opinion on their perceived benefits of the health visitor's visits, the control group became the experimental group, and the process was repeated. The health problems identified at assessment included: weight maintenance, mobility, dentition, sensory function, elimination, loneliness, performance of personal household tasks, rest and medication.

Findings indicated that the experimental group in both cases reported significant improvement in problems and that the effect of the health visitor intervention lasted after the service was withdrawn. Most patients said they enjoyed the visits and thought that they had benefited in some way, although a small minority claimed they had not. Less than half wanted the visits to continue and over a third claimed they did not. The health visitor was perceived as helpful in providing advice for health maintenance. Luker ends with a plea for service evaluation to be given a more prominent place within the health services research agenda.

Had her clarion cry been heeded the contribution of health visiting to public health and primary care research and practice would have been much clearer to articulate to policy-makers. Stronger alliances could have been forged between primary care and public health specialists, rather than health visitors working in relative isolation. Instead, many years later the jury is still out on health visiting, although some progress has been made on the evaluation side. Health visiting has been the subject of a sys-tematic review within the NHS Health Technology Assessment R & D Programme, led by another author within this collection, Jane Robinson. But the examples of good practice in targeting and tailoring services, community development outreach efforts, quantifying and qualifying the contribution to social and urban regeneration efforts are still too few. Health visiting is a case in need of radical research treatment where efforts to mainstream research within multi-disciplinary health services and public health research communities need to be strengthened.

There is a crusading quality to this paper in that it deploys rhetorical touches and turns to persuade us that it is clinical effectiveness that paves the royal road to policy and practice impact. It is bold and brave in its denunciation of special case treatment for health visiting, ducking the issues or being defensive about practice. Its message is clear and sadly remains as relevant today.

LUKER, K. (1983)

An evaluation of health visitors' visits to elderly women*

INTRODUCTION

This chapter attempts to give an overview of health visitor involvement with the well elderly. Because there is a lack of information available concerning the health visitor's independent function of 'surveillance', the literature reviewed focuses primarily on the health visitor's dependent function in assisting the general practitioner with screening programmes.

The possible benefits of health visitor visits to the elderly are discussed and the need for and problems involved in evaluating health visiting are explored. A study which attempted to evaluate the outcome of health visitor intervention on an elderly population is reported in detail.

The case is made for more research to evaluate health-care services in terms of their benefit to the client.

HEALTH OF THE ELDERLY[1]

The growing numbers of elderly people are commonly viewed by society as a problem (Wilson, 1973) and the health of the aged is one of the major concerns of the health service since large financial resources have to be devoted to their care. Moral issues are involved in devoting immense resources to the care of this age group especially when quality of life is open to question. The document *Prevention and Health Everybody's Business* (DHSS, 1976a) adopts the moral approach that resources should be available but comes out in favour of early detection of disability amongst the elderly because it is thought to be cost effective. Few studies were conducted to ascertain the health, conditions and problems of the elderly until the late 1940s. Sheldon's (1948) pioneering work put the sociological study of old age on a firm basis and the study conducted by Wedderburn and Townsend (1965) gave the first national figures concerning the welfare and living conditions of the aged. Findings of unmet socio-medical needs have subsequently been confirmed by other observers (Age Concern, 1977; Barber and Wallis, 1976; Barker, 1974; Gardiner, 1975; Hiscock *et al.*, 1973; Milne *et al.*, 1972). In general terms, these studies indicate that elderly people fail to report changes in health status most often related to hearing, vision, mobility, incontinence and dementia to the general practitioner. It would seem that the present system of patient-initiated consultation with the general practitioner coupled with the appointment system (Age Concern, 1972) is not always in the best interests of the elderly as there is a tendency for them to view change in health status as 'just old age' (Brocklehurst, 1975).

Physicians caring for the elderly have found that older people are commonly referred to them late on in their illness and have felt that more could have been done if they had sought help sooner (Anderson, 1976). The alternative to patient-initiated consultation is doctor-initiated consultation which is commonly referred to as screening or case finding, the aim being to identify treatable conditions or diseases. A number of investigators have conducted screening surveys on elderly people living at home; these surveys have uncovered a high incidence of untreated disease and unsuspected disability. In their early work, Williamson et al. (1964) showed in a random sample of 200 elderly men and women, taken from a list of three general practitioners, that the number of disabilities in males was 3.26 of which 1.8 were unknown to the general practitioner and in females the figures were 3.42 and 2.03 respectively. From this study, it became apparent that the elderly may not know when they are unwell, hence an iceberg of unreported illness may be present in the community amongst this age group. Williamson et al. (1964) suggested that since the self-reporting of illness fails to meet the needs of the elderly, periodic examination may be beneficial.

BENEFITS OF SCREENING PROGRAMMES

There have been many reports on screening programmes for the elderly in general practice (Burns, 1969; Currie et al., 1974; Lowther et al., 1970; Taylor, 1971; Thomas 1968). Without exception these studies are founded on the assumption that elderly persons will benefit from treatment of previously unreported disease conditions or from referral to another agency. Very few studies have been traced which attempt to evaluate the effect of the screening programmes in terms of the benefit of the treatments on the patient/client. The assumption upon which most screening programmes are based is that which is inherent in the medical model; namely, if a person has a disease or condition for which there is a known treatment or cure when the treatment is given the patient/client will benefit and it is this assumption which is open to question. Since there is evidence which suggests that prescribed medication taken by the elderly in itself may present a problem – studies indicate a high incidence of medication error in this age group (Anderson, 1974; Atkinson et al., 1977).

Few investigations have been designed in such a way that allow the effects of screening programmes in terms of their benefits to the patients to be evaluated. Barber and Wallis (1978) reported the difference in findings between two assessments on an elderly population. The interval between the first and second assessment varied from 6 months to 1 year. At the initial assessment patients socio-medical problems were identified by a health-visitor using a 'proforma', each patient had an average of 6.4 problems. The reassessment occurred after treatment had been given and patients were found to have fewer problems.

Williams (1974) also attempted to evaluate the effect of screening procedures in terms of benefit upon the elderly by following up patients who were screened in an earlier study (Williams *et al.*, 1972). Health visitors were used to interview the patients either at home or in the surgery. The health visitor collected the demographic data and took a medical history and a full medical examination was carried out by the doctor. The main finding of this study was that despite the presence of 450 disease conditions in a sample of approximately 300, many of the elderly people were active and enjoying life.

Involvement of health visitors in screening programmes

Many screening studies for the elderly already mentioned have employed health visitors to collect data. Health visitors have also been mentioned in these studies as useful to carry out health surveillance or health screening on behalf of the general practitioner. Health visitors involved in these studies as data collectors have worked to a disease-oriented model and not from an explicit nursing framework. Although these studies suggest referral of patients to health visitors it is not clear how the health visitor is to carry out her duty of 'surveillance'. Much is written about what health visitors should do but little about how they should do it (Hunt, 1972).

It would appear that only a small number of health visitors have written on the subject or conducted research in this field (Heath and Fitton, 1975; Hoadley, 1975; Kneer, 1975; Loveland and Hillman, 1971; Luker, 1979; Moore, 1973). Hence the literature pertinent to health visiting and the well elderly tends to focus on the health visitor's dependent function, that of assisting the doctor in screening programmes based on the traditional medical model rather than on the independent aspect of health visiting namely 'surveillance'. Therefore, little is known about what takes place after an elderly person is referred from a screening programme to the health visitor.

THE NEED FOR EVALUATION[2]

Some health visitors believe that the effects of health visiting are too subtle, intangible or elusive to be realistically assessed. If this were so there would be little reason for health visitors to offer a service, since no one, including the client, would be aware of its effects. Intangible or elusive changes can hardly be considered as worthwhile goals or reasons for continuing professional practice. Moreover in the context of the present economic climate it would seem urgent to assess the care given by health visitors in order to demonstrate its effectiveness and to justify the provision of the service.

Health visitors have been content to avoid studying the process of health visiting in terms of outcome and effectiveness by dismissing it as methodologically impractical. Researchers have focused on describing health visiting in terms of what health visitors say they do. In a study of health visitors in Berkshire, Clark (1973) decided against the method of participant observation on the premise that a third person would distort the interaction between the health visitor and client.

A good deal of the health visitor's work is carried out inside the home and as such is invisible to others. Dingwall (1977) observed that there were strong boundaries between the work of individual health visitors which were sanctioned by the concept of privacy. This privacy allows scope for variation in practice, the only public area of a health visitor's work being her records. It is contended (Luker, 1979) that personal preference on the part of the health visitor is probably the most salient variable in determining whether or not elderly people receive visits from a health visitor. Few studies have been undertaken to elicit the opinions of health visitors regarding visits to specific client groups. However, a small exploratory study was undertaken by Luker (1978) which sought the opinions of health visitors concerning visits to the elderly. There appeared to be agreement that the elderly were an 'at risk' group who should receive some priority. The health visitors did not seem to regard the elderly as part of their case load in the same way as they did the children and in one instance the records referring to the elderly were kept in a different place which symbolised their separateness from the main case load. The current policy in the study area was to visit the elderly after an event which necessitated them consulting their general practitioner from whom most referrals came. When asked about the feasibility of a specialised health visiting service for the elderly, the health visitors all considered that it would be a depressing job and that it would be difficult to find health visitors willing to do it. They stated that if everyone over the age of 75 years of age was to be visited on a regular basis a considerable number of such specialised health visitors would be needed since visits to the elderly took much longer than visits to other age groups. The comment by one respondent 'you just can't get away' summed it all up. Dingwall (1977) in his study of the social organisation of health visitor training commented that student health visitors did not like visiting the elderly because it took too long. Dingwall hypothesised that the reason they could not terminate a visit was because it had no structure, they were not in control and, to use his words, the health visitor students 'did not have an agenda' and hence the client took over. Dingwall's observations were confirmed by Luker (1978) who comments: 'Infants of six months of age and under seemed to receive the most intensive and structured visiting whereas visits to the elderly were the most aimless and unstructured.'

From Luker's (1978) observations it was apparent that health visitors on routine surveillance visits do not work from a medical model but instead from a developmental model related to chronological age. Hence, it can be argued that since the developmental needs of the elderly have not been well defined or documented then the care which they require is not known by health visitors and hence cannot be valued by them. This observation raises the question of how beneficial are health visitor visits to the elderly?

INTRODUCTION TO EVALUATION[3]

The term 'evaluation' is widely used and for the most part its meaning is taken for granted. Few attempts have been made to formulate a conceptually rigorous definition of evaluation or to analyse the main principles of its use. This lack of definition has resulted in the term being used interchangeably with other terms such as 'assessment', 'appraisal', and 'judgement'. Taking into account the common usage of the term 'evaluation', Suchman (1967), makes the distinction between 'evaluation' and 'evaluative research'. Evaluation, when used in a general way is said to refer to the everyday

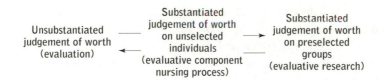

Figure 16.1   The continuum of evaluation. (Reproduced by permission of Macmillan Journals)

occurrence of making judgements of worth. 'Evaluative research' on the other hand implies utilisation of scientific methods and techniques for the purpose of making an evaluation. Suchman (1967) comments that in this sense 'evaluation' becomes an adjective specifying a type of research. The major emphasis is upon the noun 'research', and evaluative research refers to those procedures for collecting and analysing data which increase the possibility for 'proving' rather than 'asserting' the worth of some social activity. Evaluation may best be viewed as a continuum (Luker, 1981a).

The evaluation component of the nursing process can be placed almost anywhere along this continuum (Figure 16.1) depending on the way in which data are collected (systematic or otherwise) and recorded. Data which have been systematically collected and recorded during the execution of the nursing process may be used retrospectively by nurses/health visitors for research purposes. The retrospective use of the material may be referred to as 'evaluative research' because evaluation and not care giving has become the main thrust of the activity and the researcher is able to determine the population and sample to be studied.

EVALUATING THE PRACTICE OF HEALTH VISITING

Because health visiting places an emphasis on prevention it shares the problem inherent in the evaluation of all preventive techniques or programmes. Namely if something does not occur because it has been prevented how can it be measured. In a discussion on measuring the effects of prevention Lave and Lave (1977) comment that the old adage: 'an ounce of prevention is worth a pound of cure' is not an acceptable guide to the allocation of resources in the community because effective preventive techniques are lacking and therefore the adage is misleading since it places into one category 'prevention' a wide variety of programmes and activities.

In the days of the sanitary missioner through primary prevention it was possible to lower the infectious disease morbidity and mortality rates. Today in the era of the generic family visitor we are in a position of choosing from interventions which have a much lower level of effectiveness. The apparent lack of dramatic opportunities to measure the effectiveness of prevention say Lave and Lave (1977) is one estimate of how far we have come in community health.

The preventive aspects of health visiting are difficult to measure because of the long-term nature of the work and the lack of data other than for specific programmes such as immunisation and developmental screening. However, it is contended that health visitors do deal with clients and families who have tangible problems which are amenable to short-term intervention and this is probably best illustrated in the health visitor's work with the elderly. In attempting to solve short-term problems health visitors may affect the future health of the client or family in an unknown way since problems which are prevented from developing because of health visitor intervention cannot be assessed. Nevertheless, it is thought that evaluation of health visitor intervention in terms of its effect upon the client might begin in the area of tangible problems.

OUTCOME EVALUATION

To date few studies have been conducted which have attempted an evaluation of the outcome of health visitor intervention, in fact little research effort in nursing generally has been directed at evaluation, possibly because of the difficulties involved in demonstrating a cause-and-effect relationship. The usual scientific approach has been to use the experimental method which may necessitate in the context of health visiting denying a control group access to the service. Health visitors have seemed reluctant to deny their service in the interests of scientific enquiry preferring to cling to the belief that their service is without question beneficial to the client. Owing to the government recommendations that health visitors should increase their involvement with the elderly (DHSS, 1976b), it was thought that in the absence of concrete evidence of the effects of health visitor intervention with this age group an evaluation study would be timely. There were two methodological advantages in attempting to evaluate the effectiveness of health visitor intervention on an elderly population. First a knowledge of the sparseness of health visitor visits to this age group meant that it could be safely assumed that a sample of elderly people could be selected who would not have had recent contact with a health visitor. Secondly if a controlled comparison was to be made it would not be necessary to actively deny the services of a health visitor to one group, instead, they could be allowed access to the usual service which in most cases they would not receive. These advantages would not apply if an attempt was made to evaluate the effectiveness of health visitor visits to families with children under 5 years of age. However, there was one methodological disadvantage in attempting to evaluate the outcome of health visitor intervention on an elderly population in that one could reasonably expect a deterioration in health to occur in some individuals as a result of the ageing process alone. It was, however, possible to deflect this disadvantage by using an experimental design.

BACKGROUND TO THE STUDY

The study framework was generated by readings on the nursing process and by an exploratory investigation which revealed that health visitor visits to the elderly were unstructured and diffuse.

From the premise of diffuseness, it was decided to attempt to focus health visiting visits to the elderly on their actual and potential health problems. A health problem was defined as anything which might concern the subject or the health visitor about the subject's health, either at the time of the assessment or at some time in the future. Health was broadly defined to incorporate the physical and psycho-social aspects of well being. Since it was decided to focus on health, it was therefore necessary to have a framework from which to identify problems, and an assessment format incorporating the activities of daily-living approach was designed.

In order to tap the well-being aspect of health it was decided to incorporate a life satisfaction measure in the assessment format. The Life Satisfaction Index – A (LSI – A) (Neugarten *et al.*, 1961) was chosen as an appropriate and widely used instrument.

THE MAIN STUDY

The main study was planned using a two-group experimental design involving a cross-over (Figure 16.2).

In an attempt to control for as many variables as possible it was necessary to have fairly strict inclusion criteria and the criteria for inclusion into the study were as follows:

1 All subjects were registered with one group of general practitioners.
2 Sex – female.
3 Age – 70 years and over.
4 Housing – living alone.

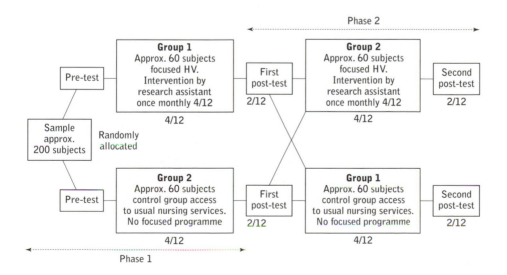

Figure 16.2   The study design. (Reproduced by permission of Macmillan Journals)

5   Mental status – no impairment on the Isaac and Walkey (1964) Mental Impairment Measure.
6   Not at present in receipt of health visiting services and should not be visited by a district nurse more than once monthly.

Approximately 230 subjects were sampled from the age/sex register of one group of general practitioners.

The subjects were randomly allocated to either the experimental or control groups before the assessment visit (pre-test). This was done in order to make the explanation of the study easier for the subjects to understand although methodologically it can be seen as a threat to internal validity.

Before the assessment visit each subject received a letter from her general practitioner, and the letter acted as identification for the researcher and also as an introduction to the subject.

The pre-test was carried out on each subject who agreed to participate and involved the completion of the assessment form and the identification of actual and potential health problems. The problems were recorded after each visit using a problem-oriented recording format modified for this study and this recording approach included a plan of action for dealing with each subject's problem.

The experimental group received focused health visitor intervention once monthly for 4 months from the research assistant, who was a health visitor employed solely to work on this study. The focus of the visit was generated by the subject's health problems.

The research assistant recorded her visits in a systematic way using the problem-oriented format, and estimated at each visit, on a separate form, whether there had been a change in the status of the problem.

The control group received no focused programme, but retained access to the usual nursing services, which in real terms meant that they did not receive any service at all.

After 4 months of focused health visiting the first post-test was carried out on both groups. This involved the completion of the assessment form including the LSI – A and changes in problem status were recorded. The experimental group were, in addition, asked their opinion about the benefits or otherwise of the health visitor's visits. The control group then became the experimental group and the whole process was repeated (Figure 16.2).

The cross-over design provided an intra-person comparison and an inter-group comparison before and after health visitor involvement on the dependent variables of problem status and life satisfaction and descriptive data were collected about subjects' perceived benefits from the programme.

FINDINGS

The findings are discussed briefly and an attempt has been made to highlight their implications for the practice of health visiting.

HEALTH PROBLEM STATUS

The type of health problems identified at the assessment visit have been subsumed under ten headings:

1 weight maintenance
2 mobility
3 dentition
4 sensory function
5 elimination
6 loneliness
7 performance of personal or household tasks
8 rest
9 medication
10 miscellaneous.

The changes in problem status after 5 months with no intervention (Group 2) are shown in Figure 16.3(a). It is apparent that the majority of problems remained as they were at the initial pre-test visit.

In contrast Figure 16.3(b) indicates the changes in problem status of Group 1, the group that received health visitor intervention and it is seen that 43 per cent of problems improved as opposed to 19 per cent in Group 2. This is a statistically significant finding below the 5 per cent level.

The cross-over in the research design (Figure 16.2) meant that the subjects in Group 2 who did not receive health visitors' visits began to receive visits after the first post-test and Figure 16.3(c) indicates how these problems changed, and the pattern is similar to that of Group 1 (Figure 16.3(b)).

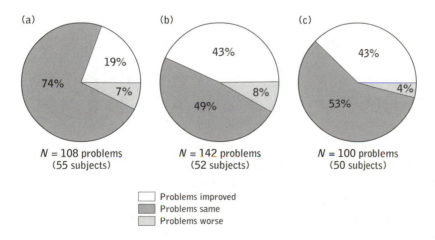

Figure 16.3 Change in problem status. (a) Problem status of Group 2 at post-test 1 (no treatment phase). (b) Problem status of Group 1 at post-test 1 (treatment phase). (c) Problem status of Group 2 at post-test 2 (treatment phase). (Reproduced by permission of Macmillan Journals)

DURATION AND EFFECT

As already mentioned, the cross-over in the research design allowed an intra-person comparison to be made and this has been demonstrated for Group 2. However, the subjects in Group 1 after the first post-test no longer received health visitor visits and at the second post-test an attempt was made to see if the effect of the health visitor visits in terms of problem improvement had been maintained. This is referred to as 'duration of effect' (Suchman, 1967).

Findings indicate in general terms that the effect of health visitor intervention can last after the service is withdrawn. This has implications for the practice of health visiting in that health visitors may be able to contemplate discharging elderly people rather than keeping them on the books indefinitely.

LIFE SATISFACTION

Life satisfaction was measured using the Neugarten *et al*. (1961) LSI – A and as such did not indicate a statistically significant change before and after health visitor intervention. This may be explained in several different ways. First, health visitors may not influence the life satisfaction of elderly women. Secondly, the instrument may have been administered at an inappropriate time in that the length of time between the last health visitor visit and the post-test varied from 2 days to 3 weeks and therefore any change in satisfaction may have been too shortlived to be reflected in the LSI – A. Thirdly, the LSI – A may have been insensitive to changes over time.

It seemed from the subjective data collected that health visitor visits did have the potential to elevate mood and hence the second explanation is favoured. It is therefore suggested that if the LSI – A is used in further research it should be administered immediately after the last health visitor visit.

SUBJECTIVE OPINION ABOUT HEALTH VISITOR VISITS

These findings relate to what the elderly women themselves said about the health visitor visits. It is not possible to share all that they said since this has been reported elsewhere (Luker, 1981c). Therefore, findings have been selected which may be of general interest.

Broadly speaking, the majority of the sample said that they enjoyed the health visitor visits and most thought they had benefited in some way. An emphasis was placed on the social aspects of the visit and there were mentions of the enjoyment inherent in 'just having a talk to somebody'.

There were, however, some mentions of the health visitors' general overseeing function. Many respondents reported that they looked forward to the day of the visit. It seemed that just having a visit to look forward to regardless of what happened may itself have been therapeutic. The notion of looking forward to the visit has been termed 'therapeutic anticipation' (Luker, 1981c). In everyday health visiting practice there appears to be a reluctance among health visitors to make appointments and it could be argued that health visitors are minimising their effectiveness by not doing so.

It is noteworthy that a small percentage of the sample reported that they did not enjoy the health visitor visits and two respondents even went so far as to say that the visit had a bad effect on them. The notion that visits from a health visitor may have a harmful or 'bad effect' on some older people is seldom addressed when contemplating routine visiting of the elderly.

Most of the respondents thought that it was a good idea for the health visitor to visit elderly people. There were many mentions of groups of people whom it was thought were in need of visits from a health visitor, namely those who are disabled, ailing or housebound, the lonely and people with no families.

The sample seemed to appreciate that health visitors were in short supply and favoured their deployment among the lonely disabled and infirm. There were many mentions by respondents who considered that there were persons worse off than themselves who were in need of health visitor services and I have termed this 'the somebody worse than me syndrome'. A typical response was: 'Oh yes, it was a good idea for health visitors to visit elderly people not so lucky as me. I have good neighbours. The health visitor can see what's going on and if somebody is not able she can tell the doctor.'

It seems that 'the somebody worse than me syndrome' might be the way that some elderly people cope with growing older, in that as long as they believe that there are people in the world worse off than themselves they are able to cope effectively with the restrictions that old age may eventually impose.

Despite the fact that the vast majority of the sample said that they enjoyed the health visitor visits and nearly two-thirds reported that they had benefited in some ways, less than half the sample reported that they would like the visits to continue and over a third said that they did not wish the visits to continue.

A number of respondents stated that they did not wish to have any further visits from a health visitor but nevertheless added that they might be glad of her services if they were ill. These elderly respondents saw the health visitor as a person who could give advice and help in times of illness rather than somebody who would give advice on how to stay healthy in old age.

IN CONCLUSION

Although the study reported here does not provide information about the full effects of health visitor intervention in that no indication has been given about the problems which were prevented from developing because of intervention, it is nevertheless hoped that the methods used and some of the issues raised will provide an impetus for further research concerning the evaluation of health visiting practice. Currently policy decisions which relate to health care are based on the logical appraisal of the options of people involved in decision-making (Reid and Holland, 1978). Thus decision-making which may result in the expenditure of large amounts of public money is commonly based on the past experience of a collection of individuals rather than on pertinent factual data. Unfortunately the findings from this study stand alone in that there are no comparable data which might assist in the interpretation of a 43 per cent problem improvement rate as either 'good' or 'bad'. This lack of comparable data points up the necessity for more research endeavour to be directed into the evaluation of health-care services, and more specifically it is contended that there is a need to focus on the benefit of the service to the client.

NOTES

* J. Wilson-Barnett (ed.) *Nursing Research: Ten Studies in Patient Care*, vol. 2, pp. 141–156. Chichester, Wiley. Reprinted with permission of John Wiley & Sons.
 1 This section reproduced by permission of the Newbourne Group.
 2 This and other material in this chapter is reproduced by permission of Macmillan Journals.
 3 This section includes material reproduced by permission of Blackwell Scientific Publications Ltd.

REFERENCES

Age Concern (1972). *Age Concern on Health*. Age Concern, London.

Age Concern (1977). *Profiles of the Elderly: Their Health and the Health Services*. Age Concern Research Publications, London.

Anderson, W. F. (1974). Administration, labelling and general principles of drug prescription in the elderly. *Gerontologica Clinica*, 16, 4–9.

Anderson, W. F. (1976). The effect of screening on the quality of life after 70 years. *Journal of the Royal College of Physicians of London*, 10, 2, 161–168.

Atkinson, L., Gibson, I. J. M. and Andrews, J. (1977). The difficulties of old people taking drugs. *Age and Ageing*, 6, 144–149.

Barber, J. H. and Wallis, J. B. (1976). Assessment of the elderly in general practice. *Journal of the Royal College of General Practitioners*, 26, 163, 106–114.

Barber, J. H. and Wallis, J. B. (1978). The benefits to an elderly population of continuing geriatric assessment. *Journal of the Royal College of General Practitioners*, 28, 192, 428–433.

Barker, J. (1974). *Hospital and Community Care for the Elderly*. Age Concern, London.

Brocklehurst, J. C. (1975). *Geriatric Care in Advanced Societies*. Blackburn Times Press, Blackburn.

Burns, C. (1969). Geriatric care in general practice. *Journal of the Royal College of General Practitioners*, 18, 88, 287–296.

Clark, J. (1973). *A Family Visitor*. The Royal College of Nursing, London.

Currie, G., MacNeill, R. M., Walker, J. G., Barnie, E. and Mudie, E. W. (1974). Medical and social screening of patients aged 70–72 by an urban general practice health team. *British Medical Journal*, 2, 108–111.

Department of Health and Social Security (1976a). *Prevention and Health Everybody's Business. A Reassessment of Public and Personal Health*. HMSO, London.

Department of Health and Social Security (1976b). *Priorities for Health and Personal Social Services in England. A Consultative Document*. HMSO, London.

Dingwall R. (1977). *The Social Organisation of Health Visitor Training*. Croom Helm, London.

Gardiner, R. (1975). The identification of the medical and social needs of the elderly in the community: A pilot survey. *Age and Ageing*, 4, 3, 81–87.

Heath, P. J. and Fitton, J. M. (1975). Survey of over-80 age grouping G.P. population based on an urban health centre. *Nursing Times Occasional Papers*, 71, 43, 109–112.

Hiscock, E., Prangnell, O. R. and Wilmot, J. F. (1973). A screening survey of old people in general practice. *The Practitioner*, 210, 1256, 271–277.

Hoadley, D. M. (1975). *Health survey into nursing and social needs of the elderly in a group general practice*. Unpublished report: West Sussex AHA.

Hunt, M. (1972). The dilemma of identity in health visiting. *Nursing Times Occasional Papers*, 71, 43, 1714–1716.

Isaac, B. and Walkey, F. A. (1964). Measurement of mental impairment in geriatric practice. *Gerontologica Clinica*, 6, 114–123.

Kneer, C. M. (1975). Country life, a survey of needs of old people in a rural area (a health visitor interviews 110 people), *Nursing Times*, 71, 43, 1714–1716.

Lave, J. R. and Lave, L. B. (1977). Measuring the effectiveness of prevention. I. *Millbank Memorial Fund Quarterly Health and Society*, Spring, 273–289.

Loveland, M. L. and Hillman, H. (1971). A survey of people over 65 years of age living alone, in contact with welfare authorities. *Health Visitor*, 44, 7, 226–229.

Lowther, C. P., MacLeod, R. D. M. and Williamson, J. (1970). Evaluation of early diagnostic services for the elderly. *British Medical Journal*, 3, 275–277.

Luker, K. A. (1978). Goal attainment: A possible model for assessing the work of the health visitor. *Nursing Times*, 74, 30, 1257–1259.

Luker, K. A. (1979). Health visiting and the elderly. *Midwife, Health Visitor and Community Nurse*, 15, 11, 457–459.

Luker, K. A. (1981a). An overview of evaluation research in nursing. *Journal of Advanced Nursing*, 6, 87–93.

Luker, K. A. (1981b). Health visiting and the elderly. *Nursing Times Occasional Papers*, 77, 35, 137–140.

Luker, K. A. (1981c). Elderly women's opinions about the benefits of health visitor visits. *Nursing Times Occasional Papers*, 11, 9, 33–35.

Milne, J. S., Maule, M. M., Cormack, S. and Williamson, J. (1972). The design and testing of a questionnaire and evaluation to assess physical and mental health in older people using a staff nurse as the observer. *Journal of Chronic Disease*, 25, 388–405.

Moore, D. M. (1973). A geriatric survey. *Health Visitor*, 46, 302–303.

Neugarten, B. L., Havighurst, R. J. and Tobin, S. S. (1961). The measurement of life satisfaction. *Journal of Gerontology*, 16, 134–143.

Reid, D. and Holland W. (1978). Measurement in health care studies, in *Health Care and Epidemiology* (eds W. Holland and L. Karhausen), Henry Kemptons, London.

Sheldon, J. H. (1948). *The Social Medicine of Old Age: Report of an Enquiry in Wolverhampton*, Oxford University Press for the Nuffield Foundation, London.

Suchman, E. A. (1967). *Evaluation Research*. Russell Sage Foundation, New York.

Taylor, G. F., Eddy, T. P. and Scott, D. L. (1971). A survey of 216 elderly men and women in general practice. *Journal of the Royal College of General Practitioners*, 21, 106, 267–275.

Thomas, P. (1968). Experience of 2 preventive clinics for the elderly. *British Medical Journal*, 2, 357–360.

Wedderburn, D. and Townsend, P. (1965). *The Aged in the Welfare State: The Interim Report of Survey of Persons aged 65 and over in Britain 1962–1963*. G. Bell & Sons, London.

Williams, E. I., Bennett, F. M., Nixon, J. V. and Nicholson, M. R. (1972). Sociomedical study of patients over 75 in general practice. *British Medical Journal*, 2, 445–448.

Williams, E. I. (1974). A follow-up of geriatric patients socio-medical assessment. *Journal of the Royal College of General Practitioners*, 24, 142, 341–346.

Williamson, J., Lowther, C. P. and Grays, S. (1966). The use of health visitors in preventive geriatrics. *Gerontologica Clinica*, 8, 362–369.

Williamson, J., Stokoe, I. H., Grays, S., Fisher, M., Smith, S., McGhee, A. and Stephenson, E. (1964). Old people at home their unreported needs. *Lancet*, 1, 1117–1120.

Wilson, M. (1973). Caring for an ageing population: The problem for society. *Nursing Times*, 69, 14, 486–488.

Chapter 17

West Berkshire perineal management trial

JENNIFER SLEEP, ADRIAN GRANT, JO GARCIA,
DIANA ELBOURNE, JOHN SPENCER, IAIN CHALMERS

Introduction

If we are asked to justify the place of research in health care, we are likely to point to its role in eliminating unnecessary procedures, procedures that may be both costly in terms of time and equipment as well as distressing or painful for patients. Midwifery has been an important area for such revelation. Within midwifery, the use of enemas and shaves as a standard preparation for delivery has declined, at least partly because of research that has demonstrated its lack of efficacy. Questions have also been posed about the possible overuse of Caesarean sections, epidural anaesthesia and various forms of foetal and maternal monitoring in the context of a growing movement to demedicalise childbirth over the last 20 or 30 years.

This paper by Jennifer Sleep and colleagues, published in 1984, looks at the use of episiotomy in spontaneous vaginal deliveries. The authors argue the need for the research into the topic by pointing to the wide variation in practice in the UK, and what they describe as a dearth of scientific evidence and consensus on its practice. Those who argue either for or against its use appear to have plausible reasons: some argue that cutting prevents potentially serious tears during delivery and complications later, while others believe that perineal tears cause fewer problems than the wounds of epi-siotomy. This difference in view, along with a reported variation in the practice – from 14 to 96% during first-time deliveries in British maternity units – set the stage for Sleep's attempt to settle the matter with a definitive experiment.

Her study uses a randomised controlled trial to compare the maternal outcomes following 'liberal' and 'restrictive' use of episiotomy. To produce useful knowledge a randomised controlled trial needs to define and reproduce a clear procedure to be applied to one group, but not another; to ensure that the group receiving the intervention and the group who remain 'untouched' are as alike as is feasible regarding characteristics deemed to be of relevance; and to have some insightful and standardised way of detecting the difference between the two groups after the intervention, sometimes without those who do the measuring knowing who has received the intervention and who has not. Added to this, of course, needs to be some consideration and comment on the applicability of the findings to practitioners attempting to make wise and scientific decisions in contexts different from those of the original experiment.

Though not as unambiguous as giving or withholding a particular drug might be, the distinction between the intervention and control group lay in the instruction given by the researchers to the midwives delivering the babies of 1000 women. For half the group, the 'control' group, the midwife was told to 'try to avoid episiotomy', only resorting to it when there were signs of foetal distress to speed delivery. The midwives delivering the other group were instructed to 'try to prevent a tear'. These instructions did produce a wide divergence in episiotomy between the groups: 10% of women in the first group compared with 51% in the latter. In this case, where there appeared to be genuine uncertainty about which approach was likely to lead to better perineal outcomes, the research team could deal with possible ethical difficulties (over denying a beneficial treatment to a group of women) by claiming that both approaches to management were aimed at 'minimising perineal trauma'.

Sleep and colleagues looked for differences in a range of both short- and medium-term maternal outcomes and in certain neonatal outcomes. Interestingly, on many measures the two groups did not differ, and perhaps the most useful finding was that severe maternal trauma was much less common overall than was expected, which might itself be seen as supporting the argument against intervention. However, four of the five women with severe tears were in the group with restricted episiotomy. Similarly, the researchers found more undamaged perineums among the restrictive group, but that group experienced more perineal and labial tears.

So, as with much research, the findings do not translate in any simple way into a directive for practice. As the authors note, their findings provide little support *either* for the free use of episiotomy *or* for arguments that restricted use of episiotomy reduces maternal problems after delivery. Perhaps clinicians are left in that position, highlighted by the champions of evidence-based practice, of being too influenced in their practice by personal witness of a very small number of misfortunes. Sleep's study is also a good example of an investigation into a nursing – in this case midwifery – intervention using, quite appropriately, an experimental design.

SLEEP, J., A. GRANT, J. GARCIA, D. ELBOURNE, J. SPENCER
AND I. CHALMERS (1984)

West Berkshire perineal management trial*

INTRODUCTION

There is a dearth of scientific evidence on which to base the practice of episiotomy.[1,2] Some people claim that the operation should be used liberally on the grounds that this will reduce both serious vaginal and perineal tears as well as longer term problems such as stress incontinence and vaginal prolapse.[3,4] Others maintain that episiotomy should be largely restricted to fetal indications because they believe that perineal tears cause women fewer problems than episiotomies done to prevent them.[5-7]

These differing views are reflected in the widely varying use of the operation; a recent survey of British maternity units reported hospital rates ranging from 14% to 96% in primiparas and from 16% to 71% in multiparas (M. J. House, personal communication). In particular, this variation is an expression of differing opinions about the use of the operation for *maternal* indications in non-instrumental delivery.

In the light of these contradictions we mounted a randomised controlled trial to compare liberal and restrictive use of episiotomy for maternal indications in otherwise normal vaginal deliveries.

PATIENTS AND METHODS

The study was conducted at the maternity unit of the Royal Berkshire Hospital in Reading; study design and protocol were approved by the hospital ethics and research committee for west Berkshire. All women booked to deliver in the hospital during the study period were given a letter in the last trimester of their pregnancies seeking their collaboration in research into delivery techniques aimed at reducing pain and discomfort after delivery. Women were eligible for entry to the study if (a) they had a live singleton fetus or at least 37 completed weeks' gestational age presenting cephalically, and (b) spontaneous vaginal delivery was expected towards the end of the second stage of labour. During the five month study period in 1982, 1077 women met these entry criteria. Of these, 77 were not recruited to the trial for the following reasons: precipitate delivery (14 cases), private patient (eight), mother's request not to be included (seven), elective episiotomy (six), other reasons (42). (During the five month period of recruitment there were 201 operative vaginal deliveries and 62 emergency caesarean sections of singleton babies of at least 37 completed weeks' gestational age presenting cephalically.)

Entry to the trial, which was signalled by opening a sealed opaque envelope, was postponed until the attending midwife had decided to 'scrub up' in expectation of a spontaneous vaginal delivery. One thousand women (93% of those who met the criteria for entry) were allocated at random to one of two management policies, both of

Table 17.1   Comparability of treatment groups

	Restrictive policy (n = 498)	Liberal policy (n = 502)
Mean (SD) maternal age, in years	26.6 (5.2)	26.7 (5.3)
No (%) primiparous	201(40.4)	219(43.6)
No (%) married	445(89.5)	435(86.7)
Mean (SD) gestational age, in weeks	39.8 (1.2)	39.8 (1.2)
Mean (SD) birth weight, in g	3393 (448)	3367 (438)
Person conducting delivery (No (%) of cases):		
Sister	163(32.7)	157(31.3)
Staff midwife	150(30.1)	161(32.1)
Student midwife	150(30.1)	155(30.9)
Medical student	26 (5.2)	25 (5.0)
Doctor	9 (1.8)	4 (0.8)

which aimed at minimising perineal trauma during spontaneous vaginal delivery. In one the midwife was instructed to 'try to avoid episiotomy,' the intention being that she should restrict episiotomy to fetal indications (fetal bradycardia, tachycardia, or meconium stained liquor) so far as possible (498 subjects). In managing the other group the midwife was instructed to 'try to prevent a tear,' the intention being that she should use episiotomy more liberally to prevent tears (502 subjects). The groups generated were similar in several important respects (Table 17.1). All 1000 women went on to have spontaneous vaginal deliveries and were delivered by people of comparable status. When performed, episiotomies were mediolateral. Perineal trauma in the two groups was repaired in a similar way by operators of similar experience, 5% of whom were senior obstetricians, 86% junior obstetricians, and 9% medical students under supervision. A continuous suture was used to repair the vagina. Interrupted stitches were used for the deeper tissues and subcuticular (40%) or interrupted sutures (60%) used to repair the perineal skin.

The consequences of the two policies were compared in terms of maternal and infant morbidity immediately after delivery and at 10 days and three months post partum.

The principal measures of outcome (with their expected incidences and methods of measurement) were as follows: (a) severe maternal trauma, predefined as extension through the anal sphincter or through to the rectal mucosa or to the upper third of the vagina (expected incidence 5%, assessed by the operator performing the repair 'blind' to the allocation); (b) Apgar score less than 7 at one minute (expected incidence 5%, assessed by the senior midwife at the delivery); (c) severe or moderate perineal pain 10 days after delivery (expected incidence 20% – standardised questionnaire administered by community midwife blind to the allocation); (d) admission to special care baby unit in first 10 days of life (expected incidence 5% – standardised questionnaire administered by community midwife blind to the allocation); (e) perineal discomfort three months after delivery (expected incidence

20% – standardised postal questionnaire self administered by the mother, in most cases blind to the allocation); (f) no resumption of sexual intercourse three months after delivery (expected incidence 5% – standardised postal questionnaire self administered by the other, in most cases blind to the allocation).

Based on these expected incidences the trial size was preset at 1000 subjects. Power calculations before the trial indicated that a trial of this size would have a 90% chance of finding a significant difference (two tailed $\alpha = 0.05$) if, in truth, the restrictive policy doubled the incidence of an outcome expected in 5% of cases, and a 95% power of detecting an increase in 50% in an outcome expected in 20% of cases. All analyses were based on the unbiased comparisons between all women randomly allocated to either the restrictive or liberal policy whether or not they sustained an episiotomy or a tear.

The follow up rate at both 10 days and three months after delivery was 89%.

The χ^2 and Student's t tests were used to compare discrete and continuous variables respectively in the two groups.

RESULTS

The episiotomy rate was 10% in the group allocated to the restrictive policy and 51% in the liberal policy group. This difference reflected the different numbers of both primiparas and multiparas in whom episiotomy was performed for maternal reasons (Table 17.2).

There was wide variation in the time interval between entry to the trial and delivery. While some babies were born immediately after the envelope had been opened, the interval was more than 20 minutes for 8% in the liberal group and 12% in the restrictive group ($\chi^2 = 3.4$; p = 0.07).

The different episiotomy rates resulted in different patterns of maternal trauma sustained at delivery. As expected, there were both more posterior tears and more intact

Table 17.2 Actual use of episiotomy. Figures are numbers of subjects (percentages in parentheses)

	Restrictive policy (n = 498)		Liberal policy (n = 502)	
Episiotomy		51(10.2)		258(51.4)
Primiparas	36(17.9)		147(67.1)	
Multiparas	15 (5.1)		111(39.2)	
Maternal indications		18 (3.6)		228(45.4)
Primiparas	12 (6.0)		130(59.3)	
Multiparas	6 (2.0)		98(34.6)	
Fetal distress		33 (6.6)		30 (6.0)
Primiparas	24(11.9)		17 (7.8)	
Multiparas	9 (3.0)		13 (4.6)	

Table 17.3   Maternal trauma at delivery. Figures are numbers of subjects (percentages in parentheses)

	Restrictive policy (n = 498)		Liberal policy (n = 502)	
Posterior trauma				
None		169(33.9)		122(24.3)
Primiparas	62(30.8)		32(14.6)	
Multiparas	107(36.0)		90(31.8)	
Episiotomy alone		45 (9.0)		227(45.2)
Primiparas	32(15.9)		125(57.1)	
Multiparas	13 (4.4)		102(36.0)	
Perineal tear alone		278(55.8)		123(24.5)
Primiparas	103(51.2)		40(18.3)	
Multiparas	175(58.9)		83(29.3)	
Episiotomy plus extension		6 (1.2)		30 (6.0)
Primiparas	4 (2.0)		22(10.0)	
Multiparas	2 (0.7)		8 (2.8)	

χ^2 test = 205.27 (3 df); p<0.0001

	Restrictive policy (n = 498)		Liberal policy (n = 502)	
Anterior trauma				
None		367(73.7)		415(82.7)
Primiparas	135(67.2)		170(77.6)	
Multiparas	232(78.1)		245(86.5)	
Labial tears		131(26.3)		87(17.3)
Primiparas	66(32.8)		49(22.4)	
Multiparas	65(21.9)		38(13.4)	

χ^2 test = 11.29 (1 df); p<0.001

perineums among those allocated to the restrictive policy. In addition, this group also sustained more anterior labial tears (Table 17.3; relative risk 1.52, 95% confidence limit 1.19–1.94).

'Severe maternal trauma' was much less common than expected. There were only four cases in the restrictive group and one in the liberal group. Both women with severe perineal injuries had been allocated to the restrictive policy; in one, a primipara, the rectal mucosa was damaged; in the other, a multipara, the anal sphincter was completely torn. In the other three cases, all primiparas, there was extension of the injury to the upper third of the vagina.

More of the women allocated to the liberal policy than to the restrictive policy required suturing (78% v 69% – χ^2 = 9.00; p<0.01); this difference was more striking in primiparas (89% v 74%) than in multiparas (69% v 66%). Apart from the four cases of severe trauma described above there was no evidence that trauma was more extensive in those women in the restrictive group who actually sustained perineal injury. Overall, women allocated to the liberal policy required 100 more packets of suture material (p<0.01) and 13 more hours of time to repair the trauma that they had sustained (p<0.01).

Table 17.4   Pain in past 24 hours 10 days post partum. Figures are numbers of subjects (percentages in parentheses)

	Restrictive policy (n = 439)		Liberal policy (n = 446)	
Mild		62(14.1)		65(14.6)
Primiparas	34(18.5)		38 (19.4)	
Multiparas	28(11.0)		27 (10.8)	
Moderate		33 (7.5)		35 (7.8)
Primiparas	19(10.3)		22 (11.2)	
Multiparas	14 (5.5)		13 (5.2)	
Severe		4 (0.9)		1 (0.2)
Primiparas	2 (1.1)		1 (0.5)	
Multiparas	2 (0.8)		0 (0.0)	
Total		99(22.6)		101(22.6)
Primiparas	55(29.9)		61 (31.1)	
Multiparas	44(17.3)		40 (16.0)	

χ^2 test = 1.91 (3 df); NS

There were no significant differences in neonatal outcome. A total of 5.4% of babies in the restrictive group and 4.6% in the liberal group had Apgar scores below 7 at one minute, and the figures for admission to the special care baby unit in the first 10 days of life were 5.7% and 7.6% respectively.

On the tenth day after delivery 3% of mothers in the restrictive group and 2% in the liberal group used oral analgesics. The incidence of pain reported by mothers was very similar in the two groups both at 10 days after delivery (Table 17.4) and at three months (Table 17.5). A similar proportion (12%) of women in each group had sought medical advice because of perineal problems. Consultation was more frequent among primiparas (19%) than multiparas (9%).

Thirty seven per cent of women allocated to the restrictive policy (33% of primiparas, 39% of multiparas) compared with 27% in the liberal group (22% of primiparas, 32% of multiparas) resumed sexual intercourse within a month after delivery (χ^2 = 8.67; p<0.01). This difference was only partly explained by the different proportions of women with intact perineums in the two groups. Overall, 90% of women had resumed sexual intercourse within three months after delivery, and the proportions were the same in the two trial groups. Of the women who had resumed intercourse, 52% in the restrictive group and 51% in the liberal group had experienced dyspareunia at some time, and 22% and 18% respectively still had this problem three months post partum. There was no difference between the two groups in the extent to which babies were being wholly or partially breast fed at 10 days (70%) and three months (48%) after delivery. Nineteen per cent of women in both groups had involuntary loss of urine three months after delivery, and 6% sometimes needed to wear a vulval pad. This problem was more common in multiparas (22%) than primiparas (15%) but did not differ significantly between the two trial groups when compared within parity strata.

Table 17.5   'Worst pain in past week,' three months post partum. Figures are numbers of subjects (percentages in parentheses)

	Restrictive policy (n = 438)		Liberal policy (n = 457)	
Mild		20(4.6)		26(5.7)
Primiparas	13 (7.6)		15(7.4)	
Multiparas	7 (2.6)		11(4.3)	
Moderate		11(2.5)		8(1.8)
Primiparas	5 (2.9)		5(2.5)	
Multiparas	6 (2.3)		3(1.2)	
Severe		2(0.5)		1(0.2)
Primiparas	0		0	
Multiparas	2 (0.8)		1(0.4)	
Total		33(7.6)		35(7.7)
Primiparas	18(10.5)		20(9.9)	
Multiparas	15 (5.7)		15(5.9)	

χ^2 test = 2.58 (3 df); NS

Analyses stratified by status of the person who had actually conducted the delivery showed that the differential effects of the policies were little affected by the experience of the attendant. Analyses stratified by time interval between entry to the trial and delivery disclosed that, although trauma was less common in those women who delivered very soon after entry to the trial, the overall effects of the two policies were still evident in these cases.

Both women who sustained severe perineal trauma had painful constipation in the immediate puerperium. Three months later one was problem free but constipation still occasionally troubled the primipara, in whom the tear had extended into the rectal mucosa; she was also one of those who did not resume sexual intercourse within three months after delivery. When contacted again 21 months after delivery she described herself as back to normal apart from a ridge along the line of the repair to the vagina, which she noticed when she inserted a tampon during her periods. It had taken 18 months for sexual intercourse to become completely comfortable. Of those whose trauma had extended to the upper third of the vagina, the one woman in the liberal group had mild perineal pain and dyspareunia when contacted three months post partum, and one of the two women in the restrictive group had dyspareunia, for which she had sought medical advice. At 21 months both were 'back to normal.' This had taken 18 months in the first case and six months in the second.

DISCUSSION

This randomised controlled trial was designed to compare two policies[8] for managing the perineum in spontaneous vaginal deliveries as they would be used in everyday practice. The research was mounted in a busy district general hospital and the deliveries performed by those who normally conduct spontaneous vaginal deliveries in the hospital. The overall episiotomy rate in the unit before the trial was 61% (52% in spontaneous vaginal deliveries) and near the middle of the range for British maternity hospitals reported by M J House (personal communication). All the episiotomies were mediolateral, which, in contrast with other parts of the world,[2] is the standard in Britain.

Ninety three per cent of eligible women were successfully recruited to the trial, and the study population may be considered to be representative of all spontaneous vaginal deliveries in the hospital. Random allocation generated two groups of women who were similar in several important respects (Table 17.1) and who were delivered by people of comparable status, 94% of whom were midwives. Although it was not possible to blind all the participants in the trial to their treatment allocation because of a prior decision to tell those who wished to know, fewer than one in 10 requested this information. Thus most women did not know their treatment allocation when completing their questionnaires. The follow up rate (89% at both 10 days and three months after delivery) was high for this type of study, and there was no evidence that those lost to follow up differed between the two groups.

The aim of both policies was to minimise maternal trauma. The reasons for the tears in the liberal group ('prevent a tear') largely reflected this – 'expected to deliver intact' (56 cases); 'tear caused by shoulder' (25); 'delivered too quickly to perform episiotomy' (43). There was good compliance with the restrictive policy. There were 18 cases (3.6%) in this group in which an episiotomy was performed for reasons other than fetal distress – 'thick perineum' or 'previous episiotomy' (11 case); 'large baby' (three); 'to prevent a tear' (four).

The overall rate of severe maternal trauma was much lower than expected from other published studies. Nevertheless, the only justification from this study for recommending an episiotomy rate as high as 50% in normal deliveries is that there were more cases of 'severe maternal trauma' among women allocated to the restrictive policy. This difference may have reflected a real effect of the restrictive policy, but despite the fact that 1000 women were entered into this trial it is still possible that the difference was due to chance. Of the five women who sustained severe trauma, two were problem free by three months and three were problem free by 21 months.

Looking at the restrictive policy in another way, it is noteworthy that despite the fact that episiotomy was used in only one in 10 women, 69% nevertheless required suturing. Similarly high rates of spontaneous trauma have been reported in other studies in developed countries.[2] In a randomised controlled trial of a birth chair for delivery[9] the episiotomy rate among those delivered in the chair (20%) was lower than in the group delivered in the conventional dorsal position (43%). The spontaneous tear rate, however, was higher in the birth chair group (52% compared with 41%) and the overall trauma rates were 72% and 84% respectively. Lower spontaneous trauma rates have been reported from other settings, and this may reflect differences in other aspects of the management of pregnancy, labour, and delivery or wider differences in social behaviour such as lifetime squatting for defecation.

In our study, restricting the use of episiotomy to fetal indications resulted in neither an increase nor a major decrease in the problems experienced by mothers in the three months after delivery; the only difference observed was a tendency for women allocated to the restrictive episiotomy policy to resume sexual intercourse sooner. These results of an experiment controlling for selection bias are in striking contrast with the findings of studies based on comparisons using observational data,[2, 5, 6] all of which suggest that the discomfort after perineal tears is considerably less than after episiotomy.

The saving in medical staff time spent suturing associated with the restrictive policy was of the same order as the saving in midwifery time managing delivery associated with the liberal policy. The more restrictive policy did, however, result in savings in suture materials (and if our results are extrapolated to the whole of England and Wales adopting a restrictive policy would save an estimated £65,000 worth of suture materials a year). It is perhaps worth noting that the episiotomy rate in spontaneous vaginal deliveries at the Royal Berkshire Hospital is now only 20%.

As expected, multiparas had fewer episiotomies, fewer anterior tears, and more intact perineums than primiparas, but they also sustained more posterior tears. They were half as likely as primiparas to have pain 10 days and three months after delivery but more likely to suffer involuntary loss of urine. When the two perineal management policies were compared within parity groups, however, the patterns of the results closely resembled that of the unstratified analysis for the total trial population; in both parity strata the incidences of pain and involuntary loss of urine associated with the two perineal management policies were very similar.

A large proportion of women (19%) had involuntary loss of urine three months after delivery, but there is no evidence from this study that liberal use of episiotomy prevents this problem. It is still possible that it may prevent stress incontinence and vaginal prolapse in the longer term, however, and we therefore plan to contact the mothers again three years after delivery.

We thank the many midwives and obstetricians in the West Berkshire Health District who worked so hard to make this study a success; the mothers who responded so enthusiastically to our requests for information about their experiences; Ann Medd for clerical work; staff midwife Anastasia Smith for help with trial coordination; and Gill Gould and Lesley Mierh for typing the manuscripts. Jennifer Sleep was Maws midwifery scholar for 1982. Additional funding for this project came from the Oxford Regional Health Authority. The National Perinatal Epidemiology Unit is supported by a grant from the Department of Health and Social Security.

NOTES

* *British Medical Journal* 289 (8): 587–590. Reprinted with permission of the BMJ Publishing Group.
  1 Russell, JK. Episiotomy. *Br Med J* 1982; 284:220.
  2 Thacker SE, Banta HD. Benefits and risks of episiotomy: an interpretative review of the English language literature, 1860–1980. *Obstet Gynecol Surv* 1983; 38:322–38.
  3 Donald I. *Practical obstetric problems*. London: Lloyd-Luke, 1979:817.

4 Flood C. The real reasons for performing episiotomies. *World Medicine*. 1982: Feb 6: 51.

5 House MJ. To do or not to do episiotomy. In: Kitzinger S, ed. *Episiotomy – physical and emotional aspects*. London: National Childbirth Trust, 1981:6–12.

6 Kitzinger S, Walters R. *Some women's experiences of episiotomy*. London: National Childbirth Trust, 1981.

7 Zander L. Episiotomy: has familiarity bred contempt? *J R Coll Gen Pract* 1982; 32:400–1.

8 Sinclair JC, Torrance GW, Boyle MH, Horwood S, Saigal S, Sackett DL. Evaluation of neonatal intensive care programs. *N Engl J Med* 1981; 305:480–94.

9 Stewart P, Hillan E, Calder AA. A randomised trial to evaluate the use of a birth chair for delivery. *Lancet* 1983; i:1296–8.

Chapter 18

Lower Medicare mortality among a set of hospitals known for good nursing care

LINDA H. AIKEN, HERBERT L. SMITH, EILEEN T. LAKE

Introduction

Demonstrating that nurses have a measurable impact on patient outcomes, an impact that can be untangled from all the other myriad and interdependent influences on patient welfare in any stay in hospital, has been, for many involved in nursing research, something of a Holy Grail. If successfully shown, the result could be increased confidence among the profession, increased recognition – and increased industrial and political bargaining power. This paper by Linda Aiken from the University of Pennsylvania, comes as close as anything to such a demonstration.

In the 1980s, the American Academy of Nursing set out to identify those US hospitals which had reputations among nurses as being good places to practice. Having been nominated by a panel of experts because of this reputation and because of their ability to recruit and retain staff, sometimes in the face of local competition, 155 hospitals agreed to provide further data to corroborate these anecdotes. The study, carried out originally in 1982, and repeated twice in that decade, identified 41 such 'magnet' hospitals, magnetic because of their tendency to attract good-quality staff. Among their key characteristics were a particular autonomy in practice and decision-making reported by nurses, good relationships with medical staff and nurse representation at high levels in these organisations. The authors of this paper note that these organisational characteristics are closely related to those said to distinguish successful major companies in other sectors.

Linda Aiken and colleagues pose the question, that must have been in the minds of many at the time, 'do these advantages for nurses, produce, in some complex way, discernibly better patient outcomes?' The paper we reproduce here would answer 'yes': magnet hospitals appear to be saving up to 9 deaths per 1000 public patients compared with similar control hospitals.

The major challenge in approaching this question is a methodological one. Trying to isolate and quantify the effect of any single variable on the final outcome of any health care episode is not to be attempted by the faint-hearted. For one thing, hospital data is notoriously inaccurate and incomplete, and needs to be handled with caution. Secondly, a large number of influences, both those related to patients and those related to the care settings and personnel, have an effect on outcome, and there are likely to be far more influences than we are aware of and can 'control for' in any analysis. Nevertheless, Aiken and colleagues approach the issue with considerable sophistication and are aided by administrative datasets that are of higher quality than those available within the UK – though even here there are variations across borders, notably between the richer coding systems available in Scotland compared with the more spartan systems in England. They matched each magnet hospital with five control hospitals, each with some similar characteristics, and compared the average mortality of the 39 magnet hospitals with the 195 controls. In their comparison, every other possible influence on patient mortality, such as the presence of multiple illnesses among the patients, or the level of qualification of medical staff needed to be taken into account. The authors found that, after such controlling, magnet hospitals did appear to produce better mortality rates among Medicare patients. The authors acknowledge that some as yet undisclosed force may have caused such a difference and that the actual causal processes of this better outcome are unknown; nevertheless, their study does have a certain common-sense appeal and a plausible hypothesis: nurses make up the largest clinical group in most health care settings and, unlike almost any other health care profession, have the opportunity for almost continuous surveillance of patients. Their own confidence, skill level and authority to make decisions would seem bound to affect, for example, how promptly complications are noted and acted upon.

Aiken and colleagues believe that the attributes of magnet hospitals can be replicated and transferred to other settings, with the possibility of improving patient outcomes – and nurse job satisfaction in the process. As we write this, a similar study is being conducted across five countries: the USA, Canada, England, Scotland and Germany. The progress of the research is being watched closely by nursing bodies because the findings, as we noted at the beginning, could be of considerable significance.

AIKEN, L., H. SMITH AND E. LAKE (1994)

Lower Medicare mortality among a set of hospitals known for good nursing care*

In this study we find that *magnet hospitals*, hospitals that embody a set of organisational attributes that nurses find desirable (and that are conducive to better patient care), have lower mortality than matched hospitals, which are similar along other organisational dimensions, but that are not known as settings that place a high institutional priority on nursing. Those familiar with the inner workings of hospitals will not be surprised there is a relationship between the practice of nursing and the mortality experience of hospital patients.[1-3] The connection between nursing and mortality rates dates as far back as the reforms in British hospitals made under Florence Nightingale during the Crimean War.[4]

Nurses are the only professional caregivers in hospitals who are at the bedside of hospital patients around the clock. What nurses do – or not do (or in some circumstances are not allowed to do) – is directly related to a variety of patient outcomes, including in-hospital deaths.[5] American physicians typically combine office and hospital-based practice, and therefore observe their hospitalised patients only periodically. Nurses are physicians' primary source of information about changes in their patients' conditions. Nurses often must act in the absence of the physician when timely intervention is required.[6] As hospital care has become increasingly complex, the exercise of professional judgment by nurses is ever more important in preventing adverse and sometimes catastrophic events.[7]

The modern hospital has been described as having two lines of authority, medicine and administration.[8] Nurses have traditionally been subordinate to both, even though they have the most direct knowledge and understanding of patient care requirements by virtue of their constant contact with patients. Lewis Thomas[9] has described nurses in contemporary hospitals as the 'glue' that keeps the highly specialised, often fragmented system of hospital care together. The potential for using nursing to improve patient outcomes is apparent in the multihospital study of variation in intensive care death rates, by Knaus and associates,[10] in which patterns of communication between nurses and physicians were the single most significant factor associated with excess mortality – more important, for example, than whether the unit had a medical director, or whether it was in a teaching hospital. Yet contemporary hospital nursing practice is most often characterised by a lack of professional autonomy, poor control over the practice setting, and inadequate provision for routine communication with physicians about crucial clinical decisions. All of these compromise the ability of nurses to exercise their professional judgment on behalf of the well-being of their patients.[8]

The degree to which hospitals empower nurses to use their professional nursing skills in a timely manner during in-patient hospital care varies. Certain forms of hospital organisation and institutional culture, ranging from unit-level specialisation (e.g., dedicated AIDS units) to the implementation of hospital-wide professional nursing practice models, do indeed result in more autonomy, control, and status for nurses.[11] We conjecture that hospitals that facilitate professional autonomy, control over practice, and comparatively good relations between nurses and physicians will be ones in which nurses are able to exercise their professional judgment on a more routine basis, with positive implications for the quality and outcomes of patient care.

In this paper we show that a group of hospitals characterised by nurses as being good places to work also achieved better patient outcomes as reflected by lower mortality. Although we cannot document the entire causal chain by which nurses affect mortality, we do review studies showing that the hospitals in which nurses prefer to work have distinct organisational features. The study provides new evidence that these features are more professional autonomy, greater control over practice environment, and better relationships with physicians. We were able to demonstrate that the superior mortality experience in the study hospitals cannot be attributed to either differential patient characteristics or other organisational features not related to nursing, but previously shown to be associated with differential hospital mortality. The proportion of physicians who are board certified, whether the hospital is a teaching facility, type of ownership, financial status, are examples of such findings.

REVIEW OF PREVIOUS STUDIES

The literature on the organisation of hospital nursing and variation in hospital mortality have developed independently of one another for the most part. Research on the organisation of nursing care primarily has been motivated by debates over the causes and potential solutions to hospital nursing shortages. The focus has been on determining how hospital work environments could be restructured to make them more desirable places for professional nurses to practice.[12–18] The dominant outcome variables studied have been nurse satisfaction, job turnover, and hospital nurse vacancy rates. Far less attention has been given to the relationship between nursing organisation and patient outcomes.

Conversely, the large literature on variations in mortality across hospitals[19–25] has concentrated on methodological issues and the association between the institutional and organisational characteristics of hospitals and their in-patient mortality. The methodological focus of the research primarily is on how to separate components of variation due to severity of illness and other characteristics of patients, from manipulable dimensions of hospital organisation. Development of measures to stage severity of illness had advanced considerably; measures of organisational dimensions have lagged by comparison.[10, 26, 27]

When institutional attributes or characteristics are the focus of hospital mortality studies, a large number of organisational correlates are examined, which sometimes includes nursing.[20, 28–33] Board certification of physicians has been found uniformly to be associated with better quality of hospital care and lower mortality.[29, 31, 34–36] The teaching status of hospitals is another variable of frequent interest. The referral patterns characteristic of such hospitals may result in a more severely ill patient population and higher mortality than at nonteaching hospitals.[37] Conversely, teaching hospital status may denote a better qualified staff, greater technological sophistication, etc., and thus be expected to yield better outcomes.[29, 38] As would be expected from such competing hypotheses, findings are inconsistent across studies, some documenting more adverse outcomes, some less and some showing no difference at teaching hospitals.[33] The ambiguity of both findings and interpretation can also be found concerning other postulated or observed correlates of mortality, including ownership, size, financial status, and urban vs. rural location.[30–35, 38]

The nursing variable in multivariate hospital mortality studies, usually registered nurse (RN) to patient ratios or RNs as a percentage of total nursing personnel, is usually found to be a significant correlate of mortality. Little substantive or analytic consideration is given to this association, which is variously interpreted as representing the effect of 'clinical skill level'[30, 31] or 'service intensity.'[32]

MAGNET HOSPITALS

Hospitals do differ from one another in their quality of nursing care. This is an important dimension of a hospital's reputation.[2, 3] Rather than undertaking a large, detailed, national study of the mortality experience of hospitals known for good nursing care, we are capitalising on the existence of a set of studies of several dozen hospitals that have been singled out as hospitals known for good nursing care for reasons other than the study of patient outcomes.

Among experts on nursing, there is general agreement on the attributes of a good nursing service.[16, 39, 40] In the early 1980s, the American Academy of Nursing (AAN) set about the task of identifying a set of hospitals with reputations as being good places in which to practice nursing.[16] These hospitals were not identified by low mortality rate, nor were they selected according to any overt organisational features. Rather, the intent of the original study was to demonstrate that hospitals differed from one another with respect to their attractiveness to nurses, and that attractive hospitals were better able to maintain low rates of nursing turnover and vacancy, which led to their eventual designation as *magnet* hospitals.

The magnet hospitals were identified in the original study as follows:[16] six AAN hospital nursing experts in each of eight regions of the country who were selected to nominate 6 to 10 hospitals that met the following three criteria: 1) nurses consider the hospital a good place to practice nursing; 2) the hospital has the ability to recruit and retain professional nurses, as evidenced by a relatively low turnover rate; and 3) the hospital is located in an area where it will have competition for staff from other institutions and agencies. A total of 165 hospitals were nominated; 155 agreed to participate in the study. Each participating hospital provided information on a range of nursing-related issues including nurse vacancy, turnover, and absentee rates; the ratio of inexperienced to experienced nurses; use of supplemental staffing agencies; nurse staffing policies, educational preparation of nurses in leadership positions; and the predominant mode of nurse organisation on the units (i.e., primary, team, functional, or other). Hospitals were then ranked according to evidence of being able to attract and retain professional nurses and to create an environment conducive to good nursing care. The top-ranked 41 institutions were subjected to a subsequent round of data collection involving interviews with staff nurses and directors of nursing. These were the hospitals that ultimately came to be designated as magnet hospitals.

The in-patient mortality rates of the hospitals were *not* considered. At that time comparative, standardised hospital rates probably were not available to either institutions or the AAN panellists. Moreover, important as they may be in the aggregate, the magnitude of mortality differences that exist among hospitals is comparatively small, and difficult for even a well-qualified observer to discern at the scene, especially when measured against a backdrop of stochastic fluctuation over time. When we subsequently compare the mortality rates of magnet hospitals with nonmagnet hospitals, we are reasonably confident that the distinction between hospital types pertains to features of the organisation of nursing, and is not in itself, another measure of hospital mortality.

The process by which these hospitals were selected does not necessarily guarantee that magnet hospitals include *all* hospitals that might meet the original specified criteria. However, the selection process appears to have been sufficiently stringent as to lead us to expect that the 41 magnet hospitals would share some common characteristics with respect to nursing that would differentiate them from the vast majority of American hospitals.

The nurses practicing in the designated magnet hospitals cited the following organisational attributes as important in making their hospitals good places to work:[15, 41–44] 1) the importance and status of nurses in the organisation as reflected in the formal organisational structure of nursing and its relationship to the organisation of the hospital, i.e., a flat organisation of the nursing department with few supervisors, and a chief nurse executive with a strong position in the bureaucratic hierarchy of the hospital; 2) nurse autonomy to make clinical decisions within their areas of competence, and to control their own practice; 3) control over the practice environment, including decentralised decision-making at the unit level, adequate staffing, a limit to the proportion of nurses who were new graduates, and established mechanisms to facilitate communication between nurses and physicians; 4) organisation of nurses' clinical responsibilities at the unit level to promote accountability and less use of 'floating' of nurses to equalise staffing across units; and 5) an established culture signifying nursing's importance in the overall mission of the institution, as reflected in salaried practice (compared to hourly wages), institutional investment in nurses' continuing education, and supervisory personnel who support nurses' decision-making responsibilities.

The original study of these hospitals was conducted in 1982.[16] A follow-up study was conducted in a geographically stratified sub-sample of the magnet hospitals in 1986,[41, 42] and again in 1989.[43, 44] At each point, the magnet hospitals were found to have maintained their ability to attract and recruit nurses, and to have retained the organisational features found in the initial study.

The organisational dimensions found to be common among the magnet hospitals are similar to those associated with lower mortality in the few previous studies on the topic, i.e., decentralised decision-making at the nursing unit level, ward specialisation, standardisation of nursing procedures, qualifications of nurses, and good relations with physicians.[10, 28, 35] What is not clear from these earlier studies is how or why these particular organisational dimensions of hospitals would be likely to affect what nurses do. Our contention is that they result in enhanced intra-organisational status for nurses that provides a level of professional autonomy and control that enables nurses to put into action what they know and can do for patients. We viewed the magnet hospitals, which are clearly at one end of the scale on which the organisation of nursing can be evaluated, as representing an opportunity to test whether there is any payoff in terms of reduced hospital mortality.

ENHANCED AUTONOMY, CONTROL, AND STATUS IN MAGNET HOSPITALS

Before tackling our primary question, we briefly explore whether the broad organisational features observed in magnet hospitals do in fact enhance the autonomy, control, and status of nurses within these hospitals. Our argument is that hospitals known to be good places for nurses to work have this reputation in part because of an organisational orientation that permits nurses to practice in an environment in which their authority is closer to their traditionally high level of responsibility. This should enhance the outcomes of patients. However, without a demonstration that autonomy, control over practice, and status of nurses are greater in the magnet hospitals, any finding of lower mortality in these hospitals is subject to skepticism, for want of an operant mechanism.

Evidence in support of the proposition that the magnet hospitals are characterised by greater nurse autonomy and control, and better relations with physicians, can be found in Table 18.1, which summarises the reports of nurses concerning the presence of various job characteristics at 25 hospitals, including 17 magnet hospitals, from two different studies. The first study is by Kramer and Hafner,[41] and involves a geographically stratified sub-sample of 16 of the original 41 magnet hospitals. Kramer generously provided to us a unit-record data tape from this study, without which the following comparison would have been impossible. The second study is by the present authors,[11] and involves a geographically stratified set of hospitals selected originally to serve as controls in a study of hospitals with specialised AIDS units. Coincidentally, it also includes two magnet hospitals from the original AAN study,[16] one of which is among the 16 magnet hospitals studied by Kramer and Hafner.[41]

In both studies, nurses at these hospitals were asked to evaluate a battery of items (the Nursing Work Index). Each nurse was asked to indicate, for each item, their agreement with the statement, 'This is present in my current job situation.' Response options were 'strongly agree,' 'somewhat agree,' 'somewhat disagree,' and 'strongly disagree.' We scored these responses, respectively, 4, 3, 2, and 1. These items included six that measured nurse autonomy, seven that measured control over the practice setting, and two that measured nurses' relations with physicians. Responses were summed across respondents to create scales, the average values of which are found, by study and hospital type, in Table 18.1.

There are two important aspects to Table 18.1. First, the magnet hospitals studied by Kramer and Hafner[41] were evaluated by the nurses in them as being significantly higher in autonomy, control, and good relations of nurses with physicians than were the eight nonmagnet hospitals for which we have comparable data. Second, this is more likely a real difference between magnet and nonmagnet hospitals than it is an artifact of different studies carried out by different researchers. The two magnet hospitals in our later study have scale scores across the three dimensions of nurse status and autonomy that are very similar to the scale scores as obtained by Kramer and Hafner several years earlier at the 16 magnet hospitals that they studied.

We conclude that the features of the hospital's reputation that are responsible for their designation as magnet hospitals proxy for organisational distinctiveness with respect to nurse autonomy, nurse control over practice, and the relations of nurses with physicians, which are all factors that should be positively related to the quality of patient care and, hence, mortality. With this as backdrop, we turn now to the question of whether magnet hospitals do indeed have lower mortality than hospitals with similar structural features, except for the organisational facilitation of professional nursing practice.

Table 18.1   A comparison of the presence of autonomy, control, and relations with physicians, as assessed by nurses, for magnet and other hospitals, from two studies

| Study | Hospital type | Number of hospitals | Number of nurses[a] | Means (and standard deviations) for scales[b] measuring the assessed presence of: | | |
				Autonomy	Control	Relations with physicians
Kramer and Hafner[41]	Magnet	16	1609	20.71 (2.08)	22.34 (2.49)	6.97 (0.91)
Aiken and Smith[11]	Magnet	2	141	20.89[c] (2.52)	23.19[c] (2.89)	6.62[c] (1.23)
	Other	8	277	17.48[d] (3.91)	17.87[d] (4.44)	5.83[d] (1.32)

[a]   Average; actual number responding may vary slightly from scale to scale.

[b]   The Autonomy scale has six items (*e.g.* 'Freedom to make important patient care and work decisions'), the Control scale has seven items (*e.g.* 'Enough time and opportunity to discuss patient care problems with other nurses'), and the Relations and Physicians scale has two items (*e.g.*, 'Physicians and nurses have good relationships'). For each item, nurses were asked to indicate the extent of their agreement that the statement is reflective of their current job situation. Item responses were 'strongly agree,' 'somewhat agree,' 'somewhat disagree,' and 'strongly disagree,' and were scored, respectively, 4, 3, 2, 1.

[c]   Does *not* differ significantly (*i.e.* P>.10) from the corresponding scale mean in the 16 magnet hospitals studied by Kramer and Hafner.[41]

[d]   Is significantly less than the corresponding scale mean in the magnet hospitals (P<.0001).

DATA AND METHODS

Our analysis of the mortality experience of Medicare patients at the magnet hospitals is based on a comparison of these hospitals with a set of hospitals not known for good nursing care, but comparable with respect to other factors thought to be correlated with hospital mortality. The 195 control hospitals, five for each magnet hospital, were selected by a multivariate matching procedure. The pool of hospitals from which these control hospitals were selected, and the method by which they were selected, are described in the following two subsections.

Magnet hospitals versus potential control hospitals

The original set of magnet hospitals was identified in 1982[16] and reexamined in 1986[41, 42] and 1989.[43, 44] Our response variable is the 1988 mortality rate (death within 30 days of admission) among hospitalised Medicare beneficiaries, as reported in the Health Care Financing Administration (HCFA) Medicare hospital mortality rate file.[45] Thirty-nine of the original 41 magnet hospitals could be found in this file; one hospital had closed, and one has a Veterans Administration hospital, which had no Medicare hospitalisations.

Potential control hospitals were sought among the 5,053 'nonmagnet' hospitals in the HCFA Medicare mortality rate file that had at least 100 Medicare discharges (because annual mortality rates are otherwise highly unreliable) and could be linked to the 1988 American Hospital Association (AHA) annual survey of hospitals.[46] The AHA annual survey of hospitals provides the most comprehensive data available on hospital organisational structure, facilities and services, beds and utilisation, finance, personnel by occupational category, medical staff, and other hospital characteristics. We compare magnet hospitals with other hospitals along a variety of dimensions; and then use these organisational characteristics to construct a matched sample of control hospitals.

The 39 magnet hospitals have lower mortality rates than the other hospitals, on the order of 20 fewer Medicare deaths per 1,000 discharges; see Variable No. 17, Table 18.2. Magnet hospitals also differ from other hospitals on a variety of organisational characteristics (Variable Nos. 1–10) that have been found to be correlated with mortality, including type of ownership (public, private non-profit, or private for-profit), teaching status (membership in the Council of Teaching Hospitals), hospital size (average daily census, total hospital beds, and volume of Medicare discharges), financial status (total hospital payroll and occupancy rate), physician credentials (the proportion of board-certified physicians on staff), resources for patient care (payroll-to-hospital-beds ratio), and technological sophistication (high technology index score).[31, 32] Magnet hospitals have significantly fewer emergency visits per average daily census (Variable No. 11). Because Medicare patients are a disproportionately small component of emergency admittances, like all of the other control variables discussed so far this variable is better conceptualised as an organisational feature of the hospital than as characteristic of the patient mix. Finally, magnet hospitals are more likely than other hospitals to be in large metropolitan areas (Variable No. 12).

There are two other dimensions on which magnet hospitals differ from other hospitals in the sample: first, they employ more registered nurses (RNs), both relative to patients (RNs/ADC) and as a proportion of all nurses (RNs/total nursing personnel); see Variable Nos. 14 and 15 in Table 18.2. Thus magnet hospitals do differ from other hospitals along the nursing organisation dimension typically operationalised in multivariate studies of differential hospital mortality.

Second, magnet hospitals have lower rates of *predicted* mortality, by a factor of 10 per 1,000 (Variable No. 16). Predicted hospital mortality rates are based on the following patient characteristics: age, sex, the presence of four comorbidities (cancer, cardiovascular disease, liver disease, and renal disease), the type and source of admission, and the presence and risk of hospitalisations within the previous 6 months. Predicted mortality is thus a proxy for patient composition. Inter-organisational variability in mortality reflects in large part differences in patient populations, with respect to both morbidity (case mix) and demographic status.[47, 48]

Construction of a matched control sample

To control for organisational differences between hospitals, we employed matching[49–51], a traditional form of adjusting for confounding variables in observational data. By analogy with experimentation, we have a key treatment – those aspects of hospital nursing organisation embodied in the 'magnet hospital' rubric – whose effects we seek to measure. Case-by-case matching across multiple dimensions is impracticable, and limited theory makes it difficult to specify a small, tractable number of important factors for which control is essential. Fortunately, recent developments in multivariate matched sampling[52] simplify the task, and allow us to control for all of the hospital characteristics in the first panel of Table 18.2 (Variables Nos. 1–12), without matching each case on each of 12 characteristics. Matching has been shown to be a robust method for reducing bias due to observed covariates[53, 54], and is intuitively easy to understand.[52] The matching procedure worked as follows:

Propensity scores

For the entire sample, a dichotomous variable (coded 1 if the hospital was a magnet hospital and 0 otherwise) was (logistically) regressed on the 12 organisational characteristics in the top panel of Table 18.2.[52] The resultant discriminant function was used to obtain, for each hospital in the sample a predicted logit (log-odds on being a magnet hospital). This predicted logit is the propensity score.

Most of the discrimination (matching) is effected by five variables: the average daily census, the occupancy rate, the number of hospital beds, the metropolitan statistical area size, and the high-technology index score. The discriminant function is not well specified from the standpoint of hypothesis testing, first because the number of predictor variables (12) is high relative to the number of hospitals being discriminated (39); second, because there is high collinearity among several of the predictor variables. However, the goals of this function are prediction (discrimination) and data reduction (creating a matching variable that is a linear combination of the original 12 control variables). Redundancy and collinearity are of little account; and, as a prediction/classification model, the estimated function works quite well: 1) the area under the receiver operating characteristic curve[55] (.904) is high; 2) at a predicted positive classification probability close to the (low) proportion of magnet hospitals in the sample (i.e., =.01), both sensitivity (percentage of magnet hospitals classified correctly) and specificity (percentage of non-magnet hospitals classified correctly) are in excess of 80%; and 3) for fairly 'thick' partitions of the predicted-probability-ordered data (e.g., 10 groups of =500 hospitals) the Hosmer-Lemeshow[56] goodness-of-fit X^2 is low and nonsignificant $X^2 = 4.05$, 8 DF, $P>.85$), strongly suggesting the classification model *not* be rejected.

Random order, nearest available pair-matching

A set of random numbers was generated, one for each of the 39 magnet hospitals.[57] Beginning with the lowest random number, and proceeding in random-number size order, each magnet hospital was matched with the non-magnet hospital in the sample with the nearest propensity score.[58] That control hospital, or 'match,' was then removed from the sample, so that no hospital served as the control for more than one magnet hospital.

Table 18.2 Characteristics of the study hospitals

Variable number	Characteristics	Magnet hospitals (n = 39)	Potential control hospitals (n = 5,053)	Matched control hospitals				
				1st (n = 39)	2nd (n = 39)	3rd (n = 39)	4th (n = 39)	5th (n = 39)
1	Ownership – percent							
	Public	7.7	28.2 [a]	2.6	12.8	0.0	5.1	10.3
	Private for-profit	7.7	14.2	18.0	5.1	12.8	12.8	2.6
	Private not-for-profit	84.6	57.7 [a]	79.5	82.1	87.2	82.1	87.2
2	Member – Council of teaching hospitals (%)	28.2	5.8 [a]	23.1	33.3	30.8	30.8	28.2
	Hospital size							
3	Average daily census (ADC)	305.5±148.9	112.0±137.6 [a]	326.2	323.5	294.1	274.6	302.9
4	Hospital beds	412.6±180.4	160.6±167.4 [a]	444.9	452.4	399.9	372.9	407.7
5	Medicare discharges	5,006±2,229	1,873±1,927 [a]	5,357	5,227	4,877	4,915	5,306
	Financial status							
6	Payroll (million dollars)	46.7±29.5	13.3±20.4 [a]	45.1	49.6	42.3	45.6	45.1
7	Occupancy rate	0.722±0.115	0.556±0.190 [a]	0.720	0.697	0.707	0.712	0.737
8	Board-certified physicians/all physicians	0.756±0.086	0.661±0.194 [a]	0.759	0.749	0.741	0.774	0.743
9	Payroll expense/hospital bed (1,000 dollars)	109±35	64±35 [a]	95 [b]	105	100	110	108
10	High-technology index score [c]	2.57±1.68	0.59±1.12 [d]	2.68	2.75	2.74	2.68	2.36
11	No. of emergency visits/ADC	117.7±69.6	181.6±144.4 [a]	121.9	127.0	96.4	127.2	129.8
12	Metropolitan statistical area size [d]	4.49±1.254	2.14±2.296 [a]	4.26	4.44	4.54	4.33	4.51
13	Propensity score	3.530±1.142	6.589±1.956 [a]	3.531	3.532	3.533	3.525	3.523

Table 18.2 (Continued)

Variable number	Characteristics	Magnet hospitals (n = 39)	Potential control hospitals (n = 5,053)	Matched control hospitals				
				1st (n = 39)	2nd (n = 39)	3rd (n = 39)	4th (n = 39)	5th (n = 39)
14	RNs/ADC	1.569±0.556	1.216±0.704[a]	1.471	1.503	1.329[b]	1.454	1.424
15	RNs/total nursing personnel	0.760±0.130	0.581±0.149[a]	0.692[b]	0.690[b]	0.682[a]	0.708[b]	0.671[a]
16	Predicted mortality	0.113±0.016	0.123±0.024[a]	0.117	0.114	0.117	0.115	0.119
17	Mortality rate	0.105±0.021	0.126±0.035[a]	0.117[b]	0.109	0.117[b]	0.111	0.006[b]

Notes: Plus-minus values are means ± standard deviation

[a] $P < .01$.

[b] $P < .05$.

[c] The High-technology index score ranges from zero to five based on the presence or absence of the following items: a cardiac-catheterisation laboratory, an extracorporeal lithotripter, a facility for magnetic resonance imaging, a facility for open-heart surgery, and organ transplantation capability.

[d] Metropolitan statistical area size is an ordinal variable with values ranging from 0 to 6 corresponding to the following Census Bureau MSA population size categories: 0 = non-metropolitan area – areas with no city with a population of 50,000 or more nor a total population of 100,000 or more; 1 = Under 100,000; 2 = 100,000 to 250,000; 3 = 250,000 to 500,000; 4 = 500,000 to 1,000,000; 6 = over 2,500,000.

Multiple controls per case

Random order, nearest available pair-matching was repeated four more times, until each magnet hospital was matched with five unique control hospitals. Variances for matched differences decline by a factor of two as the number of matched controls per treatment observation increases from one to infinity, with most of the increases in efficiency occurring in the first two to five matches. Conversely, bias *increases* with number of matches because of inappropriate matches.[59] Our analysis of these data shows that after the fifth or sixth match, bias increases dramatically. Compensating for such bias would involve proper specification of a large regression; it is to avoid this that we have limited our control to 195 (39 magnet hospitals × 5 matches per hospital) of the 5,053 potential control hospitals.

Results of the matching procedure can be described with reference to the final five columns of Table 18.2. In only one out of 60 cases (12 variables 5 matches per hospital) does a control variable in the discriminant function have a mean (or proportion) that differs significantly ($P<.05$) from the magnet hospital sample (payroll expense/hospital bed, for the first set of matches). The propensity scores (Variable No. 13), which are linear combinations of the control variables in the discriminant function, are virtually the same for magnet hospitals and matched control hospitals; there is thus no evidence that the quality of match degrades from the first to the fifth matching cycle.

Even after matching on numerous organisational characteristics, magnet hospitals clearly employ more registered nurses as a percentage of total nursing personnel (Variable No. 15; this was *not* a predictor in the discriminant function) than do their matched controls. Matching on organisational characteristics does, however, reduce differences between hospitals in patient characteristics affecting mortality. Predicted mortality rates are uniformly lower among matched control hospitals than in the potential population of controls, and in none of the five match sets is this predicted mortality significantly in excess of predicted mortality in the magnet hospital sample (Variable No. 16; also *not* a predictor in the discriminant function).

Table 18.2 shows that after equating hospitals with respect to numerous organisational features, matched hospitals still have mortality rates in excess of those in magnet hospitals, by approximately between four and 12 deaths per 1,000 (Variable No. 17). However, the precision of this estimated effect is unclear, because in only three of the five sets of matches is the difference statistically significant. In the next section, we provide results from a model that pools information on the five matches per case (magnet hospital), as well as adjusts for uncontrolled differences in patient composition (i.e., predicted mortality). We also test whether any remaining effect can be accounted for by standard organisational measures of nursing (e.g., RNs as a proportion of total nursing personnel).

RESULTS

The matching procedures previously described result in five comparison hospitals for each of our 39 magnet hospitals. In concept, our analysis is simple. We compare the average mortality of the 39 magnet hospitals with those of the 195 ($= 5 \times 39$) comparison (control) hospitals. In practice, the analysis is somewhat more complex, because having multiple controls (matches) for each magnet hospital allows us to examine whether the mortality differences between magnet and nonmagnet hospitals varies across the set of magnet hospitals. Thus, we have embedded familiar t-tests for paired comparisons in the framework of the random-effects analysis-of-variance (ANOVA). We do this by conceptualising each difference between a magnet hospital and a matched control hospital as attributable to 1) the 'general' effect of magnet hospitals on mortality; 2) an effect that is specific to a particular magnet hospital; and 3) chance error. An advantage of this general model is that it is easily extended to include control variables, such as predicted mortality (as a function of patient composition). Because the details of the statistical model will not be of interest to all readers, we have consigned them to an Appendix. Here we restrict ourselves to specific results.

The first row of Table 18.3 gives the basic ANOVA estimates (Model I). The estimate of $-.0087$ corresponds to a reduction of approximately nine deaths per 1,000 Medicare admissions. With hospital death rate averages in the order of 113 per 1,000 in the study sample, this is equivalent to an estimated 7.7% diminution in mortality.

Table 18.3 also contains estimates of the variation in mortality differences between magnet hospitals and matched control hospitals in its final two columns. There are significant differences between magnet hospitals regarding their effects on mortality, as indicated by the high level of variance between blocks of matched hospitals. This means that the average mortality reduction, of nine deaths per 1,000 Medicare admissions, blends substantial differences in effects, across magnet hospitals. Having multiple matches per magnet hospital allows us to estimate these hospital-specific effects with moderately good precision. The reliability of the estimated mortality reduction effect for specific hospitals is 0.75.

As previously detailed, hospitals appear well-matched with respect to a variety of organisational characteristics, such as size, and ownership, found by some previous studies to be related to mortality. However, as revealed in Table 18.2, the predicted mortality of magnet hospitals is somewhat lower than that of matched controls. The estimated mortality differences under Model I might reflect differences in patient composition, as measured by their functional composite, predicted mortality. Thus, in Model II of Table 18.3, we control for differences between magnet hospitals and matched control hospitals in predicted mortality. Some, but not all, of the observed mortality difference is attributable to differences in patient characteristics, as the estimate of the general magnet hospital effect on mortality shrinks from $-.0087$ to $-.0052$. The 95% confidence interval for the effect of magnet hospitals on mortality, with adjustment for hospital-specific predicted mortality, is from 0.9 to 9.4 fewer deaths per 1,000.

Controlling for differences in patient composition (i.e., predicted mortality) also substantially attenuates differences between magnet hospitals in their effect on observed mortality. A comparison, between Models I and II, of the estimated variance in effects between blocks of matched hospitals reveals that over half the original variability in estimates of mortality reduction across magnet hospitals is attributable to not having controlled for differences between hospitals in patient characteristics.

Table 18.3 Estimated parameters for three models of hospital mortality

Model	Control for predicted mortality?	Response variable	Fixed effects			Variances	
			Mean difference between magnet hospitals and matched controls γ_{00}	Between-block progression of predicted mortality difference on observed mortality differences γ_{01}	Within-block regression of predicted mortality differences on observed mortality differences γ_{10}	Between blocks of matched hospitals τ_{00}	Within blocks of matched hospitals σ^2
I	No	Mortality difference between magnet hospital and matched control hospital	−.0087 (.0032) P = .011			.00029 (χ^2 = 154) P < .001	.00048
II	Yes	Mortality difference between magnet and matched control hospital	−.0052 (.0022) P = .026	0.93 (.133) P <.001	1.01 (.074) P<.001	.00013 (χ^2 = 145) P<.001	.00022
III	Yes	Natural logarithm of the ratio of excess (observed over predicted) mortality in magnet versus control hospitals	.048 (.021) P = .034			.0139 (χ^2 = 197) P<.001	.0167

Note: 'Blocks' are a magnet hospital and its five matched control hospitals. There are 39 blocks in the analysis. For fixed effects, estimated standard errors are in parentheses. For variance components, estimated χ^2 statistics are in parentheses.

Similar results are obtained when we adjust for predicted mortality not as a covariate, but as the denominator in a measure of excess mortality (i.e., the ratio of observed to expected mortality). This is Model III, the final line of Table 18.3. In this formulation, the estimated effect of −.048 corresponds to 4.8% less excess mortality in the magnet hospitals. There is still significant variance across magnet hospitals in the extent to which their mortality differs from that of their matched controls. Excess mortality across magnet hospitals is well-measured. The reliability of estimates of hospital-specific excess mortality, under Model III, is .81.

DISCUSSION

The magnet hospitals were selected on the basis of their reputations, not on objective evidence of the presence of a unique set of organisational attributes. Their common organisational dimensions were only identified subsequently. The estimated effects on mortality might not be the same as would be found were we to: 1) enumerate the important organisational characteristics; 2) seek to identify hospitals on the basis of objective measures of those characteristics; and 3) compare them to hospitals without such characteristics. We do not know the extent to which our matched comparison hospitals share those organisational features of nursing that we have deemed conducive to lower mortality, because the only information available on the matched comparison hospitals is macro-level hospital characteristics from the AHA annual survey. However, to the extent that the control hospitals do share these characteristics, our estimates are conservative with respect to their effects on mortality.

One thing we can do to clarify these issues is to examine nursing skill mix (RNs as a percentage of total nursing personnel) in magnet and matched nonmagnet hospitals. The mix of nursing personnel is one of the distinguishing characteristics of magnet hospitals and a variable on which information is available on matched hospitals. Additionally, higher ratios of registered nurses to other nursing personnel have been associated with lower hospital mortality in other studies,[31, 35] raising the possibility that this is the major explanation for lower mortality in magnet hospitals. As noted in Table 18.2, magnet hospitals do have significantly higher ratios of RNs to total nursing personnel and slightly higher nurse to patient ratios. This provides some evidence that nonmagnet hospitals do indeed differ from magnet hospitals in nursing organisational features that comprise the 'intervention' in our quasi-experimental study design.

To test whether this particular variable provides the full explanation for the mortality effect, we extended Model II to include terms for both within-block and compositional differences in the ratio of RNs to total nursing personnel. We found no evidence that average differences between magnet hospitals and matched controls with respect to either skill mix or nurse to patient ratios, significantly affect mortality, nor do they explain any of the variability in effects across magnet hospitals. Moreover, inclusion of these variables does not significantly alter the estimate of our treatment effect ($t = 1.27, P > .10$).[59]

On the basis of this analysis, we conclude that the matched comparison hospitals are not identical in nursing organisation to the magnet hospitals. At the same time, we have also demonstrated that one of the attributes of magnet hospitals – a greater proportion of nursing service personnel being registered nurses – is not the sole explanation for their lower mortality. This finding reinforces our belief that the mortality effect derives from the greater status, autonomy, and control afforded nurses in the magnet hospitals, and their resulting impact on nurses' behaviors on behalf of patients – i.e., this is not simply an issue of the number of nurses, or their mix of credentials.

As with any observational comparison, our results are potentially subject to biases for unobserved covariates.[52] We cannot rule out the possibility that variables omitted from the analysis explain the lower mortality in magnet hospitals. If this is the case, such omitted variables will be correlated with the set of nursing variables operationalised by the magnet hospital construct. Although there may be other variables that we have not measured that affect mortality on their own account, we believe they are as likely to be functions of the within-hospital organisation of nursing as determinants of it.

We have utilised Medicare mortality data because of its availability for the hospitals of interest even though data on patients of all ages would have been preferable. It is uncertain how expanding the age range of patients on which mortality is observed would affect our findings. Mortality rates are lower among younger patients, which argues for a diminution in the size of the effect. However, within the aged Medicare population there are limits to the proportion of mortality that can be expected to be prevented by any intervention.

The practical importance of our findings is influenced by the extent to which the organisational characteristics of magnet hospitals can be replicated elsewhere. In another paper, we have demonstrated that hospital unit level reforms, such as enabling nurses to specialise, also stimulate greater autonomy, control, and intra-organisational status toward nursing. However, institution-wide professional nursing practice models (as in the magnet hospitals) stimulate them further. The authors of the original magnet hospital study[16] and researchers conducting the follow-up studies[44] believe that the attributes of magnet hospitals can be widely replicated, and we concur. The organisational attributes distinguishing magnet hospitals are almost identical to those characterising the best-run companies, and thus have potentially wide applicability across a range of organisational types.[42–44] As noted in Table 18.2, there is considerable variability among magnet hospitals in hospital size, teaching status, ownership, and financial status, all of which suggests that replication is not bound to hospital 'type.' Indeed, approximately 900 (18%) of the nonmagnet hospitals in the classification sample have combinations of organisational characteristics (teaching status, percentage of board-certified physicians, ownership, financial status, etc.) that would lead them (under certain optimal classification rules) to be predicted to be magnet hospitals.

CONCLUSION

Our narrowest conclusion is that the hospitals in the magnet hospital study have mortality rates that are lower than those among matched control hospitals, by a factor of approximately five per 1,000 Medicare discharges. This corresponds to a reduction in 'excess mortality' of 5%. The magnet hospitals do differ from their matched controls in their nursing 'skill mix,' but this is not the explanation for the mortality differential. Based on adjunct studies of the magnet hospitals, we are inclined to attribute this differential to hospital-level differences in the organisation of nursing care. Our broader conclusion is that such organisational factors are important in understanding why some hospitals achieve better patient outcomes than others. We point to the 39 magnet hospitals, that appear to be in many respects like other hospitals, except in the organisation of nursing, as evidence that further reductions in excess hospital mortality may well be within our reach.

ACKNOWLEDGMENTS

The authors thank Dr. Marlene Kramer, for data from her study of the magnet hospitals; Dr. Margaret Sovie, our colleague who was a principal researcher in the original magnet hospital study; and Deborah McIlvaine, Suzanne Cole, Linzhu Tian, and Jennifer Smith, for their research assistance.

NOTES

* *Medical Care* 32 (8): 771–787. Reprinted with permission of J.B. Lippincott Company.

1 Koska MT. Quality – thy name is nursing care, CEOs say. Hospitals 1989; 32:32.
2 Findlay S, Roberts M, Silberner J. The best hospitals, from AIDS to urology. U.S. News & World Report 1990: 108:68.
3 Sunshine L, Wright JW. The best hospitals in America. New York: Henry Holt and Co, 1988.
4 Cohen IB. Florence Nightingale. Scientific American 1984; 250:128.
5 Benner P. From novice to expert. Menlo Park, CA: Addison-Wesley Publishing, 1984.
6 Stein LI, Watts DT, Howell T. The doctor-nurse game revisited. N Engl J Med 1990; 332:546.
7 Mechanic D, Aiken LH. A cooperative agenda for medicine and nursing. N Engl J Med 1982; 307:747.
8 Mauksch HO. The organisational context of nursing practice. In: Davis Fred. The Nursing Profession: Five Sociological Essays. New York, NY: John Wiley, 1966: 190.
9 Thomas L. The youngest science: Notes of a medicine-watcher. New York: Viking Press, 1983.
10 Knaus WA, Draper EA, Wagner DP, et al. An evaluation of outcome from intensive care in major medical centers. Ann Intern Med 1986; 104:410.
11 Aiken LH, Smith HL. Effects of specialisation on the status and autonomy of nurses: Results from a natural experiment in hospital AIDS care. Paper presented at the American Sociological Association, Miami, FL, August 1993.
12 McCloskey J. Influence of rewards and incentives on staff nurse turnover rate. Nurs Res 1974; 23:239.
13 Parasuraman S, Drake BH, Zammuto RF. The effect of nursing care modalities and staff assignments on nurses' work experiences and job attitudes. Nurs Res 1981; 31:364.
14 Jacox A. Role restructuring in hospital nursing. In: Aiken LH, ed. Nursing in the 1980s: Crises, Opportunities, Challenges. Philadelphia: JB Lippincott, 1982:75.

15 Clifford JC. Fostering professional nursing practice in hospitals: the experience of Boston's Beth Israel Hospital. In: Aiken LH, Fagin CM, eds. Charting Nursing's Future: Agenda for the 1990s. Philadelphia: JB Lippincott Co, 1992:87.

16 McClure M, Poulin M, Sovie MD, et al. Magnet hospitals: attraction and retention of professional nurses. Kansas City, MO: American Academy of Nursing 1983.

17 Hinshaw AS, Atwood JR. Nursing staff turnover, stress, and satisfaction: Models, measures, and management. Annu Rev Nurs Res 1983; 1:133.

18 Orsolits M. Effects of organisational characteristics on the turnover in cancer nursing. Oncol Nurs Forum 1984;11:1.

19 Prescott PA. Vacancy, stability, and turnover of registered nurses in hospitals. Res Nurs Health 1986;9:51.

20 Moses LE, Mosteller F. Institutional differences in postoperative death rates. JAMA 1968;203:492.

21 Blumberg MS. Comments on HCFA hospital death rate statistical outliers. Health Serv Res 1987;21:715.

22 Chassin MR, Park RE, Lohr KN, et al. Differences among hospitals in Medicare patient mortality. Health Serv Res 1989;24:1.

23 Berwick DM, Wald DL. Hospital leaders' opinions of the HCFA mortality data. JAMA 1990;263:247.

24 Green J, Wintfeld N, Sharkey P, et al. The importance of severity of illness in assessing hospital mortality. JAMA 1990;263:241.

25 Green J, Passman LJ, Wintfeld N. Analysing hospital mortality: The consequences of diversity in patient mix. JAMA 1991;265:1849.

26 Knaus WA, Wagner DP, Lynn J. Short-term mortality predictions for critically ill hospitalised adults: science and ethics. Science 1991;25:389.

27 Shortell SM, Rousseau DM, Gillies RR, et al. Organisational assessment in intensive care units (ICUs): construct development, reliability, and validity of the ICU nurse-physician questionnaire. Med Care 1991;29:709.

28 Georgopoulos BS, Mann FC. The Community General Hospital. New York: Macmillan, 1962.

29 Kelly JV, Hellinger FJ. Physician and hospital factors associated with mortality of surgical patients. Med Care 1986;24:785.

30 Shortell SM, Hughes EFX. The effects of regulation, competition, and ownership on mortality rates among hospital inpatients. N Engl J Med 1988;318:1100.

31 Hartz AJ, Krakauer H, Kuhn EM, et al. Hospital characteristics and mortality rates. N Engl J Med 1989;321:1720.

32 Al-Haider AS, Wan TTH. Modeling organisational determinants of hospital mortality. Health Serv Res 1991;26:303.

33 Krakauer H, Bailey RC, Skellan KJ, et al. Evaluation of the HCFA model for the analysis of mortality following hospitalisation. Health Serv Res 1992;27:400.

34 Burstin HR, Lipsitz SR, Udvarhelyi S, et al. The effect of hospital financial characteristics on quality of care. JAMA 1993;270:845.

35 Scott WR, Forrest WH Jr., Brown BW Jr. Hospital structure and postoperative mortality and morbidity. In: Shortell SM, Brown M. eds. Organisational Research in Hospitals. Chicago, IL: Blue Cross, 1976, 72.

36 Silbert JH, Williams SV, Krakauer H, et al. Hospital and patient characteristics associated with death after surgery: A study of adverse occurrence and failure to rescue. Med Care 1992;30:615.

37 Brennan TA, Herbert LE, Laird NM, et al. Hospital characteristics associated with adverse events and substandard care. JAMA 1991;265:3265.

38 Keeler EB, Rubenstein LV, Kahn KL, et al. Hospital characteristics and quality of care. JAMA 1986;268:1709.

39 National Commission on Nursing. Summary report and recommendations. Chicago: Hospital Research and Educational Trust, 1983.

40 U.S. Department of Health and Human Services. Secretary's Commission on Nursing, Final Report. Washington, DC, 1988.

41 Kramer M, Hafner LP. Shared values: Impact on staff nurse job satisfaction and perceived productivity. Nurs Res 1989;38:172.

42 Kramer M, Schmalenberg C. Magnet hospitals: Institutions of excellence, Parts I & II. JONA 1988;18:11.

43 Kramer M. The magnet hospitals: Excellence revisited. JONA 1990;20:35.

44 Kramer M, Schmalenberg C. Job satisfaction and retention: Insights for the '90s, Parts I & II. Nursing 1991;21:50.

45 Health Care Financing Administration. Medicare hospital mortality information 1986, 1987, 1988. Washington, DC: U.S. Government Printing Office, 1989.

46 American Hospital Association. Hospital statistics, 1989 edition. Chicago: American Hospital Association, 1989.

47 Dubois RW, Brook RH, Rogers WH. Adjusted hospital death rates: A potential screen for quality of medical care. Am J Public Health 1987;77:1162.

48 Duckett SJ, Kristofferson SM. An index of hospital performance. Med Care 1978;16:400.

49 Cochran WG. The planning of observational studies of human populations (with discussion). Journal of the Royal Statistical Society, Series A. 1965;128:234.

50 Cochran WG, Rubin DB. Controlling bias in observational studies: A review. Sankhya Ser A 1973;35:417.

51 Kish L. Statistical design for research. New York: John Wiley, 1987.

52 Rosenbaum PR, Rubin DB. Constructing a control group using multivariate matched sampling methods that incorporate the propensity score. The American Statistician 1985;39:33.

53 Rubin DB. Using multivariate matched sampling and regression adjustment to control bias in observational studies. J Am Stat Assoc 1979;74:318.

54 Rubin DB. The use of matching and regression adjustments to remove bias in observational studies. Biometrics 1973;29:185.

55 Green DM, Swets JA. Signal detection theory and pychophysics. Huntington, NY: Krieger, 1974.

56 Hosmer DW Jr., Lemeshow S. Applied logistic regression. New York: John Wiley & Sons, 1989.

57 Rubin DB. Matching to remove bias in observational studies. Biometrics 1973;29:159.

58 Ury HK. Efficiency of case-control studies with multiple controls per case: Continuous or dichotomous data. Biometrics 1975;31:643.

59 Clogg CC, Petkova E, Shihadeh ES. Statistical methods for analysing collapsibility in regression models. Journal of Educational Statistics 1992;173:51.

60 Bryk AS, Raudenbush SW. Hierarchical linear models: Applications and data analysis methods. Newbury Park, CA: Sage Publications, 1992.

APPENDIX: ANALYTIC EQUATIONS
CORRESPONDING TO RESULTS

These are equations and statistical considerations pertaining to estimates reported in the Results section. This Appendix should be read in parallel with that section.

There are I = 39 magnet hospitals, each matched to J = 5 control hospitals. Let y_{ij} be the mortality rate in the jth match to the ith magnet hospital, i = 1, . . . , 39, j = 1, . . . , 5. Denote by y_{i0} the mortality rate in the ith magnet hospital. Then there are I x J = 195 pairs of mortality differences, $\Delta y_{ij} = y_{i0} - y_{ij}$.

A random-effects analysis-of-variance (Model I) for the effect of magnet hospital characteristics on mortality is

$$(A1) \quad \Delta y_{ij} = \beta_{0i} + e_{ij} \text{ and}$$
$$(A2) \quad \beta_{0i} = \gamma_{00} + u_{0i},$$

where $E(e_{ij}) = 0, Var(e_{ij}) = \sigma^2$, and $Var(u_{0i}) = \tau_{00}$. This posits a fixed effect of magnet hospitals γ_{00} across all comparisons, as well as a randomly varying effect (u_{0i}) specific to each magnet hospital and its block of five differences. Tests of the hypothesis $\gamma_{00} = 0$ are equivalent to t-tests of the difference between magnet hospitals mortality and the average mortality in matched (paired) control hospitals.[58] The test of the hypothesis $\tau_{00} = 0$ is the test of the assumption that the magnet hospital effect on mortality is common across all magnet hospitals. The reliability of β_{0i} is estimated as $\hat{\tau}_{00}/(\hat{\tau}_{00} + [\hat{\sigma}^2/n])$, where n= 5, the number of matched control hospitals in each block.

To adjust for the effects of predicted mortality, define x_{ij} as predicted mortality for the jth hospital matched to the ith magnet hospital, and x_{i0} is predicted mortality for the ith magnet hospital.

$$\text{Set } \Delta X_{ij} = x_{i0} - x_{ij} \text{ and } \Delta x_{i\cdot} = (\sum_{j=1}^{5} \Delta x_{ij})/5.$$

Model II is a random-effects egression of Δy_{ij} on both within-block (Δx_{ij}) and compositional ($\Delta x_{i\cdot}$) differences in predicted mortality:[60]

$$(A3) \quad \Delta y_{ij} = \beta_{0i} + \beta_{1i} (\Delta x_{ij} - \Delta x_{i\cdot}) + e_{ij},$$
$$(A4) \quad \beta_{0i} = \gamma_{00} + \gamma_{01}\Delta x_{i\cdot} + u_{0i}, \text{ and}$$
$$(A5) \quad \beta_{1i} = \gamma_{10} = u_{1i},$$

with Var $(u_{1i}) = \tau_{11}$ and $Cov(u_{0i}, u_{1i}) = \tau_{10} = \tau_{01}$. We were unable to reject the hypothesis that $\tau_{11} = \tau_{10} = 0$ ($\chi^2 = 3.56$, 2 DF, $P > .15$, so these terms were set equal to zero for Model II, which was re-estimated as a one-way analysis-of-covariance (ANCOVA) with random effects.[60]

Under Model II, estimates of both γ_{01} and γ_{10} (the effects of block-specific and within-block differences in predicted mortality on observed mortality) are approximately equal to one. Under the assumption that they are exactly equal to one, Model II can be re-expressed as

$$(A6)\ (y_{i0} - x_{i0}) - (y_{ij} - x_{ij}) = \gamma_{00} \div \text{variance components}$$

which is to say that the estimate of γ_{00} under Model II is essentially that which would obtain if 'excess mortality' (observed minus predicted) in magnet hospitals were compared with excess mortality in matched controls. A variant on this is to transform the response variable so as to describe excess mortality in *percentage terms*, and estimate Model III,

$$(A7)\ \ln\left[(y_{i0}/x_{i0})/(y_{ij}/x_{ij})\right] = \beta_{0i} + e_{ij},$$

with reference to equation (A2).

Chapter 19

Research for whom?

The politics of research dissemination and application

JANE ROBINSON

Introduction

In this article, Jane Robinson gives an account of the painful experience of being the bearer of bad research-based news. If anyone still believes that the scientific character of health care research means that it can be commissioned, carried out and implemented in an apolitical context, this article should disabuse them. In it, Robinson tells how, as a researcher employed by an NHS health authority in 1981, she was required to undertake an investigation into apparently high local perinatal mortality. Although, she narrates, her research adopted the current best practice and procedures, her findings that above average mortality did not appear to be explained by low birthweight or other patient factors, and, hence might be explained by the character of care received, met with professional hostility. Her research was attacked by some of the health authority's doctors as flawed and inaccurate, and she tells how the possibility that it may have held implications for practice was strongly resisted: as she says, 'there is a tendency to close ranks and to search for alternative explanations whenever a spotlight is turned on to the performance of individual groups of workers.'

The other strand of this story is the author's own frankness about her sense of grief and powerlessness to use the research findings to bring about change on behalf of the parents whose babies had died, and her guilt that she had caused upset to health authority staff who had contributed freely to the research.

Robinson draws out some of the lessons for health care – and research – practice at the beginning of the 1990s when this piece was written, before the NHS R & D initiative and before the evidence-based medicine/healthcare/nursing movements rose to prominence. Now, ten years later, the lessons are even sharper.

Research and development, critical appraisal workshops and the UK government's own health care research programmes could be an expensive masquerade, without attention to the management of any change that research findings may suggest.

There is a huge amount written about the difficulty of implementation among health care professionals. Although the reader of Robinson's article could well be forgiven for forgetting it for a moment, resistance to research findings is not the unique territory of medicine. So whether we are reading about doctors' 'resistance' or nurses' 'failure' it is important not to succumb to caricatures of either (or any other) group. It is interesting that, in the context of apparent medical power and complacency, Robinson speaks of the need to empower clinical staff so that they do not feel 'hopeless and helpless at the prospect of being able to effect structural changes in the management of their service'. It is all too easy to attribute such feelings only to nurses. At the time of writing, the situation is no less complex and impossible to generalise about than during the early 1980s when Robinson was involved in her research. We have witnessed, in the UK, the inquiry into the management of care of children receiving complex heart surgery at the Bristol Royal Infirmary, but it is impossible to know in how many other situations clinicians have not shown the extreme bravery needed to disclose apparent failures of practice. Likewise various government NHS R & D initiatives, such as the Service Delivery and Organisation programme can be seen to be employing a welcome range of research methods but, anecdotally at least, some of the changes suggested by such research findings have been rejected by certain clinicians on the grounds that they have not proceeded from sufficiently 'rigorous' research designs, i.e. from randomised controlled trials. In other words, the very mechanisms of research, can be taken up to support the status quo as well as question it. Furthermore, we should not assume that well-implemented research offers the universal solution to unsatisfactory care. It seems likely that often it is poor resourcing, poor relationships, poor management practices or flawed policy that contribute far more than ignorance to failures in care.

The second lesson concerns the welfare of the researcher. Robinson is at pains to warn the new researcher that many research questions which they may innocently pose, in higher degree work or elsewhere, are likely to have political consequences. She laments that many standard nursing research texts have been strong on technique and process, but weak on cultural and political context – though today we are hopefully better served by more sophisticated accounts. Nurse researchers' tales of harsh treatment by ethics committees, who perhaps have understanding only of a limited range of research approaches, fuel the profession's tendency to insecurity and defensiveness in the face of what is often seen as a controlling and powerful medical profession. Perhaps some of this unfair treatment can be forestalled through expert and canny presentation, but some will always remain as an unavoidable effect of the power of establishment bodies. Researchers need to develop a self-confidence to manage these situations without incurring personal damage. Robinson urges the employers of contract researchers, first to understand their own crucial responsibility to ensure that the focus and methodology of the research they commission are appropriate for the question under study, and second to support their research staff throughout the process, including its implementation. Otherwise researchers may well feel that they have been set up to fail. Academic supervisors of such research should also reflect on and include these issues as part of their supervision. It is probably not unusual that research completed for higher degrees turns out to be not a simple presentation of processes and findings, but rather a critical and, importantly, therapeutic reflection and analysis of the political and institutional problems encountered in health research.

So Robinson's paper is sobering but, as she also acknowledges, in some senses it serves to support the arguments of many policy theorists that the impact of research is, at best, indirect. It offers a frank account of what it is to be caught up in such processes of influence.

ROBINSON, J. (1994)

Research for whom? The politics of research dissemination and application*

INTRODUCTION

> Research methodologies abound in prescriptive, normative statements about how research should or should not be done. Indeed the function of most social science methods texts is to provide recipes for doing social research – and such texts are known in the trade as cookbooks. Yet all practising researchers know that social research is not like it is presented and prescribed in those texts. It is infinitely more complex, messy, various and much more interesting. These accounts do, of course, also expose the soft underbelly of social science – unprotected by the hard shell of quantitative science as normally presented to the world through those texts, books and monographs. That social science also takes place in a political context you would never guess from the methodology texts.
>
> *(Bell and Encel, 1978, pp. 4–5)*

The text from which the above quotation is taken was one of a series of edited collections which greatly helped me to make sense of the research experience described in this chapter. All of the authors included in the series struck me with their unashamed honesty about what social research (especially contract research) is *really* like. The other crucial texts included *Doing Sociological Research* (Bell and Newby, 1981), *Social Researching – Politics, Problem, Practice* (Bell and Roberts, 1984) and *Doing Feminist Research* (Roberts, 1981). How, I reflected, these accounts differed from the standard nursing research cookbooks with their preoccupation with technique and process – both apparently completely divorced from the personal, social and cultural identities of the researchers and the researched! Most of what was and is written concerning nursing research contains virtually nothing about the problems and the fascination of how we come to describe and to know the social world of which we are intrinsically a part. I was therefore delighted to receive an invitation to contribute this chapter to a book which promises to begin to set the record straight on nursing research.

The subject matter of the chapter arose from some teaching which I contributed to the MA in the Sociology of Health and Healing at the University of Warwick during the mid-1980s. One of the editors of this current edition (Richard McMahon) was a student member of that course. The messages which I tried then to convey must have struck a chord for in 1991, approximately five years later, he offered me the opportunity to record in this book some of the research experiences which I had related to his class. In trying to recall the flavour of those two sessions on policy research in health care it seemed, with all the benefits of hindsight, that I had been concerned to inject a note of caution and of realism into the whole business of applied research. In contributing to that MA course I remember feeling that I would be doing less than justice to the part time mature students (the majority of whom were nurses) if I did not sensitise them (as they embarked perhaps for the first time on a piece of research of their own) to some of the problems and the pitfalls which I had encountered as an emerging health policy analyst who also happened to be a nurse.

THE RESEARCH IN CONTEXT

At the time of those teaching sessions at Warwick I was still reeling from the impact of carrying out a highly sensitive piece of participant observation research into the problem of perinatal mortality in one health authority and I had recently been awarded a PhD (Robinson, 1986) for my account of that research experience – an account which included a multilevel description of the research context, process and product. The original research report had, however, never been published for it had been embargoed in October 1983 by the chairman of the commissioning health authority upon its one and only presentation to the closed session of a meeting of health authority members.

My reactions to this turn of events were intensely ambivalent. On the one hand they encompassed feelings of anger and grief at my powerlessness to be able to use the lessons of the research findings in order to bring about change on behalf of the parents whose babies had died and who had participated so willingly in the research process. Medical power had never seemed so omnipotent as when I realised that despite having uncovered aspects of care which raised questions about the management of some pregnancies, no one was required to consider the implications of the findings for their own professional practice. Paradoxically, on the other hand, I also felt a sense of worthlessness and guilt that I had caused hurt and upset to members of health authority staff (especially medical staff) who, like the parents, had also participated willingly in the research and who had given me open access to meetings and to medical records. This is not to suggest that nothing was achieved. As the following account shows, a working party was convened and an attempt was made to address the issues which the research raised. Yet much of the energy of that working party was devoted to denying the validity of the research observations and therefore to not accepting the need to recognise that there really was a problem about which something could be done.

One of the net results of these ambivalent feelings of impotent anger and guilt was that I found it extraordinarily painful to go back over my data in order to undertake the analyses of the policy perspectives arising from the study which were needed for the completion of the PhD. For a year I could hardly bring myself to contemplate the work and even then it was only because other people put strong pressure on me and lent me their support that the thesis itself was eventually completed. Publications proved to be equally difficult to produce, although slowly they began to emerge and over time progressed to show an interesting transition from the detail of the empirical study to the more general lessons which could be learnt from it (Robinson, 1987, 1989a, 1989b; Robinson and Allison, 1991).

REFLEXIVITY IN SOCIAL RESEARCH

It took a long period of deep personal reflection and analysis in order to understand and to come to terms with these reactions. Eventually I came to realise that such reflexivity is itself a crucial part of both the research and the learning processes which arise from it. As a result of that reflection I can now assert with reasonable confidence that feelings of guilt in situations of this nature appear to represent part of a subordination process in which the bearer of bad news is made to feel unworthy and mistaken in their conclusions. The focus of attention and the onus of proof shifts from the recipients to the bearer of the unwelcome message. In a phrase – 'If you don't like the message, shoot the messenger'. This phenomenon is now well documented in cases of 'whistle-blowing' (News Focus, 1991) but is not usually articulated in the context of research findings. This omission is a serious indictment of how research methodology and application are taught to nurses although it may help to explain why nurses so often appear to take refuge in the myth of objectivity and detachment in social research. Arguably the absence of such discussion in the context of nursing research also seriously misleads neophyte researchers into believing that research application is a simple and straightforward matter.

In the account which follows I do not believe that as a researcher I was particularly unusual or exceptional. Where I did perhaps differ was in my subsequent reactions to the experience. However painful the reflective process may have been it resulted in my becoming determined not to accept at face value the initial reactions to the research findings but to try instead to understand and to explain the phenomena. The lessons I learnt were concerned with the social and political aspects of applied research. At one level it seems perfectly obvious that if new knowledge challenges the status quo then its application will be concerned with issues of power and control. At another level it throws into question all of the current preoccupations with audit in the National Health Service and with how change is ever brought about within organisations. It is the detail of how these issues worked out in practice within one research project which I shall try to make explicit in this chapter.

The remainder of this chapter is in two parts. First, the main issues arising from the empirical research are described as a case study. Space dictates, however, that this section can only be used to convey the most minimal description of what was, in reality, an enormously detailed and complex piece of work encompassing in total two action packed years from 1981 to 1983 and then the slower part time process of writing up the PhD which took until the end of 1985. The main purpose of what I shall describe here of the actual study is to try to answer the criticisms which were received from some members of medical staff that the research findings were inaccurate. Obviously this is criticism which has to be taken seriously. For more detailed information on the broader aspects of the research the reader is directed to the original thesis (Robinson, 1986). In the second and final part of the chapter, the lessons which I have drawn from the research and which are touched on in this introductory section are developed and discussed.

THE EMPIRICAL RESEARCH

In September 1981 I was appointed to a research post in a district health authority medical department which included the following remarkable (some would say impossible) job description:

> The Research Officer is directly accountable to the District Medical Officer for the research of health problems within 'A' Health Authority in order that operational and strategic plans reflect an understanding of health care and preventive medicine needs of the community. The principal task is to introduce more precise information on the problem of perinatal mortality in order that speculative planning is reduced to the minimum. The job is concerned with the gathering and analysis of data directly from clients/patients and from health service professionals.
>
>   He/she will be responsible for the following main functions:
> a) To undertake interviews with patients/clients and professional staff in order to gather and analyse data relating to the medical, biological, social, educational, cultural and environmental factors in perinatal mortality in 'A' Health Authority.

Further clauses followed which included:

- monitoring the effects of changing policies on perinatal mortality;
- developing links with health care researchers at university, polytechnic and regional health authority levels;
- liaising with all disciplines of staff including the Planning and Information Officer;
- contributing to in-service education for a range of professionals on the implications of the research in both general and specific terms;
- generating articles on the subject of in-house research;
- undertaking similar research in other fields.

Although apparently daunting in its scope I was delighted with the opportunities which this broadbased research job offered and within the context of planning, carrying out and writing up a one year empirical study of perinatal mortality, I have no doubt that all of the objectives of that job description were fulfilled. I had had experience of two earlier pieces of research with strong policy implications, although neither was contract research (Robinson, 1979, 1980, 1982). I was absorbed already by the methodological and political problems which appear to be inherent in much policy research and also by the analytical possibilities offered through a critical approach to policy issues (Rein, 1976; Hall *et al.*, 1978; Bumer, 1982). I wanted to explore these issues further and if I needed further motivation to take the post it was that as a polytechnic (health visitor) lecturer I was intensely frustrated by the then lack of opportunity for personal research. I therefore resigned my lectureship and threw myself with excitement and enthusiasm into the challenges offered by this innovative health authority research job.

With the support of my new employers I registered simultaneously for a PhD in a university Department of Social Anthropology, Social Work and Social Policy on the understanding that I would use the empirical research as a case study of the policy implications of applied research. Despite my earlier research experience I had no anticipation that those implications would be quite so politically sensitive. I was assured of social research supervision through my supervisor Professor Olive Stevenson and I immediately set about negotiating support for the epidemiological aspects of the study. In this I was fortunate to have the interest and guidance of a professor of social medicine whose research into large volumes of historical data on perinatal mortality was to mirror some of the issues which I subsequently identified tentatively at a microscopic level (Knox, Lancashire and Armstrong, 1986). (These issues centre around the possibility of identifying unexplained variations in the performance of different obstetric units by excluding from the data certain classes of birth and on indirect standardisation for birthweight.) I was also given complete freedom to seek advice on methodological issues from a range of experts in the field, the most notable of whom were based at the National Perinatal Epidemiology Unit (NPEU) – a recently established Department of Health Research Unit – at the Radcliffe Infirmary, Oxford. It was their recommendations for research methods for local perinatal surveys which I was to follow to the letter in my study (NPEU, 1978).

The question of whether or not my findings were correct hinges on the validity of the research outcomes for each of the NPEU's four recommended inclusion criteria. Because this is such a central issue I shall discuss each in some depth together with relevant aspects of the research findings. The research methods recommended for inclusion by the NPEU were as follows:

1 All perinatal deaths within a geographically defined population

In the study referred to here this was represented by all the deaths (77) occurring between 1 January and 31 December 1982 to mothers resident within the health authority geographical boundary. This methodological device ensured that the total number of health authority births during the same period (4249) could then be used as a denominator, giving a local district perinatal mortality rate in 1982 of 18.1 per 1000 total births. Once these data were established it was then possible to identify what proportion of births to health authority resident mothers took place in different obstetric units. For example, 2428 (57%) of authority resident mothers were confined in the district maternity unit where, however, 54 (70%) of the deaths occurred. 1524 (35.9%) of births and the remaining 23 (30%) of deaths took place in three other cross-boundary hospitals. Domiciliary confinements and other hospitals accounted for the remaining 297 (7.0%) of births and there were no deaths in this latter group.

This simple but crucial aspect of epidemiological research (i.e. using a geographical population as the denominator) enables careful comparisons to be made between the characteristics and experiences of different subpopulations and eliminates the unavoidable and uninvestigatable bias which is built into studies confined to *hospital* populations. (This bias is uninvestigatable because you cannot know the boundaries and therefore the characteristics of the *total* populations from which hospitals draw their patients.) If, however, you know the distribution of certain characteristics within the total geographically defined population (the denominator) then their distribution can be compared with the same characteristics within the numerator (total perinatal deaths within that population). For example, birthweight data, which should be routinely available for all health authority births, are invalulable for such comparisons in the case of perinatal mortality.

Some detail has been given about the justification for this particular aspect of the methodology because at the end of the study some of the most bitter recriminations centred around the ways in which the babies who died were born to mothers who were 'different' to those who survived. Some medical consultants subscribed to the view that the high perinatal mortality rates experienced in their health authority arose from differences in the characteristics of the mothers for whom they were responsible (namely, that more of them came from ethnic minority groups, were poorer, less well educated, irresponsible in lifestyles and in their use of medical services than the mothers of surviving babies). They claimed, furthermore, that the health authority resident mothers who used 'their' hospital were more materially disadvantaged and booked later for antenatal care than those using the other hospitals.

These claims were not easy either to substantiate or disprove because of the unreliability of some of the data sources on which one had to depend. In particular, Hospital Activity Data which should, in theory, have provided data on numerous categories of evidence for the total population of births (including data on service utilisation and medical interventions) were found to be so incomplete as to be totally unreliable. Only data on birthweight distribution by place of birth and maternal geographical area of residence were ultimately obtained for *all* births using the Statutory Notification of Births as a data source.

Nevertheless this provided evidence that there were no significant differences in birthweight distribution between the different hospitals in the study. Indeed, if national and regional policy had been followed to the letter, one would have expected greater variation between the hospitals arising from the selection of mothers at risk of premature births for confinement in centres with neonatal intensive care facilities.

2 The generation of an appropriate control group

As stated above, in an ideal world the total population of health authority births would have been used as a denominator for a whole range of variables. However, having exhausted the potential of the data which is available for the total population, a control group provides an alternative sample population which can be used to generate further data for comparative purposes. Although the NPEU made this recommendation, no further guidance was given as to which variables to control for in the matching process between cases and controls. Surprisingly too, given the tremendous reliance on case-control trials in epidemiological research, there was very little guidance on the question of matching in the literature. In general, there appear to be an assumption that in perinatal research one controlled for factors such as age of mother, parity, social class and ethnicity. However, once these variables are matched between cases and controls they are then eliminated from any subsequent statistical analysis and this may mask important local idiosyncrasies. For example, I wanted to test out the assumption that the mothers whose babies died (the cases) were different from those whose babies survived (the controls) for a range of social, demographic and economic variables. If I had matched the social class, ethnicity, marital status and age of the control mothers with those of the case mothers, then I would have had no way of knowing whether there was any difference between the cases and the controls in these important respects. Indeed, because a vital aspect of any research lies in the nature of the questions that are selected for asking, if certain questions are eliminated by virtue of assuming *a priori* that the answers are self-evident then an important element of bias is introduced into the research infrastructure.

I consulted widely on this aspect of the methodology and concluded, somewhat arrogantly, that no one had got it *exactly* right! One perinatal epidemiologist had thought very much along the same lines and in the end a modified form of the matching used in his study was adopted (Clarke and Clayton, 1981). This involved taking the infant of the same sex born immediately prior to the perinatal death in the mother's intended place of confinement *at the time of the first antenatal booking*. The rationale behind this lay in the assumption that mothers of comparative obstetric risk would be matched – high risk mothers being booked for consultant units, lower risk mothers for general practitioner units. One could then trace the pregnancy 'careers' of the mothers through the various forms of obstetric care.

In the event, this form of matching was not ideal because 95% of mothers were booked for consultant units. Nevertheless it did enable important comparisons to be made between the units where it was discovered that policies for antenatal and intrapartum care were markedly different. It also enabled a challenge to be made to the *a priori* assumption that the mothers whose babies died were different from the control mothers on a range of social and economic variables, for *no* statistically significant differences were identified. In fact, the *total* case-control population was found to be relatively disadvantaged (for example, 25% of *all* fathers were unemployed compared with 17.2% of all males aged 16–64 in the authority for the 1981 census). The effects of the economic recession were relatively severe in the indigenous population who were mainly from social class III manual occupations and some of whose male members had recently been made redundant from heavy industries.

The number of deaths (31%) to mothers from ethnic minorities appeared to be high in comparison to the proportion in the indigenous population (11.4% from the New Commonwealth and Pakistan in the 1981 census); but not in comparison with their controls. There was an almost equal distribution of case and control mothers from ethnic minorities in each of the hospitals in the study. This distribution appeared to be representative of the varied proportions of ethnic minority mothers using the different obstetric units. However, in the absence of an appropriate population denominator for births to all residents by ethnic group the validity of this observation could not be tested. This finding was also undoubtedly skewed to some extent by variations in the age distribution between the ethnic and indigenous populations. The ethnic minority groups not only had larger proportions of younger people of childbearing age but also experienced higher fertility rates than the indigenous population. The excess of observed over expected deaths appeared to lie in the large number of lethal congenital malformations occurring amongst the ethnic minority mothers. Once again, the absence of appropriate denominator data meant that the validity of this observation could not be tested.

There were 11 illegitimate babies amongst the cases, eight amongst the controls. Eleven of the mothers (six cases and five controls) were living in apparently stable cohabitation and three were single mothers living with their own parents. Just two were living in apparently unstable social circumstances. One was a high risk mother who was in regular contact with health and social workers. Nevertheless she was the only mother in the whole survey to have concealed her pregnancy and to have received no antenatal care. (She proved highly elusive and was never interviewed properly even though I helped with the baby's funeral arrangements, including transporting the mother to hospital and to the Registrar.) For the remainder, antenatal attendance varied only slightly from the population of legitimate pregnancies. This variety in social circumstances was a powerful reminder that legally defined illegitimacy is a relatively common contemporary occurrence. Nevertheless, these births predominated amongst young mothers aged 18–19 years and evidence from the interviews suggested that the stigma associated with illegitimacy persists and that this led, on occasions, to very serious breakdowns in communication between health care professionals and the mothers themselves.

Differences in maternal age and total number of previous pregnancies between cases and controls were statistically significant ($p = 0.05$ and $p = 0.01$ respectively). These are well known indicators of increased obstetric risk and mothers in these groups should, in theory, experience increased antenatal care and surveillance but this was not always apparently the case.

One third of case mothers smoked during pregnancy compared with one fifth of controls (not significant, $p = 0.07$). While 13 (17%) of case mothers stated that they smoked more than 16 cigarettes a day before the pregnancy, four claimed to have reduced consumption or given up once pregnant. In total, 25 (32%) case mothers compared with 16 controls smoked during pregnancy. Although undoubtedly worrying, these numbers were substantially less than was widely believed by health care professionals. Indeed it was later suggested that the mothers lied about this information.

There was little evidence of mothers deliberately refraining from booking antenatal care. By 18 weeks 84.3% of cases and 85.7% of controls had attended their GP and 78% of both populations had attended hospital for the first time. A small proportion of mothers had not by then arrived in the United Kingdom or were in the Indian subcontinent on holiday.

It was concluded that no clearcut picture between cases and controls emerged for a range of social, maternal and access to service variables. The overwhelming impression was of a group of mothers many of whom (but not all) experienced some form of social and physiological disadvantage (estimated in the survey by maternal height, weight, haemoglobin estimation and morbidity in pregnancy); some lost their babies, others did not. Once in the health care system the service which some of the mothers received gave rise to more concern. This population, which was disadvantaged on a number of measures, did not always appear to receive the compensatory forms of health care recommended by the Short Committee (House of Commons, 1980). The overall picture of investigations carried out during pre-, intra- and postpartum care was of a very limited use of screening techniques and/or technological intervention even in cases where there was uncertainty about dates, maternal morbidity and/or a family history of premature labour or congenital malformation. For example seven mothers received alphafetoprotein estimation (146 did not, one (case) had amniocentesis) and 44.2% of cases did not have an ultrasound examination. The report did not suggest that these procedures should be performed routinely, it merely noted that different hospitals apparently followed different policies.

Further differences in medical intervention and attitudes were observed between staff in the four hospitals. For example, three complicating factors during labour – spontaneous rupture of membranes with delayed labour onset, intrapartum haemorhage and abnormal presentation – showed highly significant differences between cases and controls. Although such differences are predictable (these complications are inevitably associated with an increase in perinatal deaths) there were variations in the response to them by medical staff in different hospitals in the study.

Forty seven (62%) of the deaths occurred in apparently normally formed infants weighing 1000 g and above and standardisation by birthweight showed that there was an excess of observed over expected deaths in the heavier birthweight band of 2501 g and above.

Nineteen (25%) of the deaths were in babies with identified congenital malformations. Nine of these were neural tube defects which together with five survivors beyond the first week of life gave a district rate of 3.29 per 1000 births compared with 1.92 for England and Wales (1981). (This was apparently related, in part, to the absence of routine screening procedures for these conditions.)

The district perinatal rate was 6.8 points above the rate for England and Wales. Nevertheless, just two babies (both cases) were delivered by a consultant obstetrician. Consultant obstetricians were not present at any of the remaining deliveries. Twenty nine cases and 19 controls were delivered by an obstetric registrar or SHO; 44 and 56 respectively by midwives. No cases or controls had a consultant anaesthetist or pae-diatrician present at the delivery. Eighteen cases and ten controls had a paediatric registrar or Senior House Officer present.

All of the information referred to in this section was generated for both cases and controls and was obtained via the two remaining research methods recommended by NPEU which are described below.

3 A minimum data set suggested by NPEU for use by all researchers surveying perinatal death

An 18 page questionnaire was eventually developed encompassing (with some modi-fications) the NPEU recommended minimum data set plus a range of questions derived from additional sources. The questionnaire was completed mainly from med-ical records. Where necessary clarification was sought from parental interviews, health care professionals and from attendance at the perinatal review meetings held to review individual cases in each of the hospitals. (The latter varied widely in form and content and this aspect of management was eventually incorporated in the final report and in the PhD thesis.)

4 Information sought from the mother, preferably in her own home

Seventy five cases and 73 controls (a total of 96%) mothers, and many of the fathers, were interviewed; a sad experience which revealed many unexpected facets of the sit-uation. For example, the funerals of dead babies had proved to be very traumatic for many and a relatively expensive procedure for several parents (Robinson, 1987). Some of the mothers had harrowing stories to tell (not confined to cases) of seeking help when there was a feeling that all was not well, of powerlessness in the face of medical 'expertise' and of the intransigence of some doctors in their refusal to take seriously the mother's account of events.

Participant observation as a health authority employee attending perinatal review meetings, maternity liaison group meetings and interviewing the parents of cases and controls led to the conclusion that inequality lay not so much in the characteris-tics of the population whose babies died as in the treatment they or their mothers received. Attempts on the part of parents, especially mothers, to participate in their care or to communicate their worries that all was not well with their pregnancy were 'put down' by some members of medical staff. This behaviour was justified on the grounds that the mothers were either too ill educated or so irresponsible that they could not possibly know what was happening to them. On occasions quite blatant racism and 'classism' were observed.

Yet doctors working in the hospital where the largest proportion of deaths occurred were hardworking and committed. There were severe shortages of medical and mid-wifery staff; they worked in the shadow of a regional centre of excellence; and they had to cope with the persistent stigma of relatively high perinatal mortality rates. Nevertheless the authoritarian and didactic attitudes which were observed led them to 'blame the victims' rather than to examine possible modifications of their practice and to seek amelioration of staffing problems. It was concluded that technological intervention might possibly have led to a satisfactory outcome in some cases (or screened out lethal malformations) but parents generally did not have the choice. It was the absence of choice, of any feeling of partnership in care, which gave a sense of real poverty to the services which some of these parents experienced. Inequality in health meant nothing to them in terms of impersonal collective categories such as ethnicity, class or marital status. Inequality on their terms was the reality of poverty, of losing your baby, of not being able to afford the funeral and sometimes being treated as if you were feckless or stupid or uncaring. Worst of all, it could mean being denied the right to be listened to even when what you had to say might just have altered completely the subsequent course of events.

Subsequent study arising from the empirical evidence for the completion of the PhD led to the development of explanations for the phenomena encountered in this study. For example, detailed examination of the Registrar General's annual statistical reports from the 1940s onwards and of several major inquiries into maternity services and perinatal death led to the conclusion that perinatal mortality is almost invariably constructed in official statistics in such a way as to highlight the significance of social and maternal characteristics rather than the possible influence of medical care (Joint Committee, 1948; Joint Committee, 1949; Butler and Bonham, 1963; Butler and Alberman, 1969; Chamberlain et al., 1975; Chamberlain et al., 1978; DHSS, 1980; House of Commons, 1980, 1984).

The analysis of the 'social construction' of mortality rates lends powerful support to the idea that medical education leads to the socialisation of some doctors to see perinatal mortality in maternal, economic and social terms for successive medical reports on the problem have emphasised sometimes in subtle and sometimes quite direct ways the victims' contribution to the failed pregnancy (Armstrong, 1986; and Allison, 1991).

Finally, it was hypothesised that women in medicine have to fight so hard to reach the top in their careers that (paradoxically) they may have become even more didactic than male doctors (as was observed in the study).

EARLY LESSONS FROM THE RESEARCH EXPERIENCE

This study of perinatal mortality in one health authority demonstrated unequivocally the complex and often contentious nature of research which exposes hidden assumptions and explores them in a systematic way. Work of this nature (although written extremely carefully and never claiming more from the evidence than could reasonably be deduced from a one year study) was inevitably very threatening to the key actors who were directly involved. They reacted with anger and having all the power of the medical profession behind them (including the threat of the Medical Defence Union), insisted that it should only be presented in the strictest confidence to one closed health authority meeting and then embargoed. The chairman charged members with the total confidence of the report and referred it to the Maternity Services Working

Party for investigation of its policy implications. I was included in this group and so observation of later developments was possible.

The group processes during the eight months of the Working Party's existence could be divided into roughly three stages. First, there was dissipation of anger and the re-establishment and confirmation of individual and group identities. During this first period the research was attacked systematically as inaccurate yet most of the attacks were oblique, ignoring completely, for example, the hard evidence of the quantitative data. The justification for this non-scientific approach appeared to lie in the fact that as the research worker had been a nurse this exonerated anyone from taking the findings seriously.

The attack was led by a consultant member in the form of a report which ignored the carefully constructed analysis and qualified comments in the original research. A detailed response to the criticisms was presented but was completely ignored by the medical members. Nursing and midwifery members regrettably made no contribution at all, although their privately expressed anxiety about some of the issues which had been raised was common local knowledge. The capacity to ignore the arguments of the research report and to describe the findings as inaccurate was encountered through-out the meetings, although gradually as members were charged by the chairman with specific tasks the overt hostility grew less. One consultant produced a report on obstetric aspects of perinatal death which simply compared a range of subcategories of perinatal death for three (non-health authority) hospitals. The entrenched notion of looking only at hospital populations despite their acknowledged inbuilt biases was rein-forced. The idea that the women of the authority were ignorant or feckless was reiterated and, on one occasion, when protesting at the assumptions of irresponsibil-ity which were being implied I repeated the research findings of numerous failures of communication. It was claimed then that even talking to the women 'in words of two syllables' produced no effect.

Following the third meeting of the Working Party the chairman wrote a report for members. It stated that opportunities had been given for discussion of the scientific aspects of the research report and assumptions examined in order that members should be fully briefed before looking at specific programmes of action. The time had now come to decide on the tasks which the Working Party should complete within the time scale. As a way forward it was suggested that effort should be concentrated on those recommendations which could be directly implemented by the health authority and which had practical expression. Each Working Party member was then charged with individual task(s) to be completed within a specific period of time.

In this way the situation was 'moved on' from the catharsis of anger to the con-structive aspects of building new policy proposals together with strategies for their implementation. Subject areas included: medical and midwifery staffing levels; peri-natal audit; health education and communication; family planning; screening; rubella immunisation; counselling; training; provision of services; and the need for improved data collection and for research.

The second stage of the Working Party's lifespan did not produce any utopian change of attitudes. Nevertheless it became apparent that the focus of debate had shifted from the sterile and self-fulfilling defeatism of 'blaming the victims' to an examination of issues which were potentially within members' control.

At first the discussions were pessimistic. Resource constraints within the National Health Service and particularly the then current (1983) review of manpower targets led members to ask how they could possibly expect any improvement in service provision. Under the chairman's guidance, however, it was realised that unless constraints on service provision were made explicit there would be no hope of convincing others of the justice of their case.

As the members produced their individual reports for the Working Party more and more questions came to be asked, for example:

> We've always known about the low levels of midwifery staffing – but why do midwives not come and those that do come, leave?
>
> With the present system of shared care for the majority of mothers how can we (the consultants) get to know about low risk mothers who become high risk during pregnancy?
>
> Can we recommend that general practitioners should not see antenatal patients during general surgeries?
>
> Every general practitioner is an independent practitioner, you can't do anything about those who provide bad antenatal care. Can we recommend a midwife to every GP's clinic?

Perhaps the most surprising remark (given the previous hostility) was from the consultant who said:

> We need health visitors to sort out the social problems. I'm a doctor – I can't help being a doctor – and inevitably I concentrated on medical factors.

By the time of the seventh meeting sufficient evidence had been produced and collated in order for the chairman to present an interim Working Party report to the health authority. The following four areas were identified and agreed by the authority as having priority:

- the establishment of a Maternity Services Liaison Committee as recommended in *Maternity Care in Action* (DHSS, 1982); (this involved the acceptance of a lay health authority member as chairman);
- the establishment of a multidisciplinary Perinatal Review Committee;
- the advice given relating to midwifery and medical staffing levels;
- progress in health promotion in the maternity services.

In terms of participant observation this stage represented the conclusion of my connection with the health authority perinatal survey. There had been a movement, at least on paper, from apparent stalemate to a constructive approach to the problems. Preoccupation with social and maternal characteristics had been replaced, through the chairman's insistence, by attention to policy issues which members could at least hope to influence. Deeply held beliefs and attitudes would not change overnight – if at all. It would be during the third stage and beyond that the real evidence of constructive planning might be seen to be implemented. As researcher I was not privileged to observe the outcomes. Just three pieces of information were conveyed to me privately during the calendar year after my involvement ceased.

The first was a telephone message from the engineer in charge of maintenance of hospital equipment saying that servicing of fetal monitoring equipment was now routine in one of the hospitals. 'Things', he was reported to have said, 'have come out of cupboards that never saw the light of day before you came.' Nevertheless there was reason to believe that this change in practice had more to do with the appointment of new medical staff than with radical changes amongst the old.

Secondly it was learnt that a midwifery sister who had a special interest and training in bereavement counselling had been appointed.

Thirdly a verbal report was received that a consultant had stated that the continuing (relatively) adverse perinatal mortality rate for 1983 was due entirely to socioeconomic factors and that medical care was not implicated in any way!

These three observations appeared to confirm the diffuse and indirect way in which many policy theorists argue that the application of research is achieved. There was no evidence of a direct linear relationship between a recommendation and its implementation. It was abundantly clear that the presentation of knowledge was sufficient to bring about change. It was also necessary for the process to be mediated through the social networks and power structures of role holders in the authority. This process had more to do with professional politics than with the acquisition of research based knowledge. Indeed, the one recommendation which would have ensured the continuing evaluation of trends (the routine collection of statistical information on category of perinatal death by birthweight and place of delivery) was never to my knowledge acted upon.

THE CONCLUDING ANALYSIS FROM THE EMPIRICAL STUDY

Work for the PhD went on to attempt to develop explanations for the phenomena which had been observed. It was concluded that notions of 'causation' in perinatal death could not be separated from the social context in which they were constructed. That context is highly complex and its understanding requires insights into the origins and status of medical expertise; of the place of gender both in medical practice *and* in the ways in which doctors and parent communicate with each other.

Finally, the place of the nurse as researcher in a 'medical' field was explored. It was concluded that the initial, expedient appointment made in the face of public pressure to 'do something' about perinatal mortality and the lack of resources to appoint someone medically qualified had never taken account of a nurse researcher's ability to produce research of this kind. As a result there were profound differences in perception as to what constituted the nurse researcher's role. Therefore, from one point of view, when the findings of the empirical study were denounced as 'inaccurate', it appeared that this verdict was legitimated through being made by doctors whose expertise authorises them to judge. At a superficial level it was doctors saying 'This nurse is not competent'. From a social constructionist perspective of medical knowledge, however, it epitomised the appropriation of reality by a powerful sector of society. To what extent this situation could be attributed to social class differences, professional hierarchy or rivalry, or the imposition of an authoritarian medical ideology was impossible to judge.

The outcome nevertheless carried implications for policy development in the arena of perinatal mortality. Class, gender and racial discrimination will exist in different manifestations and at different times and may indeed influence individual explanations for phenomena. But this, as Popper (1945) points out, is only to be expected, for we all suffer from our own systems of prejudice. The ultimate lesson of this study was that it is only through the exposure of such individual hypothetical positions to the rigours of replication, falsification and public debate that progress towards scientific explanation can be distinguished from the pseudoscientific, however elegantly it may be disguised as 'expertise'.

LESSONS FOR THE FUTURE

There are several topical policy lessons from this research for nurses which can be extrapolated to the context of current developments in the NHS. Despite current, highly desirable concern with the development of 'audit', in practice the procedures appear to be being focused on (and controlled by) individual professional groups. Yet, as this research demonstrated, there is a tendency to close ranks and to search for alternative explanations whenever a spotlight is turned on to the performance of individual groups of workers, especially if they have the ultimate power to control events. It seems almost inevitable, therefore, that vast sums of money will be spent on going through the *motions* of audit but with no real hope of change in subsequent practice unless the really difficult issue of *change management* is taken on board at the same time.

One major lesson was that if the opportunity arose to go back and do all of the perinatal research again in the light of what has subsequently been learnt, it would be with the intention of carrying out a piece of *true* action research. This would require incorporation into the research methodology of techniques for taking members of staff along with the findings as they arose and for dealing with their feelings of threat and denial. It would need to involve helping them to recognise and to come to terms with their own stereotyped views on the nature of the problem. It would also involve empowering the staff so that they did not feel hopeless and helpless at the prospect of being able to effect structural changes in the management of their service. But all of this would require me *as the researcher* to feel confident to bring about the changes which might have a chance of becoming permanent. Yet, as I have shown, the research experience left me feeling *disempowered* and guilty at the upset I had caused. Which brings me to the final issues arising from this research experience.

No contract researcher should be left unsupported with the awesome responsibility both of doing the research and of handling the highly charged political consequences of the findings. This is a serious lesson for nurses in the context of the current NHS. Many nurses are being appointed to either purchaser or provider health service research and development posts (often with far less research training and academic supervision than I enjoyed). Without that crucial element of support many of them may come to feel that they have been set up to fail. Their immediate employers need to understand their own crucial responsibilities in ensuring first that the focus and methodology of the studies they ask for are appropriate for the questions which need to be asked and, second, that they then back the researcher all the way through the research. Structures of power and hierarchy in health care are unlikely to be swept away. Nurses need to learn to recognise them for what they are and to develop the self-confidence to manage them. This is just as important during the process of carrying out research as in any other form of organisational life.

Academic supervisors of nurse research students also need to reflect on these issues for research teaching and supervision. The majority of nurse students for higher degrees are similar to those who I taught on the Warwick MA. They are mature and experienced professionals who look to research education to provide them with rigorous and systematic techniques in order to address the specific problems which they face in their work situations. They will often wish to research issues for their dissertations such as workload measurement, the organisation of nursing work and quality assurance in health care – all issues which are likely to bring political consequences in their train. Will the day ever arise when we shall see a research supervisor or manager answering charges at the UKCC that they are in breach of the Nurses' and Midwives' Professional Code of Conduct because of failure to support a researcher in the dissemination and application of research findings? This is not as extreme a scenario as it may sound, for the whole ethos claimed to lie behind the current NHS reforms is that they will improve standards in health care and make professionals much more accountable to the customer. After all – for whose benefit are we doing all this research?

NOTES

*Robinson, J. (1994) Research for whom? The politics of research dissemination and application. In Buckeldee and McMahon (eds) *The Research Experience in Nursing*, Nelson Thornes. Reprinted with permission of Nelson Thornes.

REFERENCES

Armstrong, D. (1986) The invention of perinatal mortality. *Sociology of Health and Illness*, 8, 211–32.

Bell, C. and Encel, S. (1978) *Inside the Whale: Ten Personal Accounts of Social Research*, Pergamon, Australia.

Bell, C. and Newby, H. (1981) *Doing Sociological Research*, George Allen and Unwin, London.

Bell, C. and Roberts, H. (1984) *Social Researching: Politics, Problems, Practice*, Routledge and Kegan Paul, London.

Bulmer, M. (1982) *The Uses of Social Research. Social Investigation in Public Policy-Making*, Contemporary Social Research, No. 3, George Allen and Unwin, London.

Butler, N.R. and Alberman, E.D. (1969) *Perinatal Problems. The Second Report of the 1958 British Perinatal Mortality Survey*, E. and S. Livingstone, Edinburgh.

Butler, N.R. and Bonham, D.G. (1963) *Perinatal Mortality. The First Report of the 1958 British Perinatal Mortality Survey*, E. and S. Livingstone, Edinburgh.

Chamberlain, R., Chamberlain, G., Howlett, B. and Claireaux, A. (1975) *British Births 1970. Volume 1. The First Week of Life*, Heinemann, London.

Chamberlain, G., Phillipp, E., Howlett, B. and Masters, K. (1978) *British Births 1970. Volume 2. Obstetric Care*, Heinemann, London.

Clarke, M. and Clayton, D. (1981) The design and interpretation of case-control studies of perinatal mortality. *American Journal of Epidemiology*, 113(6), 636–45.

Department of Health and Social Security (1980) *Report of the Working Group on Inequalities in Health* (Chairman, Sir Douglas Black). HMSO, London.

Department of Health and Social Security (1982) *Maternity Care in Action – Part 1*, HMSO, London.

Hall, P., Land, H., Parker, R. and Webb, A. (1978) *Change, Choice and Conflict in Social Policy*, Heinemann, London.

House of Commons (1980) *Second Report from the Social Services Committee, Perinatal and Neonatal Mortality*, HMSO, London.

House of Commons (1984) *Third Report from the Social Services Committee, Perinatal and Neonatal Mortality Report: Follow Up*, HMSO, London.

Joint Committee of the Royal College of Obstetricians and Gynaecologists and the British Paediatric Association (1949) *Neonatal Mortality and Morbidity: Reports on Public Health and Medical Subjects No. 94*, HMSO, London.

Joint Committee of the Royal College of Obstetricians and Gynaecologists and the Population Investigation Committee (1948) *Maternity in Great Britain*, Oxford University Press, Oxford.

Knox, E.G., Lancashire, R. and Armstrong, E.H. (1986) Perinatal mortality standards: construction and use of a health care performance indicator. *Journal of Epidemiology and Community Health*, 40(3), 193–204.

National Perinatal Epidemiology Unit (1978) *An Introduction to the National Perinatal Epidemiology Unit and Annual Report for 1978*, Radcliffe Infirmary, Oxford.

News Focus (1991) Whistling down the wind. *Health Services Journal*, 101(5282), 14.

Popper, K. (1945) Against the sociology of knowledge, reprinted in Miller, D. (ed.) (1983) *A Pocket Popper*, Fontana, London.

Rein, M. (1976) *Social Science and Public Policy*, Penguin, Harmondsworth.

Roberts, H. (1981) *Doing Feminist Research*, Routledge and Kegan Paul, London.

Robinson, J.A. (1979) Inter-disciplinary in-service education (for health visitors and social workers). *Child Abuse and Neglect*, 3, 749–55.

Robinson, J.A. (1980) An evaluation of health visiting: a study of the relevance of historical and theoretical perspectives, and of its impact upon clients' perceptions and usage of the service. University of Keele. Dissertation.

Robinson, J.A. (1982) *An Evaluation of Health Visiting*, CETHV/ENB, London.

Robinson, J.A. (1986) A study of the policy implications arising from a local survey of perinatal mortality. University of Keele. Dissertation.

Robinson, J.A. (1987) A casket instead of a crib. *Senior Nurse*, 7(1), 16–18.

Robinson, J.A. (1989a) Perinatal mortality – report on a research study. *International Journal of Health Care Quality Assurance*, 2(2), 13–19.

Robinson, J.A. (1989b) The role of the social sciences in evaluating perinatal care, in *Effective Care in Pregnancy and Childbirth*, (eds. I. Chalmers, M. Enkin, and M.J. Keirse), Oxford University Press, Oxford.

Robinson, J.A., and Allison, J. (1991) *The Social Construction of Perinatal Mortality: A Case Study of Power Relationships between Primary and Secondary Care Obstetrics*. Paper given at the International Conference on Primary Care Obstetrics and Perinatal Health, S'Hertogenbosch, The Netherlands, 21–22 March 1991. In press.

Index